Innovations In Assisted Reproduction Technology

Edited by Nidhi Sharma, Sudakshina Chakrabarti, Yona Barak and Adrian Ellenbogen

Published in London, United Kingdom

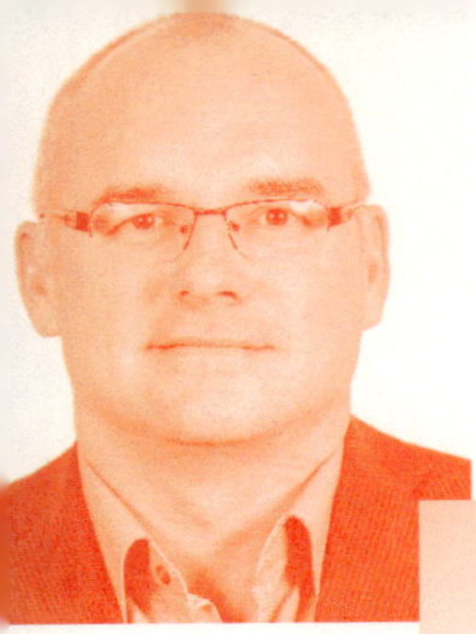
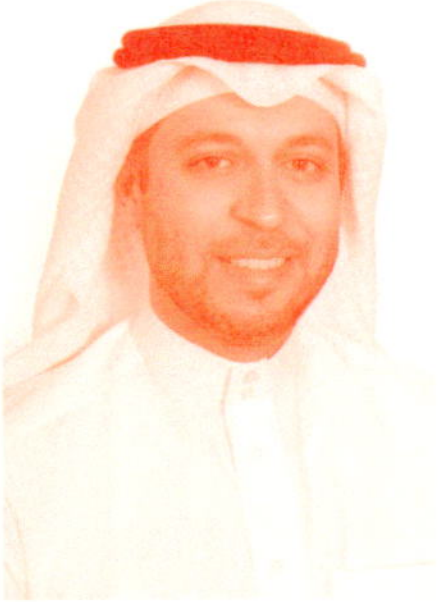
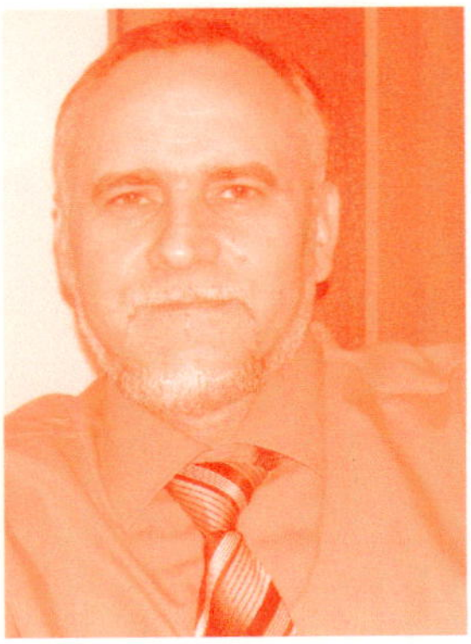
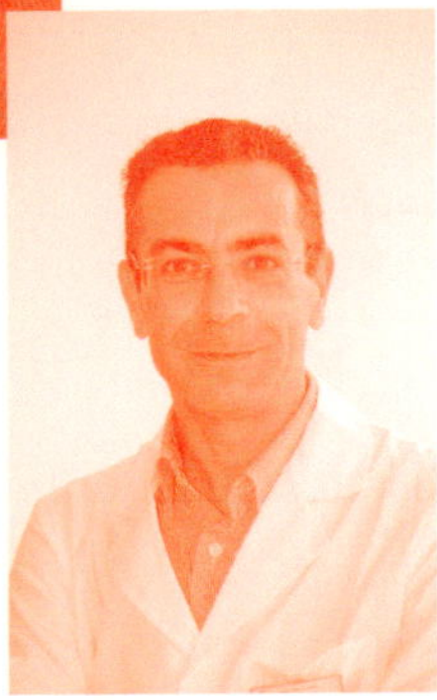
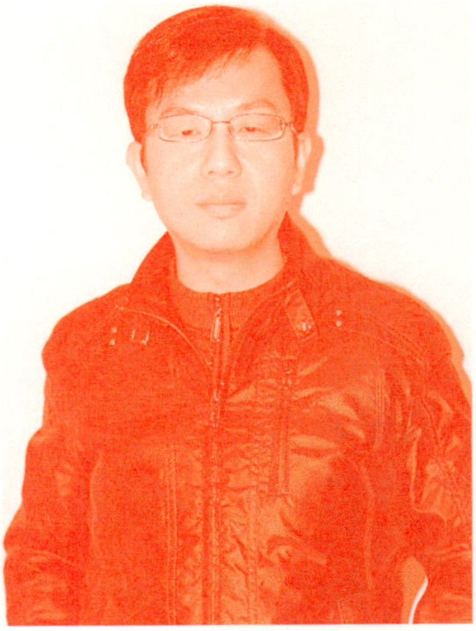
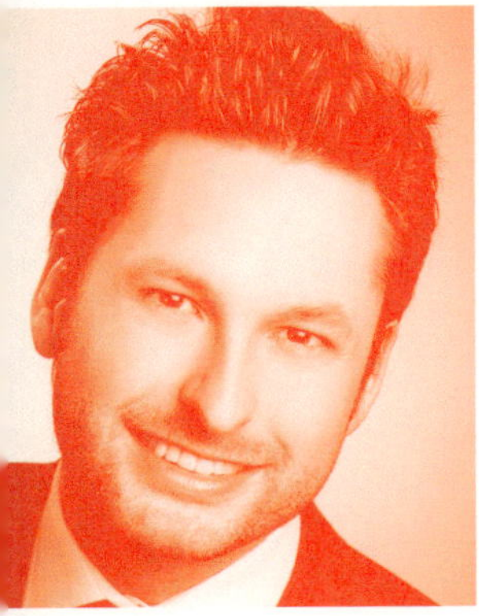
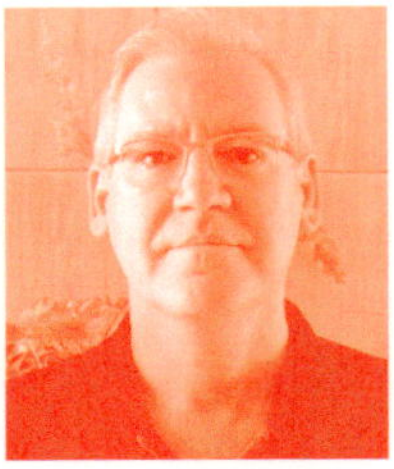

IntechOpen

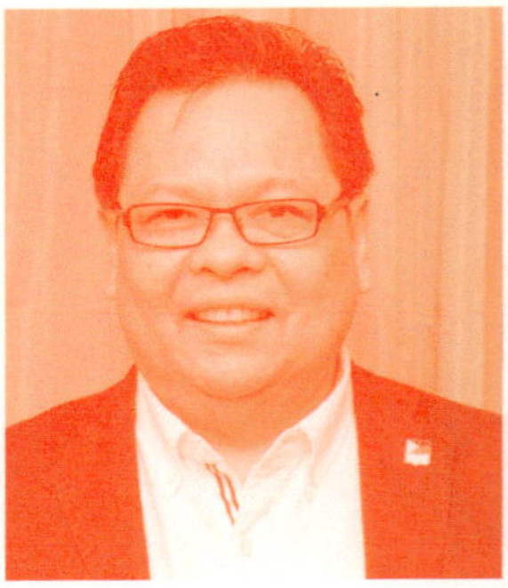
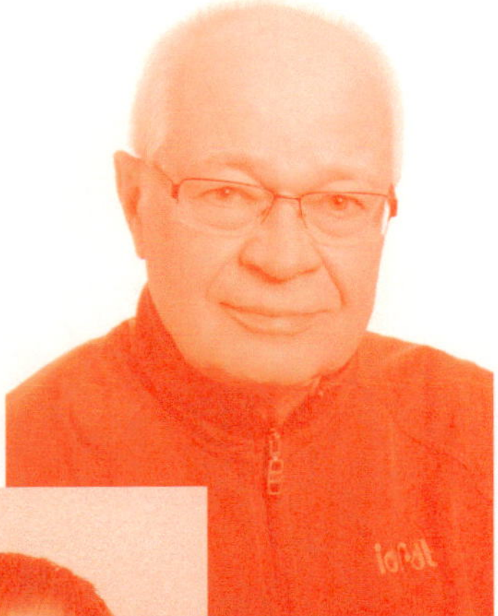
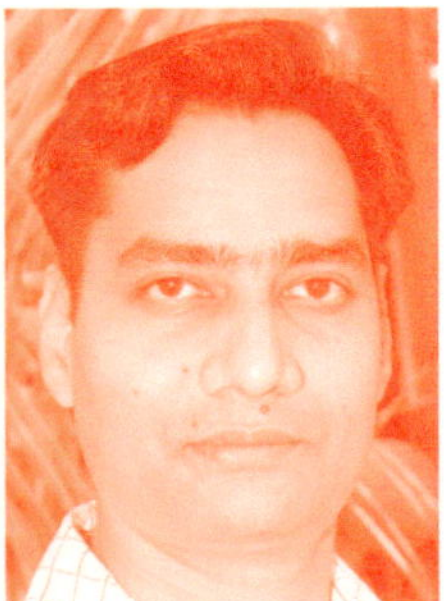
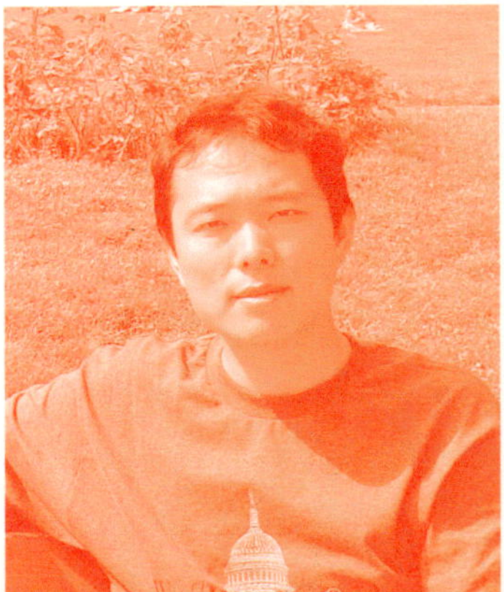
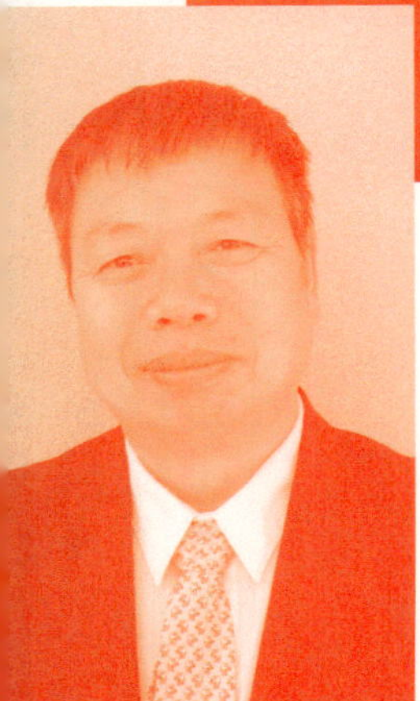
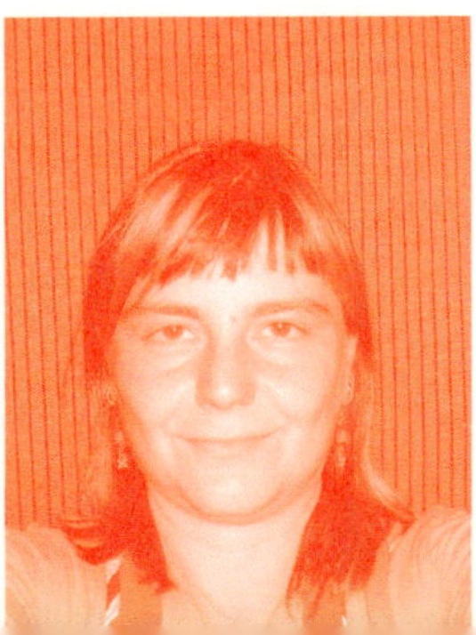

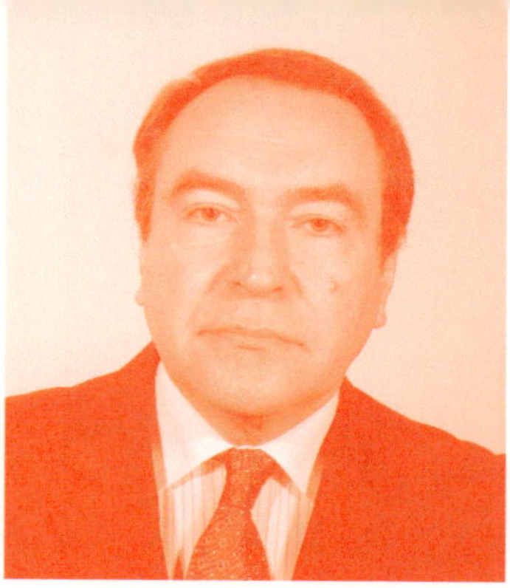
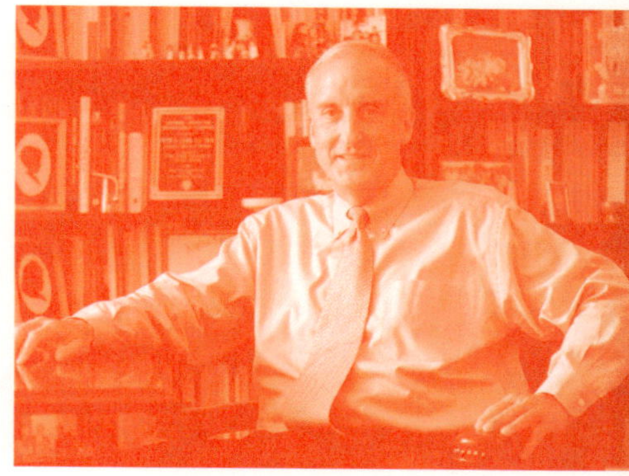
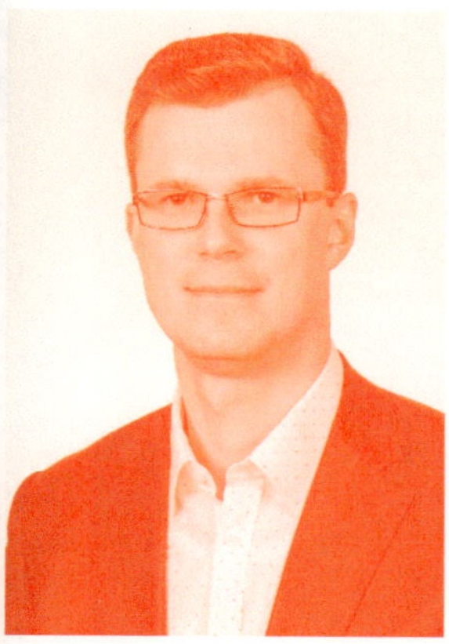
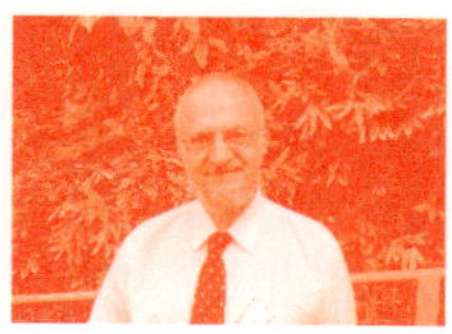
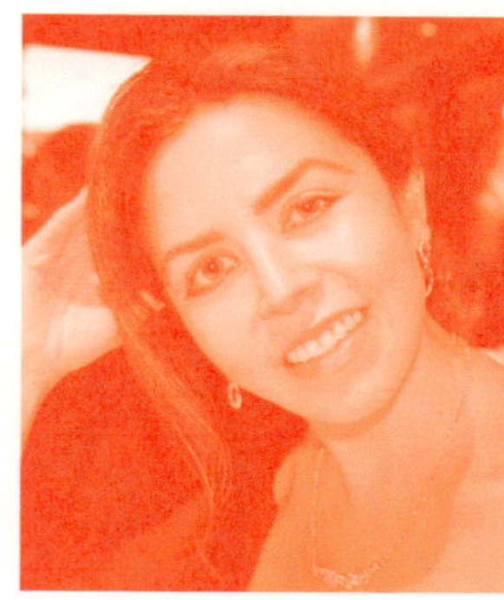

Supporting open minds since 2005

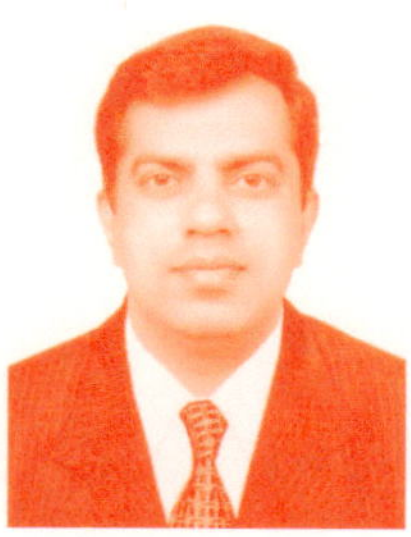
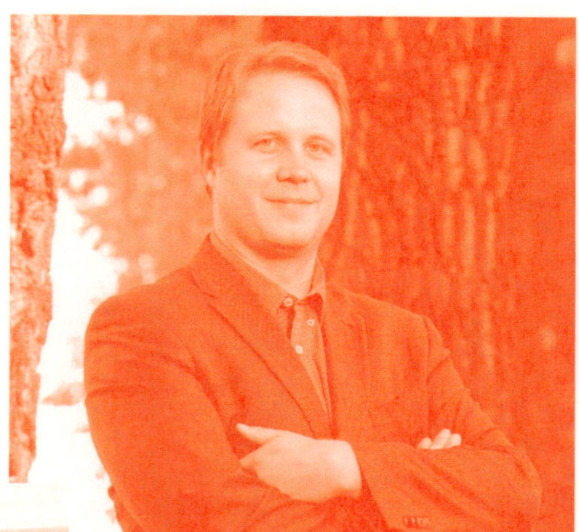
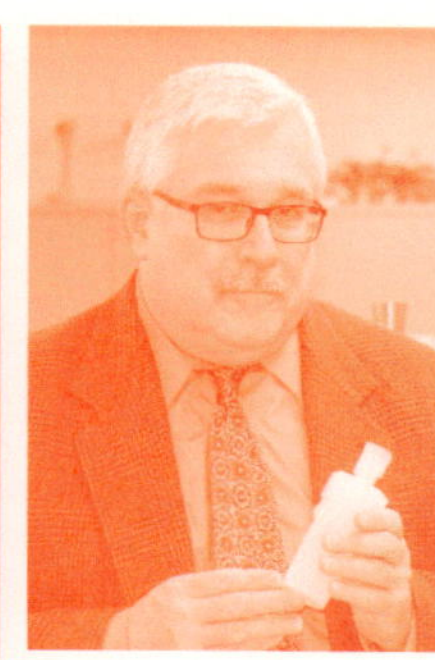
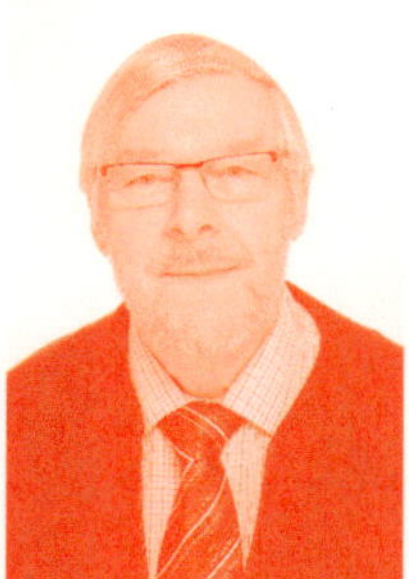
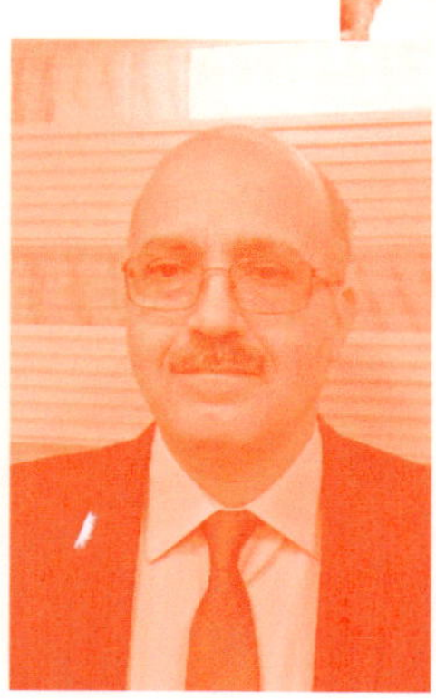
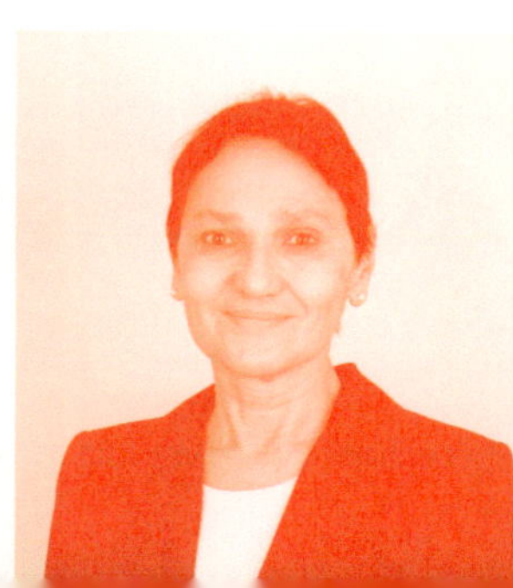
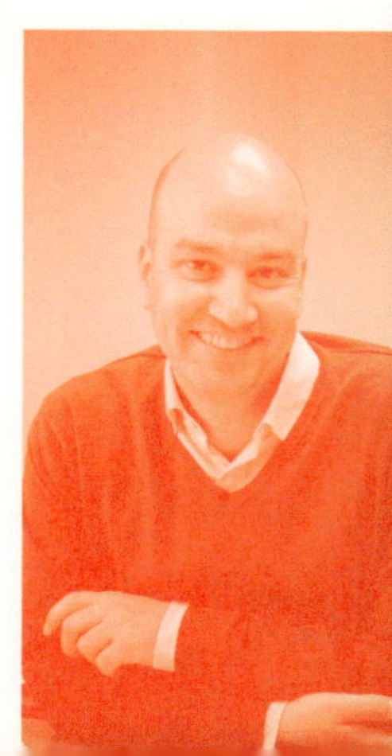

Innovations In Assisted Reproduction Technology
http://dx.doi.org/10.5772/intechopen.77538
Edited by Nidhi Sharma, Sudakshina Chakrabarti, Yona Barak and Adrian Ellenbogen

Contributors
Tanya Milachich, Desislava Dyulgerova, Dahril Dahril, Aulanni'am Aulanni'am, Widi Nugroho, Jan Tesarik, Sonu Chand Thakur, Mohd Sajad, Alexander Shpakov, Andrey Bakhtyukov, Kira Derkach, Dmitry Dar'in, Goran Mitulović, Tanja Panić-Janković, Eswari Beeram, Vinicius M. Lopes, Murilo C. Souza-Oliveira, Eduardo S. Pimentel, Amanda Evelyn C. Goulart, Natalia I. Zavattiero Tierno, Anna Luiza Moraes Souza, Jean Pierre B. Brasileiro, Valeria L. Mathias Castro, Tatianna Q. F. Ribeiro, Cristina T. Medina, Leilane G. Noleto Lima, Nidhi Sharma, Sudakshina Chakrabarti, Lauren Grimm, Angeline Beltsos, Roohi Jeelani, Amber Cooper, Justo Aznar Lucea, Julio Tudela, Mitchel C. Schiewe, Casey Zeffiro, Silvina Bocca, Helena Russell, Yona Barak, Adrian Ellenbogen

First published in London, United Kingdom, 2020 by IntechOpen
IntechOpen is the global imprint of INTECHOPEN LIMITED, registered in England and Wales, registration number: 11086078, 7th floor, 10 Lower Thames Street, London, EC3R 6AF, United Kingdom
Printed in Croatia

British Library Cataloguing-in-Publication Data
A catalogue record for this book is available from the British Library

Additional hard and PDF copies can be obtained from orders@intechopen.com

Innovations In Assisted Reproduction Technology
Edited by Nidhi Sharma, Sudakshina Chakrabarti, Yona Barak and Adrian Ellenbogen
p. cm.
Print ISBN 978-1-83880-548-7
Online ISBN 978-1-83880-549-4
eBook (PDF) ISBN 978-1-78985-871-6

For EU product safety concerns:
IN TECH d.o.o., Prolaz Marije Krucifikse Kozulić 3, 51000 Rijeka, Croatia, info@intechopen.com or visit our website at intechopen.com.

Meet the editors

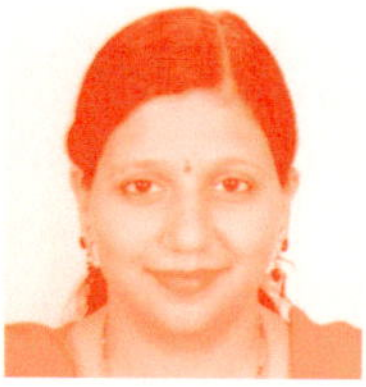

Dr. Nidhi Sharma received a MBBS and MS from Banaras Hindu University, Varanasi, India. She is a fellow of the Indian College of Obstetrics and Gynecology, fellow of assisted reproductive techniques, and Professor of Obstetrics and Gynecology at Saveetha University, India. Dr. Sharma has 80 indexed publications and has authored several chapters in textbooks. She received her PhD in Obstetrics and Gynecology from Saveetha University, India, and Diploma in IVF and Reproductive Medicine from UKSH Universitätsklilikum Schleswig-Holstein, Germany. Dr. Sharma has been a member of the teaching faculty of MBBS, MS, and PhD for 15 years. She is course coordinator and academic supervisor of BSc in Reproductive Biology, MSc in Clinical Embryology, Fellowship in Reproductive Medicine, and PhD in Reproductive Medicine at Saveetha University.

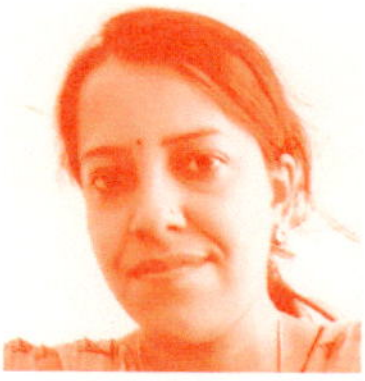

Dr. Sudakshina Chakrabarti is Associate Professor of Anatomy at Saveetha Medical College and hHospital, Chennai, India. She obtained a MBBS from Kempegowda Institute of Medical Sciences, Bangalore. Dr. Chakrabarti completed a postgraduate degree in Obstetrics and Gynecology from J.J.M Medical College, Davangere, Karnataka, India; an MD in Anatomy from Sri Ramachandra Medical College, Chennai, India; and is currently pursuing a PhD at Saveetha University, Chennai, India. She is an ACLS, BLS, and PALS instructor under the American Heart Association and involved in simulation education. She has recently completed an Advanced Course in Medical Education and is an active member of the Medical Education Unit at Saveetha Medical College and Hospital Chennai with experience in conducting faculty development programs.

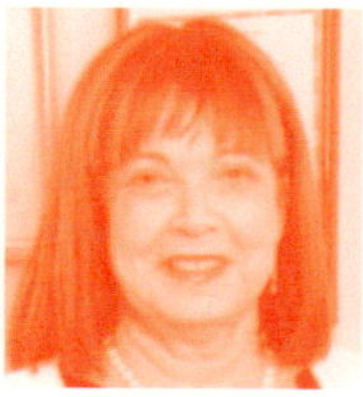

Dr. Yona Barak obtained a BSc MSc and PhD from Tel Aviv University, Department of Zoology Faculty of Life science . Both theses for these degrees dealt with in vitro maturation of mammalian oocytes. Dr. Barak established IVF laboratories and programs worldwide: one in 1984 at the Tel Aviv Medical Center where she was director of the IVF laboratory for 12 years, and one in 1986 at the Herzliya Medical Center where she served as scientific lab director for about 25 years. She established other programs in the United States, Germany, Czech Republic, Lithuania, Cyprus, Dominican Republic, India, Ukraine, Russia, and Belarus. In 2001, she established, owned, and led the InviMed clinics in Poland. Throughout her career, Dr. Barak trained many embryologists worldwide. In 1996, she established and became a lecturer and the clinical director of the MSc program of Gametology and Embryology at Bar Ilan University, Israel. From 1998 to 2003, she was a member of the Faculty Scientific Advisory Board and lecturer of the MSc course for Clinical Embryology at Danube University, Krems Austria, an international program of clinical embryology in cooperation with Bourn Hall, UK and Alpha Scientists in Reproductive Medicine. In 1996, she was elected by the members of Alpha Scientists in Reproductive Medicine as an executive board member. In 1999, she became a vice president of Alpha, and in 2001, she became president and served until 2004' and is an honorary member until today. Honorary member of embryologists in Mexico, Argentina, and Italy, and a member of the Israeli National Advisory Committee of Gynecology, Embryology and Neonatology. Dr. Barak is an active scientist who has published research in the field of assisted reproductive technologies. She is a pioneer for Hyaluronate as a replacement for polyvinylpyrrolidone (PVP) in intracytoplasmic sperm injection (ICSI); intracytoplasmic morphologically selected sperm injection (IMSI) (Breakthrough paper; 2002); in vivo maturation (IVM); human oocyte vitrification in closed systems; and more. She is owner and director of Dr. Yona Barak Laboratories for fertility services, and specializes in IMSI.

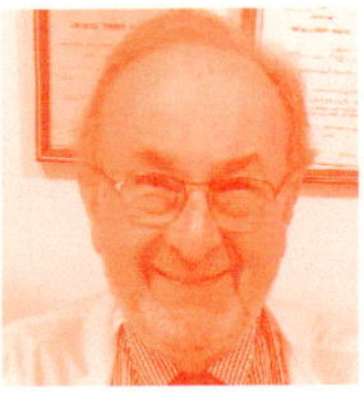

Adrian Ellenbogen, MD, is Clinical Assistant Professor in Obstetrics and Gynecology at the Rappaport School of Medicine, Technion-Institute of Technology, Haifa, Israel. He conceded fellowship at the IVF Unit, Hammersmith Hospital, London, England. He is also the founder and director (retired) of the IVF unit at Hillel Yaffe Medical Center, Hadera, Israel. In addition, he is Scientific Director for the postgraduate course in Obstetrics Gynecology and Infertility at the Rappaport School of Medicine, as well as Fertility Advisor and head of the Fertility Clinic, Meuheded Female Health Center, Bnai-Brack, Israel. Dr. Ellenbogen is a member of American Society of Reproductive Medicine, European Society of Human Reproduction, International Society for Mild Approaches in Assisted Reproduction, International Society for In Vitro Fertilization, International Federation of Fertility Society, Israeli Fertility Association, and Israeli Society of Obstetrics and Gynecology. He is an editorial board member and reviewer for the *Journal of Reproductive System and Sexual Disorders*, and a reviewer for *Fertility and Sterility* and *Harefuah*. He has published 52 papers in scientific journals, two book chapters, and has presented 33 plenary lectures in international congresses and organized 12 international scientific meetings. He has presented more than 120 lectures in international and national congresses.Dr. Ellenbogen pioneered IVF treatment with minimal stimulation and egg donation law in Israel. He has trained physicians in Israel, Dominican Republic, Poland, Macedonia, and Russia in IVF. He received the 2003 Israeli Ministry of Health and Israeli Civil Service Commission Award for Excellency in Labor, the Star Award of the American Society of Reproductive Medicine in in 2012, 2013, 2014, and 2015, and the Award of the Israeli State Physicians Association in 2018 for his contribution to the Israel medical community.

Contents

Preface

This book is the result of contributions from many authors and researchers across the globe. Divided into four sections, this volume covers all the relevant clinical aspects of infertility. The first section elaborates on the recent understanding of infertility, which has developed as a result of newer imaging tools, serum hormone detections, and chemical analysis. The second section describes the recent developments in diagnosis and treatment of infertility. The third section covers the ethical and legal aspects of assisted reproductive technology (ART). The fourth section gives recent insights into contraception.

The first chapter introduces the tools used to comprehend the physiology of reproduction. It elaborates the male factor and describes multiple environmental and epigenetic factors affecting spermatozoa and seminal plasma. The chapter also explains the etiologies and pathophysiology of diminished sperm quality. Since the etiology and pathogenesis is segregated and multifactorial, there are multitudes of resulting sperm defects. The second chapter describes these pathophysiological factors in detail. The third chapter explains the recent use of novel markers of semen analysis. The fourth chapter examines the biophysical and serum markers of oocyte reserve and quality. It also elaborates on the rational basis of drugs used for controlled hyper stimulation.

The second section discusses the newer low molecular weight ligands of gonadotropins. It explains newer laboratory techniques of omics to help readers optimize ART results. It also presents the preparation and use of autologous platelet-rich plasma to improve endometrial receptivity in recurrent implantation failures. The chapter on recurrent implantation failure helps us to understand the intricacies of embryo–endometrial interactions. The chapter also provides meticulous detail regarding the practical procedure of in vitro maturation of oocytes. The in vitro culture of oocytes is likely to open new horizons of hope for cancer patients and patients who have repeated ovarian hyper stimulation syndromes. This technology also carries potential benefits of reducing cost and time.

The chapter on bioethics weighs the ethical and legal aspects of assisted reproduction in light of religious beliefs and provides insights into how far is far enough.

This book is an attempt to identify and standardize technology that is likely to improve ART outcomes. The basic scientific knowledge is valuable, pure, and self-correcting. Future studies are likely to provide new insights, developing these new concepts even further. We wish to express our gratitude to all the authors for their time, effort, and commitment in sharing their knowledge and skills. The authors have painstakingly prepared chapters and modified and proofread drafts despite all the laboratory work. Our sincere thanks to Ms. Mia Vulovic for communicating with all authors and singlehandedly coordinating this entire effort to ensure a final book of quality. We have to acknowledge the support of our publisher IntechOpen for their continuous guidance and support. Finally, we acknowledge our families with whose support and patience we have been able to complete this book.

Nidhi Sharma and Sudakshina Chakrabarti
Saveetha Medical College and Hospital,
Chennai, India

Yona Barak
Dr. Yona Barak Laboratories,
Israel

Adrian Ellenbogen
Rappaport School of Medicine,
Israel

Section 1

Physiology

Chapter 1

The Sperm: Parameters and Evaluation

Tanya Milachich and Desislava Dyulgerova-Nikolova

Abstract

Sperm abnormalities are a major factor of human infertility. Since 1987, there are several references in different editions of World Health Organization (WHO) manual defining optimal sperm parameters. Over the years, many reproductive specialists have been constantly debating, suggesting and remodeling the frame values in those guidelines. Semen parameters have a leading role both in natural conception and assisted reproduction technologies (ART) outcomes. Deviations expressed in lower sperm count, impaired motility, abnormal morphology, and high percentage of sperm DNA fragmentation are linked to reduced chances to achieve pregnancy. In cases with low sperm count, severe oligoasthenozoospermia (OA) or azoospermia, karyotyping or evaluation with sperm aneuploidy test (SAT) could be an option and genetic counseling will be necessary if there is an obvious deviation or aberration (e.g., translocation, aneuploidy, etc.). Taking care of lifestyle factors as body mass index (BMI), diets, alcohol intake, smoking, using some additional nutrition and vitamin supplements might affect sperm parameters and contribute to the chances of a couple to conceive.

Keywords: sperm count, OAT, azoospermia, ART, karyotyping, sperm aneuploidy, DNA fragmentation, genetic testing, lifestyle

1. Introduction

The link between semen quality and fertility has been studied in humans since 1930 [1]. Semen analysis, as a standard laboratory test, gives basic information on spermatogenesis, secretory activity of the gonads and patency of the male genital tract [2]. The results obtained during the semen sample analysis could point out absence of spermatozoa, severe or mild deviation in sperm parameters or normal values for semen volume, sperm count and concentration, motility and morphology of the spermatozoa. Over the years many reproductive specialists have been constantly debating, suggesting and remodeling the frame values of the semen in reference to male fertility. Since 1987, there are several updates in different editions of World Health Organization (WHO) manuals defining the optimal sperm parameters with reference to pregnancy outcomes. The last (fifth) edition of the manual, published in 2010, defines serious decrease in cutoff values for sperm parameters related to chances of achieving pregnancy and thus its significance was widely discussed [3, 4]. One of the strong limitations of semen analysis and the defined fertility potential references in the last WHO edition is the lack of correlation with the female age, as only 30% of infertility in couples is due to male factors alone [5, 6]. The sixth edition of WHO is in discussion as some of the directions of changes would be: semen analysis references including the Asian population for reference establishment; additional separate chapters for sperm morphology and computer assisted sperm analysis (CASA); importance of microbiological assessment. Some of the inapplicable tests at the modern andrology lab tests, e.g., postcoital test, capillary tube, Hamster test, counting in glass chambers will be excluded from the manual. New techniques such as sperm DNA fragmentation tests, aneuploidy screening, acrosome reaction assay, motile sperm organelle morphology examination (MSOME), Calcium ionophore activation, Catsper channels activity examination, influence of epigenetics and miRNA will be described [7].

2. Semen sample parameters

Semen sample parameters could be influenced by various factors such as sexual abstinence periods [8, 9], gonadal activity [10], abnormal hormonal levels [11], testicle size [12], body mass index (BMI) [13–15], urogenital infections and antibiotics or anabolic substances intake [16–18], individual diet regiment [19–21], working environment and lifestyle [22–24]. Sperm parameters have a leading role both in natural conception and assisted reproduction technologies (ART) outcomes. In order to establish male fertility potential, at least two to three sperm samples in a 3-month period should be analyzed [25]. Attention to intraindividual variability in parameters has to be considered. Reports in various studies show fluctuation in sperm volume and count, concentration, motility and morphology in one individual [26–29]. There are limitations to semen analysis depending on the patient specificity and the use of good laboratory practice protocols. Only this analysis by itself has a contradictory clinical value and might not be a stand-alone predictor for male fertility [30, 31]. In conditions such as azoospermia, globozoospermia or necrozoospermia, exceptions are made and male infertility could be stated [32].

When there are no sperm cells detected through microscope observations (azoospermia), the condition needs further investigation. Performing at least two separate semen analysis is needed. Centrifugation of the whole ejaculated volume is necessary in order to detect specific conditions [33]. When several or sporadic sperm cells are routed out in the sediment of the centrifuged sample the definition would be cryptozoospermia [34].

2.1 Azoospermia

Approximately 10–15% of all infertile men are diagnosed with azoospermia. When according to laboratory test a patient is diagnosed with azoospermia, further hormonal and genetic tests along with andrology, urology, genetic consultation and ultrasound scan are needed [35].

Obstructive azoospermia (OA): could be due to obstruction in the epididymis, vas deferens or the ejaculatory duct [36]; it could also be the consequence of infections, inflammation, scrotal trauma, rare genetic conditions (cystic fibrosis), vasectomy or injury of vas deferens or previous surgery [37]. Depending on the specific case, microsurgery is an option for restoring the passage of the sperm cells. Different techniques for sperm retrieval: percutaneous epididymal sperm aspiration (PESA), microsurgical epididymal sperm aspiration (MESA), testicular sperm aspiration (TESA) or testicular sperm extraction (TESE) could be applied in order to obtain reproductive cells for further use in in vitro fertilization (IVF) or ICSI treatment [38].

Nonobstructive azoospermia (NOA): could be the consequence of hormonal imbalance [39, 40], Y-chromosome deletion or altered karyotype [41, 42], long period of toxins exposure [43], chemotherapy or radiation treatment [44], certain medications intake or varicocele [45]. Resurrecting the spermatogenesis process could be achieved depending on the factors inducing azoospermia. Another option is performing TESE and ICSI procedure when sperm cells are retrieved after the extraction. In order to suggest and apply the proper treatment for the patient with NOA, adequate genetic consulting and testing should be present [46, 47].

Oligozoospermia: the condition is characterized by reduced sperm density as sperm concentration below the fifth centile in fertile men was recently reduced from 20 to 15 million/ml [48]. In 75% of the cases with oligozoospermia the cause of infertility is considered idiopathic [49]. In men with severe oligozoospermia, concentration of less than 5×10^6 sperm/ml, possibility of residual spermatogenic function decline has been reported [50]. Fertility preservation via sperm freezing is an option. Another, yet controversial, issue reflecting in low sperm count is obesity. WHO consultation in 1997 [51] recognized obesity as a global epidemic affecting society in the developed countries [52, 53]. Studies point out correlation of obesity and overweight to increased risk of azoospermia and oligozoospermia [54] and adherence to healthy and diverse diet could improve male fertility [55].

2.2 Sperm morphology

Sperm cell morphology is strongly correlated to male reproduction. Abnormalities might affect sperm motility, sperm fertilize ability and conception. Some conditions such as globozoospermia or stunted tail sperm defects could lead to inability to father biological children as a consequence of natural conception [56–58].

Recently, the intact human flagellum has been studied using cryo-electron microscopy and tomography [59]. A novel structure—tail axoneme intra-lumenal spiral (TAILS)—was reviled and described [60]. This new discovery suggests the need of further exploration and observation of sperm structures—not only in order to connect them to sperm function but also to clarify their significance. As previous studies reported, abnormal tail structure is correlated to sperm motility disorders, as nonspecific flagellar anomalies (NSFAs) are found to be the most frequent flagellar pathology in severe asthenozoospermia, and thus reduces the chance for natural conception [61]. According to the new data revealing TAILS, the explanation to some cases considered as unexplained infertility might be reviled.

Link between sperm morphology and numerical or structural chromosome abnormalities are suggested and investigated [62–64]. In fertile men, who have different translocations the frequencies of sperm chromosomal abnormalities were high (33–92%) in comparison to those with normal karyotype [65].

Post-radiotherapy treatments also show in altered number of structural and numerical chromosome aneuploidies (from 6 to 67% respectively [65]. Studies on infertile men with teratozoospermia (<14% normal forms), globozoospermia and macrocephalic, multinucleated or multiflagellate spermatozoa show an increased incidence of sperm aneuploidy up to 50% [65, 66]. Sperm with normal chromosome constitutions can be exhibited in men with normal or abnormal sperm parameters [67, 68].

2.3 Sperm sample evaluation and references

Investigating male fertility potential initially is based on routine semen analysis. Establishment of certain values for semen in order to predict chances of conception generates the need of references for male fertility. Requirement for semen analysis and semen parameters have been set as recommended in successive editions of WHO in 1980, 1987, 1992, 1999 and 2010 [1]. The following table [69] represents changes for cut off values for semen parameters according consecutive WHO manuals:

Semen characteristics	WHO (1980)	WHO (1987)	WHO (1992)	WHO (1999)	WHO (2010)[a]
Volume (mL)	ND	≥2	≥2	≥2	1.5
Sperm count (10^6/mL)	20–200	≥20	≥20	≥20	15
Total sperm count (10^6)	ND	≥40	≥40	≥40	39
Total motility (% motile)	≥60	≥50	≥50	≥50	40
Progressive motility[b]	≥2[c]	≥25%	≥25% (grade a)	≥25% (grade a)	32% (a + b)
Vitality (% alive)	ND	≥50	≥75	≥75	58
Morphology (% normal forms)	80.5	≥50	≥30[d]	(14)[e]	4[f]
Leukocyte count (10^6/mL)	<4.7	<1.0	<1.0	<1.0	<1.0

[a] Lower reference limit obtained from the lower fifth centile value

[b] Grade a, rapid progressive motility (>25 μm/s); grade b, slow/sluggish progressive motility (5–25 μm/s); Normal, 50% motility (grades a + b) or 25% progressive motility (grade a) within 60 min of ejaculation

[c] Forward progression (scale 0–3)

[d] Arbitrary value

[e] Value not defined but strict criterion is suggested

[f] Strict (Tygerberg) criterion; *ND* not defined

Sperm sample evaluation in a modern andrology lab might be measured by the means of CASA. The use of computer aid does not exclude additional evaluation by the human eye [70, 71]. For sperm morphology evaluation, WHO [72] recommends criteria by strict morphology [73].

3. DNA fragmentation

Recently, DNA fragmentation tests have been widely incorporated in laboratory practice. DNA integrity and sperm hereditary information are essential to the offspring as male gametes has major contribution to the fertilization processes, embryo quality and embryo development even in early gestational stages [74–76]. Sperm contains almost 3000 different kinds of mRNA coded for proteins that are active in the early embryo development period. There are also some others still unknown and with no equivalent in the oocyte [77, 78].

3.1 Morphology evaluation and sperm selection in real time

Since the introduction of ICSI as routine procedure, the significance of standard semen analysis was neglected, as sperm concentration and motility have no longer such importance, since a single sperm cell has to be injected. When standard ICSI procedure under a Hoffman modulation contrast microscope, or Nomarski optics at magnification ×400 is performed visualization and assessment of sperm head (size and shape) mid-piece and tail are possible, but detailed ultrastructural morphology examination is limited [79, 80]. When conventional ICSI is performed, it would be difficult to evaluate and select morphologically normal sperm based on its detailed structural portrait: vacuolization, membrane invaginations, mid-piece thickness or deformity, etc. It is controversial whether high vacuolization in the sperm head is associated with higher DNA fragmentation and aneuploidy rate [81, 82] that may have adverse effect on embryo quality and postimplantation development and higher frequency of pregnancy loss at early gestational stages. Still, for some couples detailed sperm examination prior ICSI is preferable [83, 84].

Intracytoplasmic morphologically selected sperm injection (IMSI) is the cornerstone to sperm morphology evaluation. Based on the examination of motile sperm organelle morphology (MSOME) IMSI is the only real-time, unstained method used for selection of motile and morphologically normal spermatozoa for intracytoplasmic injection. IMSI was first introduced by Baratoov et al. [85]. MSOME selection is made under inverted light emitting microscope with Differential interference contrast or Nomarski differential interference contrast optics and digital camera at high magnification ranging from ×6600 to ×13,000. Using MSOME criteria, the motile sperm fraction and each cell malformation is evaluated according to the morphological status of six organelles comprising the acrosome, post-acrosomal lamina, neck, mitochondria, tail and nucleus. Only 33% of spermatozoa from the examined samples appeared morphologically normal according to these criteria [86].

Defects defined for each area are:

acrosomal area—lack, partial or vesiculated;

post-acrosomal lamina—lack or vesiculated;

neck—abaxial, cytoplasmic droplet.

mitochondria—lack, partial, disorganization;

tail—lack, coiled, broken, multi, short;

nucleus—small or large oval, narrow, wide or short, regional disorder, vacuoles occupying more than 4% of the nuclear area [87, 88]. However, evaluation of motile spermatozoa might differently be determined by various scientists [89].

What seems to be the most important in the observation of motile spermatozoa under high magnification in real time is evaluating the presence of vacuoles in the head of the sperm cell—number, size and location. The precise origin of the vacuoles is still unknown, but different hypothesis suggest they derived from early stages of spermatogenesis during sperm maturation and their number increase on account of vacuole area [90]. Other studies suggest that vacuoles formation in spermatozoa starts in incubation and capacitation period after ejaculation [91]. Nevertheless, high vacuolization or the presence of large vacuoles in the sperm head might be associated with increased DNA fragmentation rates and increased level of chromatin immaturity and could influence fertilization and pregnancy rates [92–94].

Sperm morphology evaluation could be based on the Cassuto and Barak Score as a precise rate system for sperm selection [94]. For the establishment of the score six parameters of the spermatozoon were taken into account: head, acrosome, vacuole, basis, insertion, and cytoplasmic droplet ("HAVBIC"). Head, vacuole, and basis were considered as major criteria for abnormalities, and acrosome, insertion, and cytoplasmic droplet are minor criteria for sperm evaluation. The following equation was developed:

$$\text{Score of spermatozoa} = (2 \times \text{Head}) + (3 \times \text{Vacuole}) + (1 \times \text{Base}) \quad (1)$$

Based on the formula, sperm cells score could vary between 0 and up to 6, and in relation to the quality three groups were differentiated:

Class 1—High-quality spermatozoa (score 4–6);
Class 2—Medium-quality spermatozoa (score 1–3); and
Class 3—Low-quality spermatozoa (score 0) [81].

Since its introduction and based on the first articles demonstrating increase in the pregnancy rates using IMSI compared to ICSI [85, 87] the method became widely incorporated in laboratory practice despite it is a time-consuming technique.

Evaluation of motile spermatozoa under high magnification is suitable for patients with high levels of DNA fragmentation sperm aneuploidy, severe oligo- or oligoasthenozoospermia and/or teratozoospermia, recurrent implantation failures or history of repeated early miscarriages, advanced female age and advanced male age [80]. Subsequent studies provided further analysis and information for the importance of the new method evaluating sperm morphology for obtaining better results in patients with male factor infertility.

There are still controversial study conclusions for the impact of IMSI procedure on *in vitro* cycle outcomes. However, what seems to benefit its practice is the better understanding of sperm morphology and function [95].

3.2 Genetics and sperm count

Y-chromosome deletion is associated with azoospermia, oligozoospermia (low sperm count) or abnormal sperm morphology and motility [96, 97]. When AZFa and AZFb deletions are detected, testicular sperm retrieval would be ineffective [98], but it is successful option for most males with AZFc deletions [99–101]. There is a case [102] reporting natural conception and Y-microdeletion passing. When diagnosed, and considering that Y chromosome infertility is inherited in a Y-linked manner, the patients should discuss and consult the specific genetic condition with genetics specialists as this could lead to infertility in the next generations [103].

Another gene that could be investigated in order to obtain the option for TESE is the Testis expressed gene 11 (TEX 11). Studies show that *TEX11* (X-linked meiosis-specific gene) is mutated in azoospermic men [104]. Sperm retrieval is not applicable for those patients [105, 106].

Congenital bilateral absence of vas deferens (CBAVD) and the lack of sperm cells in the ejaculate are superable using microsurgical TESE or PESA followed by ICSI [107]. As CBAVD has been associated with mutations in the cystic fibrosis transmembrane conductance regulator (CFTR) gene [108, 109] investigating the condition and genetic testing and consultation prior the procedures should be provided as there is a risk for the couple to have a child with cystic fibrosis [110].

In conclusion, genetic counseling as well as prenatal genetic diagnosis (PGD) or preimplantation genetic screening (PGS) should be offered as part of the fertility treatment [111, 112].

4. Cross points between cancer treatment and male fertility

Cancer healing by chemo- or radiation- therapy may disturb hormone production, ejaculation and spermatogenesis for long period of time or even permanently. These aggressive treatments could lead also to higher DNA sperm fragmentation [113, 114]. For cancer patients with assigned therapy, freezing one or several semen samples prior the start of any medicaments and manipulations (including operation, X-ray for additional diagnostics) is an option for further fertility preservation. Although cryopreservation of sperm does not guarantee preserving fertility or achieving pregnancy, it is substantial to consult and encourage the patient/couple to do it. Still, in patients with terminal loss of spermatogenesis due to cancer treatment, frozen samples are the only chance of hope to father a biological child. When a female partner is involved, counseling should consider the fact that female age is a leading factor in conception and postponing the ART or natural conception, could seriously decrease the chances of having a baby [115–119].

4.1 Using donor sperm in ART

Despite the advances of modern science and reproductive medicine, for some men, the only chance to father a child is through donated sperm [120]. In cases when after thorough examination male sterility was diagnosed [121]; severe hereditary conditions are established, or a couple with male factor infertility had numerous in vitro cycles [122] with no positive results, using donated sperm is an option. Employing donor spermatozoa in the fertility treatment could influence the couple's psychological state, the relationship between the partners and their relatives [123, 124]. In order to perceive infertility and take informed choice for further fertility treatment psychological support could be of help [125].

5. Reactive oxygen species (ROS)

Superoxide anion (O^{2-}), hydrogen peroxide (H_2O_2), hypochlorite (OHCl), and hydroxyl radical (OH) are highly reactive oxygen species (ROS) and their production occurs during normal metabolism of the cell. In semen ROS are produced mostly by the leukocytes and immature spermatozoa and are related to acrosome reaction, capacitation, mitochondrial stability, and fusion with oocyte. Imbalance between the formation of ROS and the inability of the antioxidants to neutralize the excessive production of ROS is defined as oxidative stress (OS). As seminal plasma contains antioxidants and has natural antioxidant capacity, it sustains the free radicals balance in the sperm; overproduction of ROS and OS results in lipid peroxidation, protein changes, DNA damage and sperm death, and this may affect male fertility [126, 127].

High concentrations of ROS as potential cause of male infertility have been studied since 1943 [128]. Potential internal yield of excess ROS could be consequence to damaged or abnormal spermatozoa, varicocele, cryptorchism, testicular torsion, infection, inflammation and aging. Some external factors such as exposure to toxins (toluene, methoxyethanol, sulfur dioxide), metals (cadmium) chemotherapy and ionizing radiation (cancer treatment) may also influence ROS levels and form OS.

Studies demonstrate association between elevated ROS levels and abnormal sperm concentration, motility, morphology, higher DNA damage and apoptosis. Comparison between infertile men and donors showed that excess ROS values had a sensitivity of 68.8% and specificity of 93.8% in correlation with poor semen parameters and could result in infertility [129, 130].

It is important to understand the physiological role of ROS as they are relevant to sperm capacitation, hyperactivation and sperm-egg fusion formation. ROS are involved in intracellular cyclic adenosine monophosphate (cAMP) increase followed by protein Kinase A activation and elevation of tyrosine phosphorylation. These changes lead to sperm capacitation and hyperactivation, sperm membrane becomes unstable and initiates acrosome reaction (releasing enzymes contained in the acrosome—nonzymogen acrosin, proacrosin, inhibitor-bound acrosin, hyaluronidase, acid phosphatase, beta-glucuronidase, beta-glucosidase, beta-N-acetylglucosaminidase, beta-galactosidase and beta-N-acetylgalactosaminidase) which allows the binding of sperm cell to oocytes zona pellucida (ZP) [131].

Imbalanced ROS levels could compromise semen quality and functions and keeping them in normal concentration is considered essential to fertility. Oxidative stress and nutritional status are of importance to every person as antioxidant deficiency and malnutrition may alter the health in general. ROS are also related to various respiratory and cardiovascular diseases, neurodegenerative, digestive disorders and even cancer. The clinical importance of OS in relation to fertility is thoroughly studied. The clinical awareness of nutritional balance in disease occurrence, progression and outcome is still limited, but the need of balanced diet nutrients and antioxidants is urged and necessary [132, 133].

6. Processing sperm samples *in vitro*

The ability of a men to become biological father is not only a consequence of normal sperm count but is also linked to the normal function of the male reproductive tract and sperm activity. Failure in sperm production or low sperm count and motility, poor morphology, disturbance in sperm movement and progressive passage through the cervical mucus, uterus, ampulla of the oviducts, capacitation and acrosome reaction, binding zona peluccida, etc. can result in male infertility.

To overcome male infertility in ART different protocols for sperm processing have been developed. There are still many debates on the exact influence of specific techniques used for sperm processing and their benefit to achieve pregnancy. Selecting a proper technique must be strongly individual according the couple's infertility history and ART treatment plan along with semen quality. Isolating an optimal fraction (higher count with progressive movement, morphologically normal rates) of spermatozoa gives the opportunity for selection and usage of the spermatozoa with a better fertilizability and higher chances to contribute for a viable fetus, for intrauterine insemination (IUI), IVF or ICSI.

Two of the most explored methods for sperm processing in ART—density gradient centrifugation (DGS) and swim-up (SU)—are investigated in details. Compared to fresh sample, the processed one has lower DNA fragmentation rates [134, 135] and lower concentration of ROS regardless which method was used [136, 137].

As there are studies exploring telomere length in reproductive cells (oocytes and spermatozoa) and their connection to infertility, shorter telomeres in spermatozoa might be assumed as a factor causing idiopathic infertility [138]. Truncated telomeres and altered DNA integrity in sperm could negatively influence fertilization, pronuclei formation, embryo morphology and quality and thus could compromise blastocyst formation and implantation. Spermatozoa obtained by either DGC or SU have longer telomeres compared sperm cells in the raw semen [139].

Some substances such as pentoxifylline (methylxanthine derivate primarily used in intermittent claudication and other vascular disorders treatment) might enhance the motility and quantity of motile sperm after processing. By using pentoxifylline primarily on samples with poor quality increased sperm viability in infertile men with oligoasthenozoospermia, was observed. Samples obtained by PESA or TESE could also be improved by implementing this xanthine derivative in cultural media and thus improve sperm motility [140].

Sperm preparation methods along with technical advantages of MSOME allow the selection of sperm cells, with best predictive values, for ART treatments. There are some limitations related to each method used and that is now an open field to research and establish new noninvasive protocols for sperm selection in the routine practice.

7. Conclusion

Spermatogenesis is a complexed process of division and formation of male reproductive cells. It is highly sensitive to various internal (hormonal regulation, transmitters, growth factors) and external (nutritive substances, therapeutics, drugs, hormones and their metabolites, different toxic substances or X-radiation, increased temperature) factors [141]. Given that the time frame for formation of every new generation of spermatozoa takes approximately 3 months, it should be considered that unfavorable effects purge would be the consequence to time consuming treatment or lifestyle changes.

Modern day society—environment, lifestyle and diet are suspected to be harmful to different processes in the organism such as spermatogenesis and could negatively affect the quality and quantity of life through human lifespan including the ability to reproduce. Considering that sex formation takes place during early fetal development attention to mother's nocuous habits, lifestyle, and environmental specifics should be advert. Events during pregnancy could also influence male fertility later in life [142]. In some specific cases, when there was a long exposure to high dosage of toxins, chemotherapy or radiotherapy, spermatogenesis regeneration would most probably take years or may never be restored. Healthy life style along with regular medical check and tests could indicate on time and even prevent urological or fertility problems.

Acknowledgements

The authors wish to thank their IVF unit colleagues at Ob/Gyn Hospital "Dr. Shterev" for most helpful discussions while summarizing this chapter.

Conflict of interest

The authors report no financial or commercial conflicts of interest.

Appendix: this appendix presents the definitions of terms/notations used through the report

AMA	advanced maternal age
ART	assisted reproduction technology
BMI	body mass index
CASA	computer assisted sperm analysis
cAMP	cyclic adenosine monophosphate
CBAVD	congenital bilateral absence of vas deferens
CFTR	cystic fibrosis transmembrane conductance regulator gene
DGC	density gradient centrifugation
ICSI	intracytoplasmic sperm injection
IMSI	intracytoplasmic morphologically selected sperm injection
IUI	intrauterine insemination
IVF	in vitro fertilization
MESA	microsurgical epididymal sperm aspiration
MSOME	motile sperm organelle morphology examination
NOA	nonobstructive oligoasthenozoospermia
OA	oligoasthenozoospermia
OS	oxidative stress
PESA	percutaneous epididymal sperm aspiration
PGD	preimplantation genetic diagnosis
PGS	preimplantation genetic screening extraction
ROS	reactive oxygen species
SAT	sperm aneuploidy test
SU	swim up
TAILS	tail axoneme intra-lumenal spital
TESE	testicular sperm
TEX 11	testis expressed gene
WHO	World Health Organization
ZP	zona pellucida
H_2O_2	hydrogen peroxide
O^{2-}	superoxide anion
OHCl	hypochlorite
OH	hydroxyl radical

Author details

Tanya Milachich* and Desislava Dyulgerova-Nikolova
SAGBAL "Dr. Shterev", Sofia, Bulgaria

*Address all correspondence to: tanya_ivf@yahoo.com

References

[1] Andrade-Rocha FT. On the origins of the semen analysis: A close relationship with the history of the reproductive medicine. Journal of Human Reproduction. 2017;**10**(4):242-255. DOI: 10.4103/jhrs.JHRS_97_17

[2] Vasan SS. Semen analysis and sperm function tests: How much to test? Indian Journal of Urology. 2011;**27**(1):41-48. DOI: 10.4103/0970-1591.78424

[3] Murray KS, Andrew J, McGeady J, Reed ML, Kuang WW, Nangia AK. The effect of the new 2010 World Health Organization criteria forsemen analyses on male infertility. Fertility and Sterility. 2012;**98**(6):1428-1431. DOI: 10.1016/j.fertnstert.2012.07.1130. [Epub: 24 August 2012]

[4] Alshahrani S, Aldossari K, Al-Zahrani J, Gabr AH, Henkel R, Ahmad G. Interpretation of semen analysis using WHO 1999 and WHO 2010 reference values: Abnormal becoming normal. First International Journal of Andrology Andrologia. 2018;**50**(2):e12838. DOI: 10.1111/and.12838

[5] Patel A, Leong JY, Ramasamy R. Prediction of male infertility by the World Health Organization laboratory manual for assessment of semen analysis: A systematic review. Arab Journal of Urology. 2018;**16**:96-102. DOI: 10.1016/j.aju.2017.10.005. eCollection 2018 Mar

[6] Esteves SC, Zini A, Aziz N, Alvarez JG, Sabanegh ES Jr, Agarwal A. Critical appraisal of World Health Organization's New reference values for human semen characteristics and effect on diagnosis and treatment of subfertile men. Urology. 2012;**79**:16-22. DOI: 10.1016/j.urology.2011.08.003. [Epub: 08 November 2011]

[7] Baldi E, Festin MP. WHO manual: Status report and who perspectives. Abstracts of the 10th Congress of the European Academy of Andrology. Andrology. 2018;**6**(Suppl 2):23

[8] Sorena K, Craig JR, Zhang C. Impacts of abstinence time on semen parameters in a large population-based cohort of subfertile men. Urology. 2017;**108**:90-95

[9] De Jonge C, LaFromboise M, Bosmans E, et al. Influence of the abstinence period on human sperm quality. Fertility and Sterility. 2004;**82**(1):57-65

[10] Mahdi MA, Shwish DL, Almhmdi NA. Evaluation of the impact of the level of (Testosterone, Luteinizing Hormone, Follicle-Stimulating Hormone and Prolactin) on some semen parameters in infertile males. Tikrit Journal of Pure Science. 2018;**23**(7). ISSN: 18131662

[11] Miller MR, Mannowetz N, Iavarone AT, et al. Unconventional endocannabinoid signaling governs sperm activation via the sex hormone progesterone. Science. 2016;**352**(6285):555-559. DOI: 10.1126/science.aad6887

[12] PapeMøller A. Ejaculate quality, testes size and sperm competition in primates. Journal of Human Evolution. 1988;**17**(5):479-488

[13] Veleva L, Milachich T, Bochev I. Relationship of somatic indicators with motility and velocity parameters of sperm movement. Reproductive Health. 2015;(22):9-13

[14] Sermondade N, Faure C, Fezeu L, et al. BMI in relation to sperm count: An updated systematic review and collaborative meta-analysis. Human Reproduction Update. 2013;**19**(3):221-231. DOI: 10.1093/humupd/dms050

[15] Andersen JM, Herning H, Aschim EL, Hjelmesæth J, Mala T,

Hanevik HI, et al. Body mass index is associated with impaired semen characteristics and reduced levels of anti-Müllerian hormone across a wide weight range. PLoS One. 2015;**10**(6):e0130210. DOI: 10.1371/journal.pone.0130210

[16] Rusz A, Pilatz A, Wagenlehner F, et al. Influence of urogenital infections and inflammation on semen quality and male fertility. The World Journal of Urology. 2012;**30**(1):23-30. DOI: 10.1007/s00345-011-0726-8. [Epub: 12 July 2011]

[17] Keck C, Gerber-Schäfer C, Clad A, Wilhelm C, Breckwoldt M. Seminal tract infections: Impact on male fertility and treatment options. Human Reproduction Update. 1998;**4**(6):891-903. DOI: 10.1093/humupd/4.6.891

[18] Ochsendorf FR. Sexually transmitted infections: Impact on male fertility. Andrologia. 2008;**40**(2):72-75. DOI: 10.1111/j.1439-0272.2007.00825.x

[19] Salas-Huetos A. Adherence to the Mediterranean diet is positively associated with sperm motility: A cross-sectional analysis. Scientific Reports. 2019;**9**. DOI: 10.1038/s41598-019-39826-7. Article number: 3389

[20] Nassan FL et al. Diet and men's fertility: Does diet affect sperm quality? Fertility and Sterility. 2018;**110**(4):570-577. DOI: 10.1016/j.fertnstert.2018.05.025

[21] Luque EM, Tissera A, Gaggino MP, Molina RI, Mangeaud A, Vincenti LM, et al. Body mass index and human sperm quality: Neither one extreme nor the other. Reproduction, Fertility and Development. 2015;**29**:731-739. DOI: 10.1071/RD15351

[22] Sharma R, Harlev A, Agarwal A, Sandro C, Esteves SC. Cigarette smoking and semen quality: A new meta-analysis examining the effect of the 2010 World Health Organization laboratory methods for the examination of human semen. European Urology. 2016;**70**(4):635-645. DOI: 10.1016/j.eururo.2016.04.010. [Epub: 21 April 2016]

[23] Gaskins AJ, Mendiola J, Afeiche M, et al. Physical activity and television watching in relation to semen quality in young men. British Journal of Sports Medicine. 2015;**49**:265-270. DOI: 10.1136/bjsports-2012-091644. [Epub: 04 February 2013]

[24] Lähdetie J. Occupation- and exposure-related studies on human sperm. Journal of Occupational and Environmental Medicine. 1995;**37**(8):922-930. DOI: 10.1016/j.fertnstert.2005.06.048

[25] Keel AB. Within- and between-subject variation in semenparameters in infertile men and normal semen donors. Fertility and Sterility. 2006;**85**(1):128-134

[26] World Health Organization. WHO laboratory manual for the examination of human semen and sperm-cervical mucus interaction, 3rd ed. Cambridge: Cambridge University Press; 1992

[27] Ossenbuhn S. Exogenous influences on human fertility: Fluctuations in sperm parameters and results of in-vitro fertilization coincide with conceptions in the normal population. Human Reproduction. 1998;**13**(8):2165-2171. DOI: 10.1093/humrep/13.8.2165

[28] Ombelet W, Maes M, Vandeput H, et al. Chronobiological fluctuations in semen parameters with a constant abstinence period. Archives of Andrology. 1996;**37**(2):91-96. DOI: 10.3109/01485019608988508

[29] De Giorgi A, Volpi R, Tiseo R, et al. Seasonal variation of human semen parameters: A retrospective study in Italy. Chronobiology International. 2015;**32**(5):711-716. DOI: 10.3109/07420528.2015.1024315. [Epub: 04 May 2015]

[30] Moazzam A, Choudhary MN, Muhammad I, et al. From basic to contemporary semen analysis: limitations and variability. The Journal of Animal & Plant Sciences. 2015;**25**(2):328-336. ISSN: 1018-7081

[31] Wang C, Swerdloff RS. Limitations of semen analysis as a test of male fertility and anticipated needs from newer tests. Fertility and Sterility. 2014;**102**(6):1502-1507. DOI: 10.1016/j.fertnstert.2014.10.021

[32] Sikka SC, Hellstrom WJG. Current updates on laboratory techniques for the diagnosis of male reproductive failure. Asian Journal of Andrology. 2016;**18**:392-401. DOI: 10.4103/1008-682X.179161

[33] World Health Organization. WHO Laboratory Manual for the Examination and Processing of Human Semen. 5th ed. Geneva: World Health Organization; 2010

[34] Karabulut S, Keskin İ, Kutlu P, Delikara N, Atvar Ö, Öztürk MI. Male infertility, azoozpermia and cryptozoospermia incidence among three infertility clinics in Turkey. Turkish Journal of Urology. 2018;**44**(2):109-113. DOI: 10.5152/tud.2018.59196

[35] Practice committee of the American Society for Reproductive Medicine in collaboration with the Society for Male Reproduction and Urology. Evaluation of the azoospermic male: A committee opinion. Fertility and Sterility. 2018;**109**(5):0015-0282. DOI: 10.1016/j.fertnstert.2018.01.043

[36] Cornud F, Belin X, Delafontaine D, et al. Imaging of obstructive azoospermia. European Radiology. 1997;7:1079. DOI: 10.1007/s003300050258

[37] Schlegel NP. Causes of azoospermia and their management. Reproduction, Fertility and Development;**16**(5):561-572. DOI: 10.1071/RD03087

[38] Baker K, Sabanegh E Jr. Obstructive azoospermia: reconstructive techniques and results. Clinics (Sao Paulo). 2013;**68**(Suppl 1):61-73. DOI: 10.6061/clinics/2013(sup01)07

[39] Kumar R. Medical management of non-obstructive azoospermia. Clinics (Sao Paulo). 2013;**68**(Suppl 1):75-79. DOI: 10.6061/clinics/2013(Sup01)08

[40] Emokpae MA, Uadia PO, Mohammed AZ, Omale-Itodo A. Hormonal abnormalities in azoospermic men in Kano, Northern Nigeria. The Indian Journal of Medical Research. 2006;**124**:299-304

[41] Nagvenkar P, Desai K, Hinduja I, Kusum Zaveri K. Chromosomal studies in infertile men with oligozoospermia & non-obstructive azoospermia. The Indian Journal of Medical Research. 2005;**122**:34-4234

[42] Xie C, Chen X, Liu Y, Wu Z, Ping P. Multicenter study of genetic abnormalities associated with severe oligospermia and non-obstructive azoospermia. Journal of International Medical Research. 2018;**46**(1):107-114. DOI: 10.1177/0300060517718771

[43] Benoff S, Jacob A, Hurley IR. Male infertility and environmental exposure to lead and cadmium. Human Reproduction Update. 2000;**6**(2):107-121. DOI: 10.1093/humupd/6.2.107

[44] Boekelheide K. Mechanisms of toxic damage to spermatogenesis. JNCI Monographs. 2005;**2005**(34):6-8. DOI: 10.1093/jncimonographs/lgi006

[45] Weedin JW, Khera M, Lipshultz LI. Varicocele repair in patients with nonobstructive azoospermia: A meta-analysis. The Journal of Urology. 2010;**183**(6):2309-2315. DOI: 10.1016/j.juro.2010.02.012. [Epub: 18 April 2010]

[46] Hamada AJ, Esteves SC, Agarwal A. A comprehensive review of genetics and genetic testing in azoospermia. Clinics (São Paulo, Brazil). 2013;**68**(Suppl 1):39-60. DOI: 10.6061/clinics/2013(sup01)06

[47] Wosnitzer MS. Genetic evaluation of male infertility. Translational Andrology and Urology. 2014;**3**(1):17-26. DOI: 10.3978/j.issn.2223-4683.2014.02.04

[48] World Health Organization. World Health Organization Laboratory Manual for the Evaluation and Processing of Human Semen. 5th ed. Cambridge, UK: Cambridge University Press; 2010

[49] Punab M, Poolamets O, Paju P, et al. Causes of male infertility: A 9-year prospective monocentre study on 1737 patients with reduced total sperm counts. Human Reproduction. 2017;**32**(1):18-31. DOI: 10.1093/humrep/dew284

[50] Song S-H, Bak CW, et al. Natural course of severe oligozoospermia in infertile male: Influence on future fertility potential. Journal of Andrology. 2010;**31**(6). DOI: 10.2164/jandrol.110.010199. [Epub: 29 July 2010]

[51] World Health Organization. Obesity: Preventing and Managing the Global Epidemic, Report of a WHO Consultation (WHO Technical Report Series 894). Geneva, Switzerland: World Health Organization; 2000

[52] Caballero B. The global epidemic of obesity: An overview. Epidemiologic Reviews. 2007;**29**(1):1-5. DOI: 10.1093/epirev/mxm012

[53] Craig JR et al. Obesity, male infertility, and the sperm epigenome. Fertility and Sterility. 2017;**107**(4):848-859. DOI: 10.1016/j.fertnstert.2017.02.115

[54] Sermondade N, Faure C, Fezeu L, et al. Obesity and increased risk for oligozoospermia and azoospermia. Archives of Internal Medicine. 2012;**172**(5):440-442. DOI: 10.1001/archinternmed.2011.1382

[55] Salas-Huetos A, Bulló M, Salas-Salvadó J. Dietary patterns, foods and nutrients in male fertility parameters and fecundability: A systematic review of observational studies. Human Reproduction Update. 2017;**23**(4):371-389. DOI: 10.1093/humupd/dmx006

[56] Dam AH, Feenstra I, Westphal JR, Ramos L, van Golde RJ, Kremer JA. Globozoospermia revisited. Human Reproduction Update. 2007;**13**(1):63-75. DOI: 10.1093/humupd/dml047. [Epub: 28 September 2006]

[57] Vicari E, Perdichizzi A, De Palma A, Burrello N, D'Agata R, Calogero AE. Globozoospermia is associated with chromatin structure abnormalities: Case report. Human Reproduction. 2002;**17**(8):2128-2133. DOI: 10.1093/humrep/17.8.2128

[58] Baccetti B et al. Notulae seminologicae. 2. The 'short tail' and 'stump' defect in human spermatozoa. Andrologia: First International Journal of Andrology. 1993;**25**(6):331-335. DOI: 10.1111/j.1439-0272.1993.tb02736.x

[59] Koning RI, Koster AJ. Cryo-electron tomography in biology and medicine. Annals of Anatomy—Anatomischer Anzeiger. 2009;**191**(5):427-445. DOI: 10.1016/j.aanat.2009.04.003

[60] Zabeo D, Heumann JM, Schwartz CL, Suzuki-Shinjo A, Morgan G, Widlund Per O, et al. A lumenal interrupted helix in human sperm tail microtubules. Scientific Reports. 2018;**8**:2727. DOI: 10.1038/s41598-018-21165-8

[61] Chemes HE, Sedo CA. Tales of the tail and sperm head aches: Changing concepts on the prognostic significance of sperm pathologies affecting the

head, neck and tail. Asian Journal of Andrology. 2012;**14**(1):14-23. DOI: 10.1038/aja.2011.168

[62] Wyrobek AJ, Bruce WR. The induction of sperm-shape abnormalities in mice and humans. In Chemical Mutagens: Principles and Methods for Their Detection Vol. 5. Hollaender A, de Serres FJ. New York, Plenum; (1978): 257-285.

[63] Martin RH, Rademaker A. The relationship between sperm chromosomal abnormalities and sperm morphology in humans. Mutation Research. 1988;**207**(3-4):159-164

[64] Ray P, Toure A, Metzler-Guillemain C, et al. Genetic abnormalities leading to qualitative defects of sperm morphology or function. Clinical Genetics. 2017;**91**(2):217-232. DOI: 10.1111/cge.12905, Special Issue: A Special Issue on Genetics and Human Reproduction. [Epub: 09 December 2016]

[65] Sun F, Ko E, Martin RH. Is there a relationship between sperm chromosome abnormalities and sperm morphology? Reproductive Biology and Endocrinology. 2006;**4**(1):1. DOI: 10.1186/1477-7827-4-1

[66] Devillard F, Metzler-Guillemain C, Pelletier R, DeRobertis C, Bergues U, Hennebicq S, et al. Polyploidy in large-headed sperm: FISH study of three cases. Human Reproduction. 2002;**17**(5):1292-1298. DOI: 10.1093/humrep/17.5.1292

[67] Boushaba S, Belaaloui G. Sperm DNA fragmentation and standard semen parameters in Algerian infertile male partners. The World Journal of Men's Health. 2015;**33**(1):1-7. DOI: 10.5534/wjmh.2015.33.1.1

[68] Belloc S, Benkhalifa M, Cohen-Bacrie M, Dalleac A, Chahine H, Amar E, et al. Which isolated sperm abnormality is most related to sperm DNA damage in men presenting for infertility evaluation. Journal of Assisted Reproduction and Genetics. 2014;**31**(5):527-532. DOI: 10.1007/s10815-014-0194-3

[69] Menkveld R, Wong WY, Lombard CJ, Wetzels AMM, Thomas CMG, Merkus H, et al. Semen parameters, including WHO and strict criteria morphology, in a fertile and subfertile population: An effort towards standardization of in-vivo thresholds. Human Reproduction. 2001;**16**(6):1165-1171. DOI: 10.1093/humrep/16.6.1165

[70] Engel KM, Grunewald S, Schiller J. Automated semen analysis by SQA Vision® versus the manual approach—A prospective double-blind study. Andrologia. 2019;**51**(1):e131490. DOI: 10.1111/and.13149

[71] Dearing C, Jayasena C, Lindsay K. Can the Sperm Class Analyser (SCA) CASA-Mot system for human sperm motility analysis reduce imprecision and operator subjectivity and improve semen analysis? Human Fertility. Published online May 6, 2019:1-11. DOI: 10.1080/14647273.2019.1610581

[72] World Health Organization. WHO Laboratory Manual for the Examination of Human Semen and Sperm-Cervical Mucus Interaction. 4th ed. Cambridge: Cambridge University Press; 1999

[73] World Health Organization. WHO Laboratory Manual for the Examination and Processing of Human Semen, 5th ed. Geneva: World Health Organization; 2010

[74] Kim SM, Kim SK, Jee BC, Kim SH. Effect of sperm DNA fragmentation on embryo quality in normal responder women in in vitro fertilization and intracytoplasmic sperm injection. Yonsei Medical Journal. 2019;**60**(5):461-466. DOI: 10.3349/ymj.2019.60.5.461

[75] Sedó CA, Bilinski M, Lorenzi D, et al. Effect of sperm DNA fragmentation on embryo development: Clinical and biological aspects. JBRA Assisted Reproduction;**21**(4):343-350. DOI: 10.5935/1518-0557.20170061

[76] Esquerré-Lamare C, Walschaerts M, Chansel Debordeaux L, et al. Sperm aneuploidy and DNA fragmentation in unexplained recurrent pregnancy loss: A multicenter case-control study. Basic and Clinical Andrology. 2018;**28**:4. DOI: 10.1186/s12610-018-0070-6. [Epub: 02 April 2018]

[77] Krawetz SA. Paternal contribution: New insights and future challenges. Nature Reviews. Genetics. 2005;**6**(8):633-642. DOI: 10.1038/nrg1654

[78] Bukowska D, Kempisty B, Piotrowska H, Sosinska P, Wozna M, Ciesiolka S, et al. The structure and role of mammalian sperm RNA: A review. Veterinární Medicína. 2013;**58**(2):57-64. DOI: 10.17221/6696-VETMED

[79] Berkovitz A, Eltes F, Lederman H, Peer S, Ellenbogen A, Feldberg B, et al. How to improve IVF–ICSI outcome by sperm selection. Reproductive Biomedicine Online. 2006;**12**(5):634-638. DOI: 10.1016/s1472-6483(10)61191-1

[80] Yona B, Ellenbogen A. Interacytoplasmic morphologically selected sperm injection: A tool for selecting the best sperm in real time. 2018. DOI: 10.5772/intechopen.73388 In book: Spermatozoa - Facts and Perspectives. License CC BY 3.0

[81] Gosálvez J et al. Single sperm selection and DNA fragmentation analysis: The case of MSOME/IMSI. Natural Science. 2013;**5**(7A):7-14. DOI: 10.4236/ns.2013.57A002

[82] Ebner T, Shebl O, Oppelt P, Mayer RB. Some reflections on intracytoplasmic morphologically selected sperm injection. International Journal of Fertility & Sterility. 2014;**8**(2):105-112

[83] Delaroche L, Yazbeck C, Gout C, KahnV, OgerP, RougierN. Intracytoplasmic morphologically selected sperm injection (IMSI) after repeated IVF or ICSI failures: A prospective comparative study. European Journal of Obstetrics, Gynecology, and Reproductive Biology. 2013;**167**(1):76-80. DOI: 10.1016/j.ejogrb.2012.11.011. [Epub: 29 December 2012]

[84] Boitrelle F, Guthauser B, Alter L, Bailly M, Bergere M, Wainer R, et al. High-magnification selection of spermatozoa prior to oocyte injection: Confirmed and potential indications. Reproductive Biomedicine Online. 2014;**28**(1):6-13. DOI: 10.1016/j.rbmo.2013.09.019. [Epub: 28 September 2013]

[85] Bartoov B, Berkovitz A, Eltes F. Selection of spermatozoa with normal nuclei to improve the pregnancy rate with intracytoplasmic sperm injection. The New England Journal of Medicine. 2001;**345**(14):1067-1068. DOI: 10.1056/NEJM200110043451416

[86] Lo Monte G, Germond M, Marci R. Focus on intracytoplasmic morphologically selected sperm injection (IMSI): A mini-review. Asian Journal of Andrology. 2013. DOI: 10.1038/aja.2013.54

[87] Bartoov B, Berkovitz A, Eltes F, Kogosowski A, Menezo Y, Barak Y. Real-time fine morphology of motile human sperm cells is associated with IVF-ICSI outcome. Journal of Andrology. 2002;**23**(1):1-8. DOI: 10.1002/j.1939-4640.2002.tb02595.x

[88] Antinori M, Vanderzwalmen P, Barak Y. IMSI as a valuable tool for sperm selection during ART. In: Racowsky C, Schlegel P, Fauser B,

Carrell D, editors. Biennial Review of Infertility. Vol. 2. Boston, MA: Springer; 2011. pp. 363-276. DOI: 10.1007/978-1-4419-8456-2_19

[89] Tanaka A, Nagayoshi M, Tanaka I, Kusunoki H. Human sperm head vacuoles are physiological structures formed during the sperm development and maturation process. Fertility and Sterility. 2012;**98**:315-320. DOI: 10.1016/j.fertnstert.2012.04.034. [Epub: 22 May 2012]

[90] Leahy T, Gadella BM. Sperm surface changes and physiological consequences induced by sperm handling and storage. Reproduction. 2011;**142**:759-778. DOI: 10.1530/REP-11-0310. [Epub: 29 September 2011]

[91] Boitrelle F, Ferfouri F, Petit JM. Large human sperm vacuoles observed in motile spermatozoa under high magnification: Nuclear thumbprints linked to failure of chromatin condensation. Human Reproduction. 2011;**26**(7):1650-1658. DOI: 10.1093/humrep/der129. [Epub: 02 May 2011]

[92] Sellami A, Chakroun N, Zarrouk SB, Sellami H, Kebaili S, Rebai T, et al. Assessment of chromatin maturity in human spermatozoa: Useful aniline blue assay for routine diagnosis of male infertility. Advances in Urology. 2013;**2013**:578631. DOI: 10.1155/2013/578631

[93] Vanderzwalmen P, Hiemer A, Rubner P, et al. Blastocyst development after sperm selection at high magnification is associated with size and number of nuclear vacuoles. Reproductive Biomedicine Online. 2008;**17**(5):617-627. DOI: 10.1016/s1472-6483(10)60308-2

[94] Cassuto NG et al. A new real-time morphology classification for human spermatozoa: A link for fertilization and improved embryo quality. Fertility and Sterility;**92**(5):1616-1625. DOI: 10.1016/j.fertnstert.2008.08.088. [Epub: 05 November 2008]

[95] Tosti E, Ménézo Y. IMSI, useful, useless or harmful? Fertilization: In vitro. 2012;**2**:e115. DOI: 10.4172/2165-7491.1000e115

[96] Akınsal EC, Baydilli N, Dündar M, Ekmekçioğlu O. The frequencies of Y chromosome microdeletions in infertile males. Turkish Journal of Urology. 2018;**44**(5):389-392. DOI: 10.5152/tud.2018.73669

[97] Elfateh F, Rulin D, Xin Y, Linlin L, Haibo Z, Liu RZ. Prevalence and patterns of Y chromosome microdeletion in infertile men with azoospermia and oligzoospermia in Northeast China. Iranian Journal of Reproductive Medicine. 2014;**12**(6):383-388

[98] Liu T, Song YX, Jiang YM. Early detection of Y chromosome microdeletions in infertile men is helpful to guide clinical reproductive treatments in southwest of China. Medicine (Baltimore). 2019;**98**(5):e14350. DOI: 10.1097/MD.0000000000014350

[99] Liu X.G, Hu H.Y, Guo Y.H, Sun Y.P. Correlation between Y chromosome microdeletion and male infertility. Genetics and Molecular Research 15 (2): 2016 DOI 10.4238/gmr.15028426

[100] Hopps CV, Mielnik A, Goldstein M, Palermo GD, Rosenwaks Z, Schlegel PN. Detection of sperm in men with Y chromosome microdeletions of the AZFa, AZFb and AZFc regions. Human Reproduction. 2003;**18**(8):1660-1665. DOI: 10.1093/humrep/deg348

[101] Brandell RA, Mielnik A, Liotta D, Ye Z, Veeck LL, Palermo GD, et al. AZFb deletions predict the absence of spermatozoa with testicular sperm extraction: Preliminary report of

a prognostic genetic test. Human Reproduction. 1998;**13**(10):2812-2815. DOI: 10.1093/humrep/13.10.2812

[102] Kuhnert B, Gromoll J, Kostova E, Tschanter P, Luetjens CM, Simoni M, et al. Case report: Natural transmission of an AZFc Y-chromosomal microdeletion from father to his sons. Human Reproduction. 2004;**19**(4): 886-888. DOI: 10.1093/humrep/deh186

[103] Dohle GR, Halley DJJ, Van Hemel JO, van den Ouwel AMW, Pieters MHEC, Weber RFA, et al. Genetic risk factors in infertile men with severe oligozoospermia and azoospermia. Human Reproduction. 2002;**17**(1):13-16. DOI: 10.1093/humrep/17.1.13

[104] Yatsenko AN, Georgiadis AP, Röpke A, et al. X-linked TEX11 mutations, meiotic arrest, and Azoospermia in infertile men. The New England Journal of Medicine. 2015;**372**:2097-2107. DOI: 10.1056/NEJMoa1406192

[105] Tang L, Zeng W, Clark RK, Dobrinski I. Characterization of the porcine testis-expressed gene 11 (Tex11). Spermatogenesis. 2011;**1**(2):147-151. DOI: 10.4161/spmg.1.2.16680

[106] Yang F, Silber S, Leu AN, Oates RD, Marszalek JD, Skaletsky H, et al. TEX 11 is mutated in infertile men with azoospermia and regulates genome-wide recombination rates in mouse. EMBO Molecular Medicine. 2015;**7**(9). DOI: 10.15252/emmm.201404967

[107] Samli H, Samli MM, Yilmaz E, Imirzalioglu N. Clinical, andrological and genetic characteristics of patients with congenital bilateral absence of vas deferens (CBAVD). Archives of Andrology. 2006;**52**(6):471-477. DOI: 10.1080/01485010600691993

[108] Anguiano A, Oates RD, Amos JA, et al. Congenital bilateral absence of the vas deferens. A primarily genital form of cystic fibrosis. Journal of the American Medical Association. 1992;**267**:1794-1797

[109] Kanavakis E et al. Cystic fibrosis mutation screening in CBAVD patients and men with obstructive azoospermia or severe oligozoospermia. Molecular Human Reproduction. 1998;**4**(4): 333-337. DOI: 10.1093/molehr/4.4.333

[110] Pauer HU, Hinney B, Michelmann HW, et al. Relevance of genetic counselling in couples prior to intracytoplasmic sperm injection. Human Reproduction. 1997, 1997;**12**(9):1909-1912. DOI: 10.1093/humrep/12.9.1909

[111] Harton GL, Magli MC, Lundin K, Montag M, Lemmen J, Harper JC. ESHRE PGD consortium/embryology special interest group—Best practice guidelines for polar body and embryo biopsy for preimplantation genetic diagnosis/screening (PGD/PGS). Human Reproduction. 2011;**26**(1):41-46. DOI: 10.1093/humrep/deq265

[112] Harper J, Geraedts J, Borry P, et al. Current issues in medically assisted reproduction and genetics in Europe: Research, clinical practice, ethics, legal issues and policy. Human Reproduction. 2014;**29**(8):1603-1609. DOI: 10.1093/humrep/deu130. [Epub: 08 July 2014]

[113] Smit M, van Casteren NJ, Wildhagen MF, Romijn JC, Dohle GR. Sperm DNA integrity in cancer patients before and after cytotoxic treatment. Human Reproduction. 2010;**25**(8):1877-1883. DOI: 10.1093/humrep/deq104

[114] Paoli D, Pallotti F, Andrea Lenzi A, Lombardo F. Fatherhood and sperm DNA damage in testicular cancer patients. Frontiers in Endocrinology. 2018;**9**:506. DOI: 10.3389/fendo.2018.00506

[115] Leridon H. Can assisted reproduction technology compensate for the natural decline in fertility with age? A model assessment. Human Reproduction. 2004;**19**(7):1548-1553. DOI: 10.1093/humrep/deh304

[116] Sauer VM. Reproduction at an advanced maternal age and maternal health. Fertility and Sterility. 2015;**103**(5):1136-1143. DOI: 10.1016/j.fertnstert.2015.03.004

[117] Ferrazzi E, Brembilla G, Cipriani S. Maternal age and body mass index at term: Risk factors for requiring an induced labour for a late-term pregnancy. European Journal of Obstetrics & Gynecology and Reproductive Biology. 2019;**233**:151-157. DOI: 10.1016/j.ejogrb.2018.12.018. [Epub: 20 Dec 2018]

[118] Wie HJ, Pak SE, Kim RY. Gestational age-specific risk of stillbirth during term pregnancy according to maternal age. Archives of Gynecology and Obstetrics. 2019;**299**(3):681-688. DOI: 10.1007/s00404-018-5022-z. [Epub: 21 December 2018]

[119] Pinheiro RL, Areia AL, Pinto AM, Donato H. Advanced maternal age: Adverse outcomes of pregnancy, a meta-analysis. Acta Medica Portuguesa. 2019;**32**(3). DOI: 10.20344/amp.11057. [Epub: 29 Mar 2019]

[120] Gudeloglu A, Parekattil SJ. Update in the evaluation of the azoospermic male. Clinics (Sao Paulo). 2013;**68**(Suppl 1):27-34. DOI: 10.6061/clinics/2013(sup01)04

[121] Practice Committee of the American Society for Reproductive Medicine. Diagnostic evaluation of the infertile male: A committee opinion. Fertility and Sterility. 2015;**103**(3):e18-e25. DOI: 10.1016/j.fertnstert.2014.12.103. [Epub: 15 Janaury 2015]

[122] Gorrill MJ, Burry KA, Patton PE. Pregnancy outcomes using donor sperm insemination after failed in vitro fertilization with intracytoplasmic sperm injection cycles in couples with complex infertility disorders. Fertility and Sterility. 2003;**80**(4):936-938. DOI: 10.1016/s0015-0282(03)01120-8

[123] Schover LR, Collins R, Richards S. Psychological aspects of donor insemination: Evaluation and follow-up of recipient couples. Fertility and Sterility. 1992;**57**(3):583-590. DOI: 10.1016/s0015-0282(16)54904-8

[124] Edelmann RJ, Humphrey M, Owens DJ. The meaning of parenthood and couples' reactions to male infertility. The British Journal of Medical Psychology. 1994;**67**(Pt 3):291-299. DOI: 10.1111/j.2044-8341.1994.tb01797.x

[125] Fisher JR, Hammarberg K. Psychological and social aspects of infertility in men: An overview of the evidence and implications for psychologically informed clinical care and future research. Asian Journal of Andrology. 2012;**14**(1):121-129. DOI: 10.1038/aja.2011.72

[126] Agarwal A, Ahmad G, Sharma R. Reference values of reactive oxygen species in seminal ejaculates using chemiluminescence assay. Journal of Assisted Reproduction and Genetics. 2015;**32**(12):1721-1729. DOI: 10.1007/s10815-015-0584-1. [Epub 02 October 2015]

[127] Wagner JH, Cheng W, Ko EY. Role of reactive oxygen species in male infertility: An updated review of literature. Arab Journal of Urology. 2018;**16**(1):35-43. DOI: 10.1016/j.aju.2017.11.001

[128] MacLeod J. The role of oxygen in the metabolism and motility of human spermatozoa. American Journal of Physiology. 1943;**138**:512-518. DOI: 10.1152/ajplegacy.1943.138.3.512

[129] Agarwal A, Sharma RK, Sharma R, Assidi M, Abuzenadah AM, Alshahrani S, et al. Characterizing semen parameters and their association with reactive oxygen species in infertile men. Reproductive Biology and Endocrinology. 2014;**12**:33. DOI: 10.1186/1477-7827-12-33

[130] Ko EY, Sabanegh ES Jr, Agarwal A. Male infertility testing: Reactive oxygen species and antioxidant capacity. Fertility and Sterility. 2014;**102**:1518-1527. DOI: 10.1016/j.fertnstert.2014.10.020

[131] Sabeti P, Pourmasumi S, Rahiminia T, Akyash F, Talebi AR. Etiologies of sperm oxidative stress. The International Journal of Reproductive BioMedicine (Yazd). 2016;**14**(4): 231-240

[132] Liu Z, Zh R, Zhang J, Chuang CC, Kandaswamy E, Zhou T, et al. Role of ROS and nutritional antioxidants in human diseases. Frontiers of Physiology. May 2018;**17**(9):477. DOI: 10.3389/fphys.2018.00477eCollection 2018

[133] Poljsak B. Strategies for reducing or preventing the generation of oxidative stress. Oxidative Medicine and Cellular Longevity. 2011. Article ID 194586, 15 p. DOI: 10.1155/2011/194586

[134] Rougier N. Changes in DNA fragmentation during sperm preparation for intracytoplasmic sperm injection over time. Fertility and Sterility. 2013;**100**(1):69-74. DOI: 10.1016/j.fertnstert.2013.03.005

[135] Quinn M, Jalalian L, Riberio S, et al. Microfluidic sorting selects sperm for clinical use with reduced DNA damage compared to density gradient centrifugation with swim up in split semen samples. Human Reproduction. 2018;**33**(8):1388-1393. DOI: 10.1093/humrep/dey239

[136] Agarwal A, Ikemoto I, Loughlin KR. Levels of reactive oxygen species before and after sperm preparation: Comparison of swim-up and L4 filtration. Archives of Andrology. 1994;**32**(3):169-174. DOI: 10.3109/01485019408987783

[137] Li Z, Zhou Y, Liu R, et al. Effects of semen processing on the generation of reactive oxygen species and mitochondrial membrane potential of human spermatozoa. Andrologia: First International Journal of Andrology;**44**(3):157-163. DOI: 10.1111/j.1439-0272.2010.01123.x

[138] Thilagavathi J, Kumar M, Mishra SS, Venkatesh S, Kumar R, Dada R. Analysis of sperm telomere length in men with idiopathic infertility. Archives of Gynecology and Obstetrics. 2013;**287**:803-807. DOI: 10.1007/s00404-012-2632-8

[139] Zhao F, Yang Q, Shi S, Luo X, Sun Y. Semen preparation methods and sperm telomere length: density gradient centrifugation versus the swim up procedure. Scientific Reports. 2016;**6**:39051. DOI: 10.1038/srep39051. [Epub: 13 December 2016]

[140] Ghasemzadeh A, Karkon-Shayan F, Yousefzadeh S, Naghavi-Behzad M, Hamdi K. Study of pentoxifylline effects on motility and viability of spermatozoa from infertile asthenozoospermic males. Nigerian Medical Journal. 2016;**57**(6):324-328. DOI: 10.4103/0300-1652.193857

[141] Holstein AF, Schulze W, Davidoff M. Understanding spermatogenesis is a prerequisite for treatment. Reproductive Biology and Endocrinology. 2003;**1**:107. DOI: 10.1186/1477-7827-1-107

[142] Sharpe R. Environmental/lifestyle effects on spermatogenesis. Philosophical Transactions of the Royal Society of London. Series B, Biological Sciences. 2010;**365**(1546):1697-1712. DOI: 10.1098/rstb.2009.0206

Chapter 2

Insights of Sperm Pathology and Its Association with Infertility

Mohd Sajad and Sonu Chand Thakur

Abstract

This section considers the structural characteristics of spermatozoon, its assembly, composition, and mechanism behind regulation of their peculiar function. The spermatozoon is tremendously peculiar cell with an arrangement of structural characteristics which furnish it with remarkable capability of carrying the genome of male to the egg. A variety of genes are only expressed in spermatids and result in the formation of proteins that are very crucial and distinctive to spermatozoa. These proteins package the DNA, form the head of sperm, account the component of matrix and enzymes of acrosome, construct the flagellar structure, and work as ion channels that are associated in modulating the motility of sperm and also become adenylyl cyclase which yields cyclic adenosine monophosphate (cAMP) to induce signaling effect which regulates the function of spermatozoon. These proteins are critical essential to sperm and, sometimes, mutation inhibits their synthesis or disrupts their function which leads to male infertility. Researchers are trying to identify those proteins that are significant for proper function of sperm through gene knockout approach in mice that are probable to be necessary in humans as well. However, various questions still persist regarding the spermatozoon composition, organization, and function and need to be answered.

Keywords: sperm, spermatogenesis, ROS, infertility, oxidative stress, motility

1. Introduction

Male reproductive function can be divided into three subdivision: (i) hormonal balance of male reproductive function (ii) spermatogenesis, development of sperm; and (iii) fulfill of male sexual act.

Spermatogenesis begins within the seminiferous tubules of testis through the successive mitotic, meiotic and post meiotic phases which results in the formation of spermatozoon, the end product of this process. To expand the spermatogonial population, the germ line stem cell during the mitotic phase undergo a series of division which culminates into two meiotic division and formation of haploid spermatids without the replication of DNA. For the development of male gametes these two phases are very significant. During this phase the remodeling of spermatids occurs extensively into sperm by acrosome formation, condensation of nucleus, development of flagella and loss of cytoplasm. The head and flagellum are the two-substantial component of sperm. These two components are joined together by a connective piece. The head carries the nucleus, cytoskeleton element and cytoplasm. It comprises various types of enzymes homogeneous to lysosomes of a typical cell, including hyaluronidase (having the ability to digest proteoglycan filaments of tissue) and powerful proteolytic enzymes which can digest proteins having an important role in the process of oocyte fertilization. The flagellum is divided into three regions: mid piece, principle piece and terminal piece. A central complex of microtubules covered by outer dense forms the axoneme. Mitochondria are present in the mid piece which surrounds the outer dense fibers and neighboring axoneme. The principle part of the flagellum is mostly comprised by the existence of fibrous sheath which surrounds the dense fibers and axoneme. In higher vertebrates these dense fibers and fibrous sheath are developed due to internal fertilization and these are cytoskeletal material of sperm flagellum [1]. The plasma membrane as in sperm head surrounds the flagellum tightly and contains scattered cytoplasm. Invertebrate's sperm usually have an acrosome in the head region and mitochondria and an axoneme in the flagellar region but the accessory or additional cytoskeletal elements are absent [2]. To achieve the fertilization the acrosome, have an enzyme which plays a key role to penetrate into egg. The flagellum of the sperm contains the source of energy that generates sperm motility required to reach the egg. All these characteristics of sperm are necessary to deliver the genetic material exists in sperm nucleus to egg. After that, zygote is formed by the fusion of haploid pronuclei of male and female, and thus development initiates. In most mammals, the nucleus of haploid sperm carries the sex chromosome decides the sex of resulting animals [3]. The genome of both maternal and paternal parents is essentially required to proceed the normal development, generally due to distinctive genes imprinting in males and females during gametogenesis [4, 5].

This chapter gives center of attention on the unique features of mammalian spermatozoa with especial consideration to molecules presently known that enrich to the structure and function of sperm. The main topics contemplated are; physiology of male sexual organ, spermatogenesis, sperm count, heritable effect on human sperm structure, regulation of sperm motility, effect of oxidative stress on male reproductive system, sources of reactive oxygen species in seminal plasma, physiological role of ROS in seminal plasma, consequence of Oxidative Stress on male Reproductive System, management and prevention of oxidative stress, correlation between biology of male reproduction and sleep and role of inflammation in infertility.

2. Physiology of male sexual organ

The favorable outcome of male reproductive system depends mainly upon the cohesive function of vast array of tissues. It comprises of assembly of sperm in the testes, sperm maturation in epididymis, secretion of seminal fluid by addition sex glands, deliver sperm into the reproductive tract of female, erection of penis, emission and final ejaculation. Fertilization of the egg requires the motility of sperm, successful capacitation and acrosomal reaction. These entire needs are dependent directly or indirectly on the secretion of testosterone hormone by the Leydig cells. The testis of male is comprised of up to 900 coiled seminiferous tubules, in which the sperm is formed and each seminiferous tubule exceeds up to 1 meter long in average. The sperm then discharged into one more coiled tube which is about 6-meter long known as epididymis. The epididymis enlarges into vasa deferens that infiltrates into prostate gland. There are two seminal vesicles and the material (Is secreted) from both the ampulla and seminal vesicles. The excretion from both the prostate gland and seminal vesicles enters into the ejaculatory duct through the body of prostate gland and then vacant into the internal urethra. Mucus released from urethral gland and more from bilateral bulbourethral glands which is located near to urethra is supplied to urethra [6].

3. Spermatogenesis

The process of spermatogenesis takes place in each of the testis tubules. In this process the spermatozoa are produced by the population of germ cells (spermatogonia) through process of mitosis and meiosis. This entire spermatogenesis process starts during the onset of puberty and last till the old age. This process involved various stages starting with germ cells formation in the germinal epithelium and followed by continuous development into primary and secondary spermatocytes. These spermatocytes finally developed into functional spermatozoa. Spermatogenesis is extremely well-ordered process; male germ cells proliferate and differentiate rapidly and the modulation of spermatogenesis occurs at the extra testicular and intra testicular level and can be dispersed ubiquitously. As aforementioned, spermatogonia originated from the primordial germ cells that migrate into the genital ridge of the indifferent gonads, during embryo development and are present in two to three layers in seminiferous tubules. At puberty, the spermatogonia starts mitotic division, proliferate and differentiate continuously to form mature sperm cells [7] (**Figure 1**).

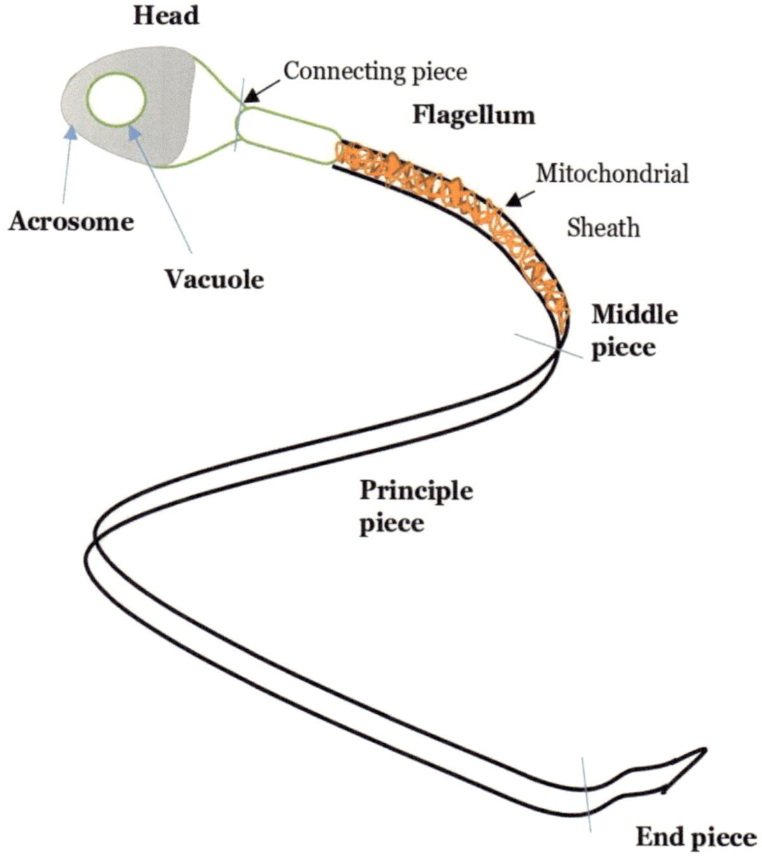

Figure 1.
General characteristics of germ.

3.1 Steps of spermatogenesis

The process of spermatogenesis starts at an average age of 12–13 years, continues throughout the remaining life, and markedly decreases during the older age. During the initial stage of spermatogenesis, the spermatogonia shift toward the central

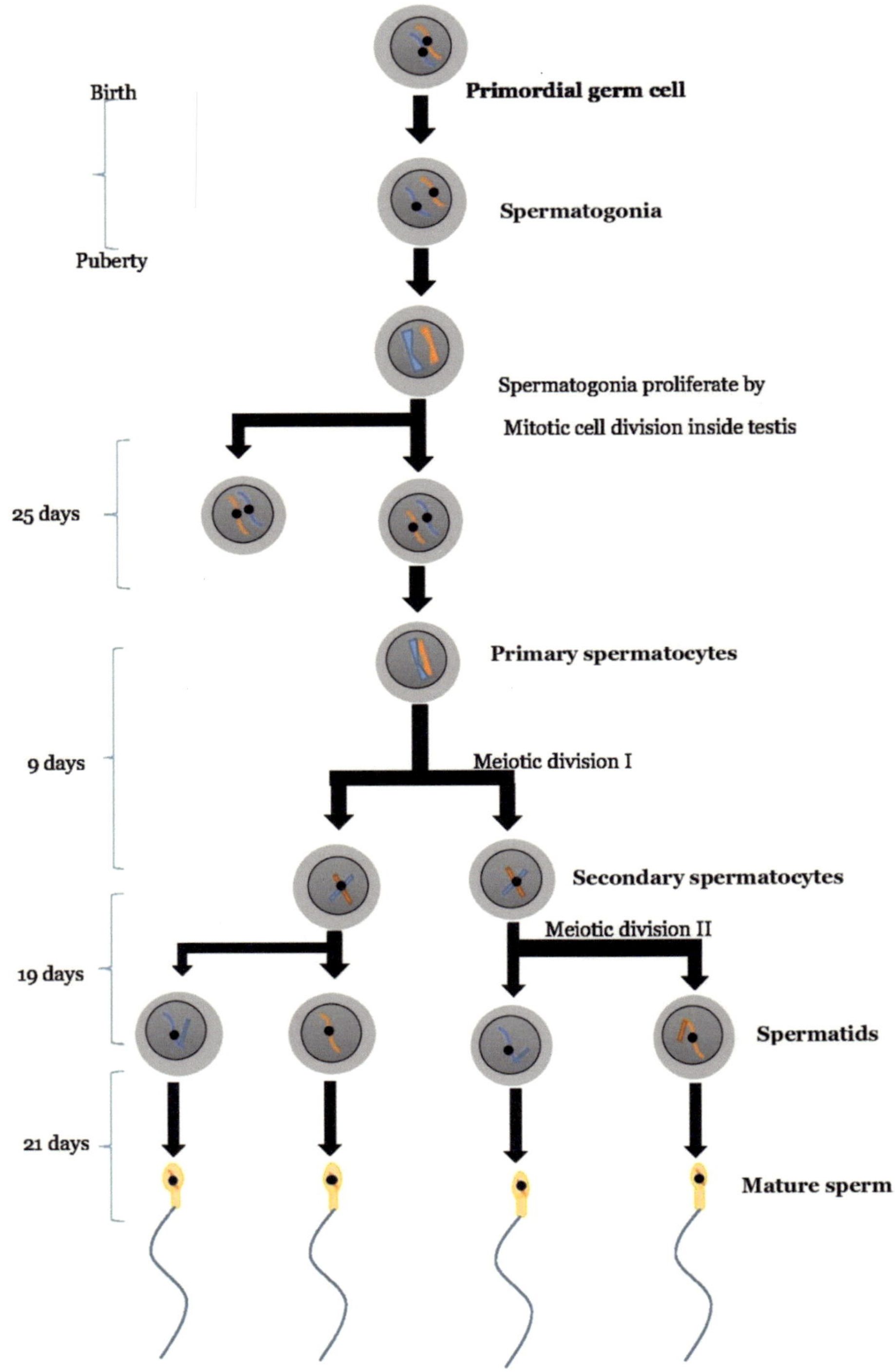

Figure 2.
Steps of spermatogenesis.

lumen of seminiferous tubules. The Sertoli cells are part of a seminiferous tubule and support the process of spermatogenesis. Its main function is to nourish the developing sperm cells throughout the stages of spermatogenesis. Sertoli cells control the entry and exit of nutrients, hormones and other substances into the tubules of the testis. The Sertoli cells are also responsible for establishing and maintaining the spermatogonial stem cell niche, which ensures the renewal of stem cells and the differentiation of spermatogonia into mature germ cells, that progress stepwise through the long process of spermatogenesis, ending in the release of spermatozoa.

3.2 Meiosis

Spermatogonia which are able to pass across Sertoli cell layer change and grow in size progressively into primary spermatocytes. The two secondary spermatocytes are formed by meiotic division from the primary spermatocytes. These secondary spermatocytes, also divide to produce spermatids that transform into sperm after a period of time. During the process of spermatocyte to spermatid stage transformation, the 23 pair of chromosomes (46 chromosome total) of spermatocytes also divides, and as a result, 23 chromosomes go to one spermatid and the rest 23 chromosomes to the other spermatid. It takes about 74 days to complete the entire process of spermatogenesis, from spermatogonia to spermatozoa [6] **Figure 2**. Suggested: Round and elongated spermatids will differentiate into mature spermatozoa, by the process of spermiogenesis.

4. Sperm motility

Motility of sperm cells is provided by the back-and-forth movement of tail and it results from rhythmic longitudinal sliding motion between the anterior and posterior tubules [8]. Different molecular markers of sperm, such as mitochondrial membrane potential (MMP), DNA fragmentations and ROS have presently concluded as reliable estimators of sperm function that can be used to evaluate the quality of the sperm [9]. Due to the overloading of ROS, osmatic stress is increased which in turn decreases the MMP and increases the fragmentation of DNA, affecting the viability of sperm [10]. It is broadly accepted that motility of sperm mainly depends upon ATP which is produced by the mitochondria. The latest is located in mid piece of spermatozoa, which explains the correlation between motility and mitochondrial membrane potential [11, 12].

4.1 Sperm count: how much is considered normal?

The spermatozoon is the cell of male reproductive system. Sperm count, also known as sperm concentration, is the parameter to measure the number of sperm cells in the ejaculate. During each coitus the quantity of ejaculated semen in average, is about 3.5 milliliters, and 120 million sperm might be present in average in each milliliter of semen. However, in normal males this count can vary from 35 to 200 million. In several milliliters of each ejaculated semen, an average of total of 400 million sperms might be present. When the sperm count is less than 20 million in 1 milliliter (ml), it might point to infertility. A relatively high sperm count might elevate the chances of conception [6].

There are several causes of infertility in males such as genetic factors like cryptorchidism, congenital absence of vas deferens, karyotype abnormalities and some acquired factors like trauma, varicocele, medication, urogenital infection, inflammation, testicular torsion and idiopathic factors.

Semen deficiencies are termed as

a. Oligospermia or oligozoospermia—lower than normal number of spermatozoa in semen.

b. Aspermia—complete lack of semen.

c. Azoospermia—absence of sperm cells in semen.

d. Hypospermia—reduction in the seminal volume.

e. Teratospermia—abnormal morphology of sperm cells.

f. Asthenozoospermia—reduced motility of sperm.

4.1.1 Oligospermia

Oligospermia, is one of male infertility causes, defined as low concentration of sperm cells in the ejaculate. Semen with decreased concentration of sperm may often depict considerable abnormalities in morphology and motility of spermatozoa. Low sperm count may be due to an endocrinopathy such as varicocele, prolactinoma or it may be a genetic cause. In about 6 and 15% of patients with severe low sperm count or azoospermia (respectively), microdelitions can be found in azoospermic factor (AZF) region of Y chromosome. AZF refers to one of several proteins or their genes, which are coded from the AZF region located in the human male Y chromosome. Deletions in this region are associated with inability to produce sperm. Subregions within the AZF region are AZFa, AZFb and AZFc, located in the long arm of Y chromosome [13]. By cytogenetic analysis, chromosomal abnormalities were detected in 2% of men having low sperm count and 15–20% with no sperm count. These abnormalities include translocation of nonsex chromosome and Klinefelter syndrome [14].

4.1.2 Asthenozoospermia

Asthenozoospermia, low sperm motility, could be derived due to:

A. Inborn metabolic deficiency (such as Kartagener's syndrome or immotile cilia syndrome—ICS).

B. Abnormal ultrastructure of the sperm flagellum: as primary ciliary dyskinesia; spermatozoa consist of altered peri-axonemal structure but have normal axoneme. Densed individual fibers are extended abnormally along the axoneme, location and number of longitudinal columns of fibrous sheath are modified and change in the order of termination of these structures [15].

Sperm with the following syndromes: abnormal axoneme, partial or complete lacking of dynein (a family of cytoskeletal motor proteins that move along microtubules in cells and convert the chemical energy stored in ATP to mechanical work), lack of central sheath and lack of inner arms might be unable to show motility;

C. Necroozospermia—binding of antisperm antibodies or an increase in white blood cell concentration in the ejaculate, which later results in the overproduction of reactive oxygen species, might lead to damages in the spermatozoa [16].

D. Dysplasia of fibrous sheath spermatozoa: spermatozoa with very short, thick, rigid and immotile tail, mainly due to disorganized and hyperplastic fibrous sheath [17, 18].

5. Heritable effect on human sperm structure

The hereditary condition which causes the defects in the flagella of sperm is termed as Kartagener's syndrome, immotile cilia syndrome (ICS), or primary ciliary dyskinesia (PCD). It often leads to chronic respiratory problems, male sterility and situs inversus [19]. These states are linked directly or indirectly with the autosomal recessive traits. The aforementioned conditions make the flagella unable to show normal movement. Sperm with these syndromes have abnormal axoneme lacking dynein arm partially or completely, lack of central sheath, lack of inner arms [20]. Due to variety of defects presented in sperm and cilia, many genes are mutated and contribute to the syndrome [21]. Another flagellar defect characterized by severe asthenozoospermia is familiar as dysplasia of fibrous sheath. In this type of disorder, the sperm have disorganized and hyperplastic fibrous sheath, and very short, thick, rigid and immotile tail [17, 18]. Another flagellar defect which appears in sperm cells of infertile men is known as flagellar dyskinesia [15]. This type of defect was observed in brothers and has been suggested that it arises due to the genetic abbreviation [22]. The sperm consist of altered peri-axonemal structure but have normal axoneme. Densed individual fibers are extended abnormally along the axoneme location and number of longitudinal columns of fibrous sheath are modified and else, there are changes in the order of termination of these structures [15].

6. Regulation of sperm motility

Sperm depicts two kinds of motility:

a. Progressive motility—typical for newly ejaculated sperm.

Spermatozoa acquire the ability of progressive motility in the epididymis. Relatively symmetrical motion of flagella which leads to forward movement has been shown in this type of motility [23].

b. Hyperactivated motility—after sometimes either in reproductive tract of female or in culture, sperm achieves the hyperactivated motility that is characterized by whip like beating of flagellum, asymmetrical flagellar bends and circular swimming [24].

6.1 Activation of motility

It is broadly acquired that precious motility of sperm is the chief component of fertility of male. During the beginning of progressive motility and origin of hyper activation of sperm, key factors are involved. These key factors are calcium (Ca^{2+}), cyclic adenosine monophosphate (cAMP) and bicarbonate (HCO_3^-). Olfactory and GABA receptors are the possible candidates which trigger the progressive and hyperactivated motility of sperm.

6.2 Role of calcium in motility

Calcium plays a key role in sperm function by different aspects. Recent studies have been demonstrated that in knockout mice there are at least four components participate in the intracellular regulation of calcium level and initiation of sperm motility. These are CatSper1, CatSper2, $Ca_v2.3$ and PMCA4. CatSper1 are localized in the principle piece of sperm and it is a voltage gated Ca^{2+} channels of the testis. Lacking or any mutation in CatSper1 gene reduces the progressive motility and causes infertility. A sperm cell that lacks the CatSper1 showed progressive motility but failed to develop hyperactivated motility [25]. CatSper2 present in flagellum shows similarity to CatSper1 and it is also a voltage-gated ion channel. Sperm of mice having knockout CatSper2 gene depict decreased flagellar amplitude and also failed to develop hyperactivated motility [26]. Disruption of gene for PMCA4, that have Ca^{2+}/calmodulin dependent ATPase activity involve in efflux of Ca^{2+}, also causes infertility in men. In developing sperm cells and sperm flagellum the cyclic nucleotide gated Ca^{2+} channels are present. The role of these channels is to regulate the influx of calcium in various micro domains of the flagella [26].

6.3 cAMP and motility

During sperm motility regulation, cAMP is the second key messenger. Adenylate cyclase converts the ATP into cAMP. Thus, the level of cAMP increases and in turn activates the cAMP dependent kinase A (PKA) which phosphorylates the serine and threonine residues in the flagellum, which ultimately causes the phosphorylation of tyrosine residues in the proteins [27, 28]. In most cells the adenylyl cyclase is activated by G protein in response to external stimuli. In mouse sperm the plasma membrane bounds (mACs) activated by G protein take a part in the acrosome reaction, and in chemotaxis and hyperactivation in human sperm [29]. It was

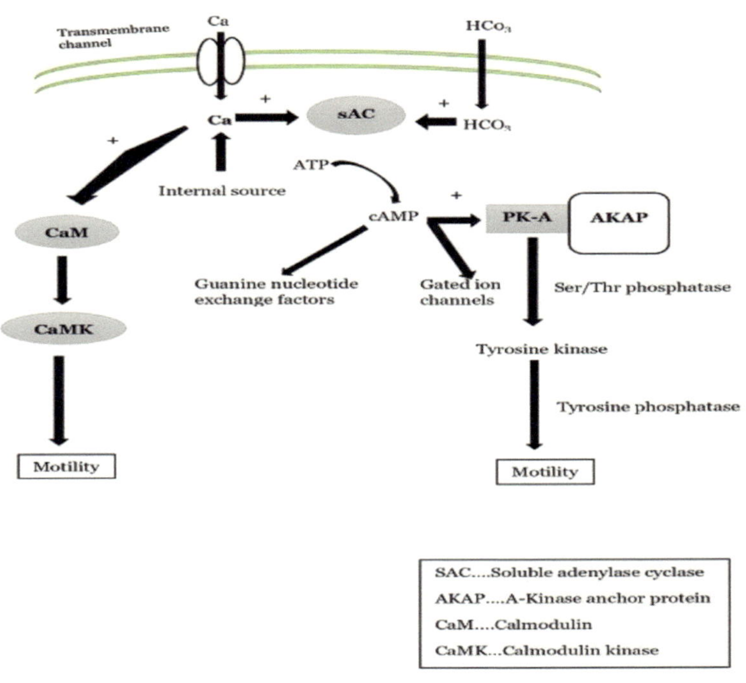

Figure 3.
Signalling pathway showing regulation of motility of sperm in mammals.

demonstrated that HCO_3^- and Ca^{2+} are inculpated in cAMP regulated activation of sperm motility. The activity of soluble adenylyl cyclase is augmented by HCO_3^- with increased activation of enzymes (adenylyl cyclase) and by reducing the substrate inhibition that happens at higher concentration of ATP-Mg^{2+}. Due to low level of HCO_3^-, activity of soluble adenylyl cyclase would be reduced in sperm by substrate inhibition stored in epididymis [30].

6.4 PKA and motility

PKA causes the phosphorylation of tyrosine residue of flagellar proteins. The proteins anchoring with PKA site (AKAP3, AKAP4 and TAKAP-80) in the fibrous sheath, point out that the main role of this structure is to bind PKA in the principle piece of flagellum [31]. Regulatory and catalytic subunits are present in PKA holoenzyme. Four genes (RIα, RIβ, RIIα and RIIβ) are present in regulatory subunits (R subunit) in human and mouse; three catalytic (C subunit) Cα, Cβ and Cγ in human, and two C subunit Cα and Cβ in mice. The cAMP binding site are present in R and C subunits. C subunits is released when cAMP binds to R subunits and their catalytic site is activated by cAMP. The R and C subunits are involved in the motility of sperm (**Figure 3**).

7. Effect of oxidative stress on male reproductive system

Oxidative stress is a state which causes disproportion between systemic reactive oxygen species and detoxifying capability of biological system to neutralize the reactive intermediates, also called antioxidant defenses. Spermatozoa have antioxidant defense mechanism that quench the ROS and therefore protects the cells of gonads and mature spermatozoa from oxidative damage [32]. Statistics from United States depicted that the major cause of male infertility is ROS. In 30–40% of infertile men's seminal plasma, there is an increase in the level of ROS [33]. In spermatozoa ROS are generated by two methods.

1. At the level of sperm plasma membrane—by nicotinamide adenine dinucleotide phosphate oxidase system.

2. At the level of mitochondria—by nicotinamide adenine dinucleotide-dependent oxidoreductase reaction [34].

The production of ROS at the level of mitochondria is the chief source. Large concentration of mitochondria is present in spermatozoa because of a constant need of energy to spermatozoa for motility. In semen, presence of nonfunctional spermatozoa considerably increases the level of ROS that in turn impair the function of mitochondria and motility of sperm. In human spermatozoa, ROS which is produced in large concentration is O_2^-. It reacts with itself to generate H_2O_2 by dismutation. H_2O_2 and O_2^- generates most destructive and reactive OH^- by Haber-Weiss reaction in the presence of iron and copper. OH^- affects the function of sperm by disrupting the fluidity of membrane [35, 36]. Recent studies depicting that O_2 production in spermatozoa showed the presence of calcium dependent NADPH oxidase also called NOX5 has been residing in acrosomal and midpiece region of spermatozoa [37]. Initially the NOX5 resides in human testis. It is activated upon binding of calcium to its cytosolic domain and causes conformational changes in cells [35]. ROS is generated during the normal metabolism of cells. Under physiological conditions the mitochondrial respiration is the chief source of superoxide anion radicals. Quality of sperm and function is affected by the high concentration of ROS and is potentially toxic.

8. Sources of reactive oxygen species in seminal plasma

The production of ROS in the seminal plasma originated from different endogenous and exogenous pathways. Ejaculate of human contains varieties of mature and immature cells, epithelial cells, leukocytes and round cells. Of these, leukocytes, immature spermatozoa, macrophages and neutrophils are considered to be the main endogenous source. Others life style practices as: excessive alcohol consumption, smoking and environmental factors (e.g., toxins and radiations) may contribute to exogenous ROS production [38–40].

8.1 Endogenous sources of ROS

8.1.1 Leukocytes

Peroxidase-positive leukocytes include polymorphonuclear leukocytes in about 50–60% and macrophages 20–30%. Peroxidase-positive leukocytes originates in large proportion from prostrate and seminal vesicles of male. These main sources of ROS are activated by different intracellular and extracellular responses such as inflammation and infection. The latest can produce 100 times reactive oxygen species than normal and also increase the secretion of NADPH through hexose monophosphate shunt [41, 42]. There is a decrease in the level of antioxidant superoxide dismutase and an increase in the concentration of proinflammatory cytokines, which can lead to the increased level of ROS and respiratory burst ultimately leading to formation of oxidative species OS. OS will than cause the damage of sperm if the concentration of seminal leukocytes is abnormally high [43]. Although in phagocytic clearance and immuno surveillance of unhealthy (abnormal) sperm, leukocytes and ROS play a decisive role. Inflammatory changes are depicted in the testes of smokers due to increased concentration of leukocyte activated free radicals. These leukocytes overcome the protective action of antioxidants and lead to oxidative stress. OS causes severe single and double stranded breaks in DNA by changing sperm chromatin integrity, modification of bases, deletions and rearrangement of chromosome [7].

8.1.2 Immature spermatozoa

During the process of spermatogenesis, the developing spermatozoa expel their cytoplasmic content to prepare itself for the process of fertilization. Due to the arrest in spermiogenesis, the abnormal spermatozoa retained excess of cytoplasm around the midpiece. This condition is referred as excess residual cytoplasm (ERC). By virtue of hexose monophosphate shunt the ERC activates the NADPH system, which is used as a source of electron by spermatozoa for production of ROS and OS [30]. Therefore, ERC affects the morphology, motility and fertilization potential of sperm which can lead to infertility [44].

8.1.3 Varicocele

Varicocele is a condition of abnormal enlargement of vein in scrotum, i.e., in the plexus pampiniformis situated throughout the spermatic cord. It is considered to be an etiology of male infertility, because varicocele is found in 19–40% of male partners in infertile couples. Current evidence suggested that oxidative stress is the central element contributing to infertility in men with varicocele [45]. Varicocele arises when damage occurs in valves into the spermatic vein(s) resulting in dysfunction and retrograde blood flow into scrotum from abdomen creating an inappropriate environment for development of sperm. Several studies reveal that oxidative stress also leads to varicocele in male, which occurs due to decrease in the concentration of antioxidants. It results in the deterioration of structure of cell membrane and in the DNA integrity. Nitric oxide is a lipophilic molecule which is presented in the spermatic vein of varicocele patient. Both NO and superoxide might cause a damage in spermatozoa [46].

8.2 Exogenous sources of ROS

8.2.1 Radiation

Radiation, a natural source of energy, has a considerable effect on humans. Several studies have been depicted that radiation emitted from mobile phone increases the concentration of ROS in human semen resulting in impaired sperm quality [47, 48]. *In vitro* studies showed that in human, spermatozoa electromagnet radiation urges the production of ROS and damages of DNA. These changes further diminish the vitality and motility of sperm cells [49]. Due to the presence of varieties of charged molecules in the cytosol the flow of electron along the internal membrane of cells can be negatively affected by these radio frequency electromagnet radiations, and therefore interferes with the functions of the cell and the organelles [50].

8.2.2 Toxins

Toxins which are discharged from industrial products and structural materials accumulates in the body of human and increases the production of ROS in the testes. This might result in the negative impact on the structure and function of sperm [51]. Phthalates which are found in the plastics objects used for industrial and domestic's purpose have been found to impair the spermatogenesis process and causes DNA damages in spermatozoa. Moreover, it has been studied that those laborers who were continuously exposed to metal toxins such as chromium, mercury, manganese and cadmium were more probable to have diminished quality of sperm, sperm count, density and volume [50].

8.2.3 Smoking

Tobacco is familiar to be one of the major causes of worldwide death. It has been reported that more than 4000 toxic chemical compounds have been present in cigarettes which includes nitrosamines, alkaloids and inorganic molecules. In the semen of smokers some of those chemicals were depicted to be the source of imbalance between antioxidant and ROS [41]. This disproportion between the ROS level and antioxidant adversely affects the overall quality of semen. It has been depicted that smoking increases by 48% the concentration of seminal leukocytes and 107% the ROS level in semen [52]. Due to the substantial increase in the level of 8-OHdG which is also a biomarker of oxidative damage, a decrease of the antioxidant level in seminal plasma, like vitamin C and vitamin E occurs, thus causing more risk of oxidative damage [40]. A study performed on smokers found an increased concentration of lead and cadmium in their semen and blood, which led to increase the production of ROS with a decrease in the motility of the sperm [53]. Moreover, the spermatozoa of smoker were substantially more prone to acid mediated denaturation as compare to nonsmoker spermatozoa which led to DNA strand break [54]. Furthermore, it was shown that prolonged smoking damages sperm DNA and apoptosis which results in male infertility.

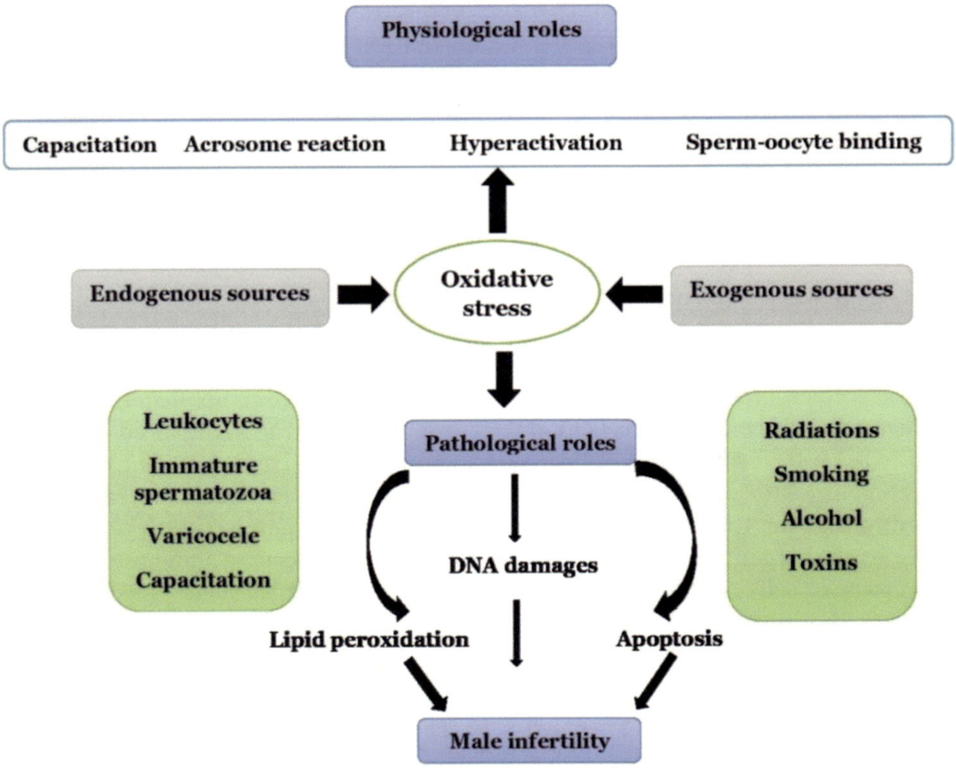

Figure 4.
Demonstration of various factors responsible for male infertility (origin).

8.2.4 Alcohol consumption

Alcohol is widely known as the inducer of ROS and it interferes with the antioxidant defense mechanism of the body, mainly in the liver. Acetaldehyde which is the byproduct of ethanol metabolism, may react with protein and lipids forming the ROS, and may lead to damages in DNA, protein and lipids at the molecular level. The excessive consumption of alcohol is linked with a decrease in the concentration of normal sperm in asthenozoospermia patients [55] (**Figure 4**).

9. Physiological role of ROS in seminal plasma

Physiological level of ROS plays a significant task in the physiological process such as capacitation, hyperactivation, acrosomal reaction, fusion of sperm and oocyte in order to assure the proper fertilization [56].

9.1 Capacitation

When spermatozoa pass the epididymis, it is supposed to be mature and their activity is checked by different inhibitory factors which are produced by genital duct epithelia. However, at that time sperm is unable to fertilize the ova. Ejaculated mammalian spermatozoa should reside in the female genital tract for several hours before gaining their fertilizability. In humans however, sperm must move out of the seminal plasma immediately after ejaculation and appear in the fallopian tube within minutes. As soon as sperm cells are moving out of the ejaculate and passing the cervical mucus, they undergo several biochemical changes collectively called capacitation. These changes involve molecules absorbing on, or integrating into, the sperm plasma membrane during epididymal maturation. The removal or alteration of these molecules prepares the sperm toward successful binding, penetration and fertilization with the egg [57]. During the process of capacitation a production of ROS occurs in spermatozoa that initiates various molecular modifications. Firstly, there is an increase in cAMP; in various organisms and varieties of life processes, this cAMP pathway is necessary because it might activate various enzymes and might regulate the expression of genes [58]. cAMP activates the protein kinase A and causes the phosphorylation of PKA substrate like arginine, serine and threonine. This successively leads to the phosphorylation of MEK, threonine-glutamate-tyrosine, and tyrosine phosphorylation of fibrous sheath proteins. This cAMP increase makes the hyperactivation of sperm. Only the hyperactivated spermatozoa undergo acrosomal reaction due to increased motility and acquired all those properties which are necessary for fertilization [59, 60].

9.2 Hyperactivation

Hyperactivation is the peculiar condition of sperm motility. The hyperactivation process is significant for lucrative fertilization and it regarded a subcategory of capacitation. Hyperactivated sperm have characteristics of asymmetric flagellar movement, high amplitude, side to side head displacement and also a nonlinear motility [61].

9.3 Acrosome reaction

Hyperactivated spermatozoon binds to zona pellucida after passing the cumulus oophorus, starting the exocytotic discharge of hyaluronidase and proteolytic enzymes, sperm acrosome reaction (AR) induced by oocyte investment, is a prerequisite event for the spermatozoa. It is obligatory for the sperm cell to enable to penetrate the zona pellucida (ZP) and to fuse with the oocyte. Progesterone (P_4), secreted by cumulus cells, is an important cofactor for the occurrence of this exocytosis event. The AR results from the fusion between outer acrosomal and plasma membranes leading to inner acrosomal membrane exposure. Binding of agonists, P_4 or ZP_3 glycoprotein, to plasma membrane sperm receptors activates intraspermatic signals and enzymatic pathways involved in the AR. Among the proteins or glycoproteins described as potential sperm receptors for ZP, G_i/G_o protein-coupled and tyrosine kinase receptors have been described. ZP- and P_4-promoted AR is mediated by an obligatory intracellular calcium increase, appearing first at the acrosome equatorial segment and spreading throughout the head. The plasma membrane channels involved in calcium entry are operated by a plasma membrane depolarization and protein phosphorylation mediated by protein kinase C and tyrosine kinase protein. Part of the calcium increase could also be due to intracellular store release through nucleotide (cAMP)-gated channels. Besides adenylate cyclase and phospholipase C activations, intracellular calcium increase also stimulates phospholipase A2 and actin depolymerization, leading to membrane fusion [62]. The sperm cell crosses the physical barrier of zona pellucida and within few minutes it fuses with the oocytes. ROS is involved in the action of the spermatozoa by phosphorylating three plasma membrane proteins [63].

9.4 Sperm-oocyte fusion

High concentration of docosahexaenoic acid (DHA) plays a considerable part in maintaining the fluidity of the membrane of spermatozoa. ROS enhances the fluidity of membrane and sperm-oocyte fusion rate, during the process of capacitation and acrosomal reaction. Throughout the entire capacitation process, ROS hinder the protein tyrosine phosphate activity and arrest the dephosphorylation and turnoff the phospholipase A_2. PLA_2 increases the fluidity of the membrane by cleaving the secondary fatty acid from the triglycerol backbone of membrane phospholipid [64, 65].

10. Management and prevention of oxidative stress

Sperm DNA of healthy males is protected from osmotic stress by two mechanisms;

1. Tightly packed and coiled DNA so that the genetic material is less exposed to ROS [66].

2. Production of ROS is minimized by natural antioxidant present in seminal plasma and spermatozoa.

Enzymatic and nonenzymatic antioxidant like superoxide dismutase (SOD), Catalase, Vitamin C, Vitamin E and Carotenoids react with ROS and neutralize it, thus prevent the onset of osmatic stress and also preserves the function of sperm [67] (**Table 1**).

Antioxidant	Mechanism of action	Effect
Superoxide dismutase	Neutralizes the superoxide anions	Prevents lipid peroxidation.
GSH/GPX	Scavenges the free radicals	Prevents the lipid peroxidation and enhance the sperm membrane characteristics.
Catalase	Splits down the H_2O_2 into H_2O and O_2.	Also arrests the lipid peroxidation.
Vitamin C	Counteracts free radicals	Protects the viability and motility of sperm.
Vitamin E	Counteracts free radicals	Blocks the lipid peroxidation and enhance the activity of other antioxidant.
Carotenoids	Suppresses the singlet molecular O_2.	Blocks the lipid peroxidation.
Carnitine	Acts as energy source and neutralize the free radical.	Prevents the damage of DNA and lipid peroxidation.
Cysteines	Elevates the concentration of GSH synthesized.	Inhibits lipid peroxidation.
Pentoxifylline	Prevents the breakdown of cAMP and quench the formation of proinflammatory factors.	Inhibits lipid peroxidation.

Table 1.
Procedure of action and consequences of different antioxidants.

11. Correlation between biology of male reproduction and sleep

The whole process of spermatogenesis is controlled by hypothalamic pituitary gonadal axis. Hypothalamus secretes GnRH that stimulates the anterior pituitary to secrete LH and FSH. FSH act on the testicular tissue and LH triggers the secretion of testosterone in the testis by Leydig cells. Maximum level of testosterone secretion occurs during sleep. This nocturnal rise in testosterone secretion appears at the same time with the beginning of resting eye movement sleep and it is not concerned with the change in the level of melatonin [68]. In male reproductive system, prolactin hormone secreted by anterior pituitary o has also a key role. Prolactin increases in Leydig cells the utterance of LH receptors at physiological level. The latest leads to increased secretion of testosterone promoting spermatogenesis. The increasing pervasiveness of 24/7 constant distribution of entertainment, disrupts the circadian rhythm and impair the duration and quality of sleep on population level. The schedule of sleep and wake is delayed by the use of electronic devices at night time. More over blue light emitted by LED reduces the secretion of melatonin and thus decreases the prolonged, objective and subjective sleepiness. Sleep restriction disrupts the level of gonadal hormone. The level of testosterone is reduced in 10 volunteer's healthy males in 1 week of restricted sleep. While in another examination of sleep restriction of 4–5 hours in 15 men is also associated with reduction in the level of testosterone. Effect of sleep restriction and resting eye movement deprivation was analyzed by Alvarenga et al. on parameter of sperm and expression of testis specific genes in male rat. Both sleep restriction (SR) and rapid eye movement sleep deprivation (RSD) group has decreased viability of sperm [69].

12. Inflammation and infertility

Inflammation is a complexed process of response to tissue damage and injury. It starts with the aggregation of leukocytes and more plasma molecules to infection site. Several factors may be responsible for inflammation in reproductive tract of male. (i) Blockage of ejaculatory duct (ii) epididymitis that causing pain, swelling in scrotal area, penile leakage and presence of blood in urine (iii) sexual transmitted diseases by several agents like *E. coli* (iv) Urethritis (v) testicular torsion is another pathology affects the fertility in male. It occurs due to abnormality in supportive tissue of testis and causing the testis to pervert inside the scrotum which result in severe swelling and pain [70]. During the process of inflammation, the quality of semen is reduced due to abnormal function of accessory glands, sperm transport hindrance and spermatogenesis dysregulation [71, 72]. Cytokines which are either secreted by activated cells or secreted after receiving stimulus might assist help in normal function of reproductive system [73, 74]. Testicular macrophage is the chief source of cytokine in male but Leydig and Sertoli cells are also depicted to secrete cytokines. Two types of changes are seen due to inflammation in male genitalia; an increase in secretion of seminal fluid leads to redness, local heat and depletion in velocity of seminal flow. Cytokines (TNF-α, IL-6, and IL-1) induce the oxidative damages that impair the quality of semen and have bad impact on fertility of male. Raised level of few cytokines in male semen also disrupts the quality, density and morphology of sperm. The increased level of TNF-α is linked with low sperm count, motility and morphology of sperm. In semen raised level of TNF-α induced apoptosis due to proliferation and differentiation of B-cell, T- cell and NK cells. At the site of inflammation, the blood vessels are dilated permitting the leukocytes in high concentration to migrate out of blood and bind with vascular endothelium. Accumulation of local fluid due to increased permeability causes pain and swelling. So different types of disorders either due to hormonal imbalance, physical or physiological problems lead to infertility in male [7].

13. Summary

Vast array of knowledge about the structural and functional characteristics of spermatozoa has been obtained in last few decades. This study provides an information about the molecular composition and mechanism of function responsible behind the unique features of spermatozoa. No doubt that the function of spermatozoa is to carry the haploid genome of male and deliver it to the oocyte, so that it can fuse with haploid genome of female to begin the development of future generation. In the last decade the most substantial approaches in knowledge regarding spermatozoa have come by using many tools of molecular biology and proteomics to recognize the gene and protein controlling composition of spermatozoa and using gene targeting method for ascertaining the function of particular gene in sperm. A few of these advances are;

a. Determination of calcium channels that helps in motility of sperm.

b. Identification of activated adenylyl cyclase.

c. Phosphorylation of tyrosine flagellar proteins during capacitation.

d. Finding the role of heredity on the structure and function of sperm.

About 15% of couples are diagnosed as infertile and in these cases, male contributes 40%. Osmatic stress has been recognized as the inducer of male fertility due to dysfunction of sperm. It has been depicted that antioxidant defense mechanism is disrupted by the production of ROS in large concentration, while only a little concentration of ROS is demanded for normal function of sperm. This augmented production of ROS has negative impact on spermatozoa quality and damage their capacity of fertilizing the egg. ROS itself and their metabolites can cause the death of cells by attacking DNA, proteins and lipids, impair the function of the enzymes, creating irreparable damage and ultimately results to diminish in semen parameter concerned with infertility of male. So, an enhanced knowledge is also needed about the composition, organization and function of spermatozoon so that highly specific approaches are to be developed to regulate the function of sperm and essential for determining the environmental effect on male fertility.

Author details

Mohd Sajad and Sonu Chand Thakur*
Centre for Interdisciplinary Research in Basic Sciences, Jamia Millia Islamia University, New Delhi, India

*Address all correspondence to: sthakur@jmi.ac.in

References

[1] Baccetti B. Evolutionary trends in sperm structure. Comparative Biochemistry and Physiology. A, Comparative Physiology. 1986;**85**(1):29-36

[2] Roosen-Runge E. The process of spermatogenesis in mammals. In: Developmental and Cell Biology Series. Vol. 10. CUP Archive; 1977

[3] Segal S. Sexual differentiation in vertebrates. In: MBL Lectures in Biology, vol. 7: The Origin and Evolution of Sex. 1985. pp. 263-270

[4] Surani MA, Allen ND, Barton SC, Fundele R, Howlett SK, Norris ML, et al. Developmental consequences of imprinting of parental chromosomes by DNA methylation. Philosophical Transactions of the Royal Society B. 1990;**326**(1235):313-327

[5] Kelly TL, Trasler JM. Reproductive epigenetics: Section Editors: Roderick R. McInnes, e-mail: mcinnes@ sickkids.on.ca Jacques Michaud, e-mail: jmichaud@ justine.umontreal.ca. Clinical Genetics. 2004;**65**(4):247-260

[6] Hall JE. Guyton and Hall Textbook of Medical Physiology e-Book. Elsevier Health Sciences; 2010

[7] Azenabor A, Ekun AO, Akinloye O. Impact of inflammation on male reproductive tract. Journal of Reproduction and Infertility. 2015;**16**(3):123

[8] Roqueta-Rivera M, Stroud CK, Haschek WM, Akare SJ, Segre M, Brush RS, et al. Docosahexaenoic acid supplementation fully restores fertility and spermatogenesis in male delta-6 desaturase-null mice. Journal of Lipid Research. 2010;**51**:360-367

[9] Wang X, Sharma RK, Sikka SC, Thomas AJ Jr, Falcone T, Agarwal A. Oxidative stress is associated with increased apoptosis leading to spermatozoa DNA damage in patients with male factor infertility. Fertility and Sterility. 2003;**80**:531-535

[10] Ghaleno LR, Valojerdi MR, Hassani F, Chehrazi M, Janzamin E. High level of intracellular sperm oxidative stress negatively influences embryo pronuclear formation after intracytoplasmic sperm injection treatment. Andrologia. 2014;**46**:1118-1127

[11] Marchetti C, Obert G, Deffosez A, Formstecher P, Marchetti P. Study of mitochondrial membrane potential, reactive oxygen species, DNA fragmentation and cell viability by flow cytometry in human sperm. Human Reproduction. 2002;**17**:1257-1265

[12] Wang X, Sharma RK, Gupta A, George V, Thomas AJ, Falcone T, et al. Alterations in mitochondria membrane potential and oxidative stress in infertile men: A prospective observational study. Fertility and Sterility. 2003;**80**(Suppl 2):844-850

[13] Repping S, Skaletsky H, Lange J, Silber S, van der Veen F, Oates RD, et al. Recombination between palindromes P5 and P1 on the human Y chromosome causes massive deletions and spermatogenic failure. The American Journal of Human Genetics. 2002;**71**(4):906-922

[14] Yen and Jaffe's Reproductive Endocrinology, Physiology, Pathology and Clinical Management. 6th ed. Saunders Elsevier

[15] Serres C, Feneux D, Jouannet P. Abnormal distribution of the periaxonemal structures in a human sperm flagellar dyskinesia. Cell Motility and the Cytoskeleton. 1986;**6**(1):68-76

[16] Ortega C, Verheyen G, Raick D, Camus M, Devroey P, Tournaye H. Absolute asthenozoospermia and ICSI: What are the options? Human Reproduction Update. 2011;**17**(5):684-692

[17] Chemes HE, Rawe VY. Sperm pathology: A step beyond descriptive morphology. Origin, characterization and fertility potential of abnormal sperm phenotypes in infertile men. Human Reproduction Update. 2003;**9**(5):405-428

[18] Chemes HE. Phenotypes of sperm pathology: Genetic and acquired forms in infertile men. Journal of Andrology. 2000;**21**(6):799-808

[19] Rossman CM, Forrest JB, Lee RM, Newhouse AF, Newhouse MT. The dyskinetic cilia syndrome; abnormal ciliary motility in association with abnormal ciliary ultrastructure. Chest. 1981;**80**(6 Suppl):860-865

[20] Afzelius BA, Eliasson R. Flagellar mutants in man: On the heterogeneity of the immotile-cilia syndrome. Journal of Ultrastructure Research. 1979;**69**(1):43-52

[21] Afzelius BA. Genetical and ultrastructural aspects of the immotile-cilia syndrome. American Journal of Human Genetics. 1981;**33**(6):852

[22] Escalier D. New insights into the assembly of the periaxonemal structures in mammalian spermatozoa. Biology of Reproduction. 2003;**69**(2):373-378

[23] Yanagimachi R. Mechanisms of fertilization in mammals. In: Fertilization and Embryonic Development In Vitro. Boston, MA: Springer; 1981. pp. 81-182

[24] Suarez SS, Ho HC. Hyperactivated motility in sperm. Reproduction in Domestic Animals. 2003;**38**(2):119-124

[25] Carlson AE, Westenbroek RE, Quill T, Ren D, Clapham DE, Hille B, et al. CatSper1 required for evoked Ca^{2+} entry and control of flagellar function in sperm. Proceedings of the National Academy of Sciences. 2003;**100**(25):14864-14868

[26] Quill TA, Sugden SA, Rossi KL, Doolittle LK, Hammer RE, Garbers DL. Hyperactivated sperm motility driven by CatSper2 is required for fertilization. Proceedings of the National Academy of Sciences. 2003;**100**(25):14869-14874

[27] Leclerc P, De Lamirande E, Gagnon C. Cyclic adenosine 3′, 5′ monophosphate-dependent regulation of protein tyrosine phosphorylation in relation to human sperm capacitation and motility. Biology of Reproduction. 1996;**55**(3):684-692

[28] Si Y, Okuno M. Role of tyrosine phosphorylation of flagellar proteins in hamster sperm hyperactivation. Biology of Reproduction. 1999;**61**(1):240-246

[29] Spehr M, Schwane K, Riffell JA, Barbour J, Zimmer RK, Neuhaus EM, et al. Particulate adenylate cyclase plays a key role in human sperm olfactory receptor-mediated chemotaxis. The Journal of Biological Chemistry. 2004;**279**(38):40194-40203

[30] Kuno N, Kadomatsu K, Fan QW, Hagihara M, Senda T, Mizutani S, et al. Female sterility in mice lacking the basigin gene, which encodes a transmembrane glycoprotein belonging to the immunoglobulin superfamily. FEBS Letters. 1998;**425**(2):191-194

[31] Carr DW, Stofko-Hahn RE, Fraser ID, Bishop SM, Acott TS, Brennan RG, et al. Interaction of the regulatory subunit (RII) of cAMP-dependent protein kinase with RII-anchoring proteins occurs through an amphipathic helix binding motif. The Journal of Biological Chemistry. 1991;**266**(22):14188-14192

[32] Henkel RR. Leukocytes and oxidative stress: Dilemma forsperm

function and male fertility. Asian Journal of Andrology. 2011;**13**:43-52

[33] Lanzafame FM, La Vignera S, Vicari E, Calogero AE. Oxidative stress and medical antioxidant treatment in male infertility. Reproductive Biomedicine Online. 2009;**19**:638-659

[34] Henkel RR. Leukocytes and oxidative stress: Dilemma for sperm function and male fertility. Asian Journal of Andrology. 2011;**13**(1):43

[35] Chen SJ, Allam JP, Duan YG, Haidl G. Influence of reactive oxygen species on human sperm functions and fertilizing capacity including therapeutical approaches. Archives of Gynecology and Obstetrics. 2013;**288**:191-199

[36] Sikka SC. Relative impact of oxidative stress on male reproductive function. Current Medicinal Chemistry. 2001;**8**:851-862

[37] Sabeur K, Ball BA. Characterization of NADPH oxidase 5 in equine testis and spermatozoa. Reproduction. 2007;**134**:263-270

[38] Gharagozloo P, Aitken RJ. The role of sperm oxidative stress in male infertility and the significance of oral antioxidant therapy. Human Reproduction. 2011;**26**:1628-1640

[39] Choudhary R, Chawala VK, Soni ND, Kumar J, Vyas RK. Oxidative stress and role of antioxidants in male infertility. Pakistan Journal of Physiology. 2010;**6**:54-59

[40] Esteves SC. Effect of cigarette smoking on levels of seminal oxidative stress in infertile men: A prospective study. International Brazilian Journal of Urology. 2002;**28**:484-485

[41] Lavranos G, Balla M, Tzortzopoulou A, Syriou V, Angelopoulou R. Investigating ROS sources in male infertility: A common end for numerous pathways. Reproductive Toxicology. 2012;**34**:298-307

[42] Agarwal A, Saleh RA, Bedaiwy MA. Role of reactive oxygen species in the pathophysiology of human reproduction. Fertility and Sterility. 2003;**79**:829-843

[43] Lu JC, Huang YF, Lü NQ. WHO laboratory manual for the examination and processing of human semen: Its applicability to andrology laboratories in China. Zhonghua NanKe Xue. 2010;**16**:867-871

[44] Hampl R, Drábková P, Kanďár R, Stěpán J. Impact of oxidative stress on male infertility. Ceská Gynekologie. 2012;**77**:241-245

[45] Shiraishi K, Matsuyama H, Takihara H. Pathophysiology of varicocele in male infertility in the era of assisted reproductive technology. International Journal of Urology. 2012;**19**:538-550

[46] Santoro G, Romeo C, Impellizzeri P, Ientile R, Cutroneo G, Trimarchi F, et al. Nitric oxide synthase patterns in normal and varicocele testis in adolescents. BJU International. 2001;**88**(9):967-973

[47] Agarwal A, Deepinder F, Sharma RK, Ranga G, Li J. Effect of cell phone usage on semen analysis in men attending infertility clinic: an observational study. Fertility and Sterility. 2008;**89**:124-128

[48] Aitken RJ, Bennetts LE, Sawyer D, Wiklendt AM, King BV. Impact of radio frequency electromagnetic radiation on DNA integrity in the male germline. International Journal of Andrology. 2005;**28**:171-179

[49] De Iuliis GN, Newey RJ, King BV, Aitken RJ. Mobile phone radiation induces reactive oxygen species production and DNA damage in human

spermatozoa in vitro. PLoS One. 2009;**4**:e6446

[50] Jurasović J, Cvitković P, Pizent A, Colak B, Telisman S. Semen quality and reproductive endocrine function with regard to blood cadmium in Croatian male subjects. Biometals. 2004;**17**:735-743

[51] Esfandiari N, Saleh RA, Blaut AP, Sharma RK, Nelson DR, Thomas AJ Jr, et al. Effects of temperature on sperm motion characteristics and reactive oxygen species. International Journal of Fertility and Women's Medicine. 2002;**47**:227-233

[52] Saleh RA, Agarwal A, Sharma RK, Nelson DR, Thomas AJ Jr. Effect of cigarette smoking on levels of seminal oxidative stress in infertile men: A prospective study. Fertility and Sterility. 2002;**78**:491-499

[53] Kiziler AR, Aydemir B, Onaran I, Alici B, Ozkara H, Gulyasar T, et al. High levels of cadmium and lead in seminal fluid and blood of smoking men are associated with high oxidative stress and damage in infertile subjects. Biological Trace Element Research. 2007;**120**:82-91

[54] Jarow JP. Semen quality of male smokers and nonsmokers in infertile couples. The Journal of Urology. 2003;**170**:675-676

[55] Agarwal A, Prabakaran SA. Mechanism,measurement,andprevention of oxidative stress in male reproductive physiology

[56] Saleh RA, Agarwal A. Oxidative stress and male infertility: From research bench to clinical practice. Journal of Andrology. 2002;**23**(6):737-752

[57] Ickowicz D, Finkelstein M, Breitbart H. Mechanism of sperm capacitation and the acrosome reaction: Role of protein kinases. Asian Journal of Andrology. 2012;**14**(6):816-821. DOI: 10.1038/aja.2012.81

[58] Tsai WW, Niessen S, Goebel N, Yates JR 3rd, Guccione E, Montminy M. PRMT5 modulates the metabolic response to fasting signals. Proceedings of the National Academy of Sciences of the United States of America. 2013;**110**:8870-8875

[59] Kothari S, Thompson A, Agarwal A, du Plessis SS. Free radicals: Their beneficial and detrimental effects on sperm function. Indian Journal of Experimental Biology. 2010;**48**:425-435

[60] De Lamirande E, O'Flaherty C. Sperm activation: Role of reactive oxygen species and kinases. Biochimica et Biophysica Acta. 2008;**1784**:106-115

[61] Suarez SS. Control of hyperactivation in sperm. Human Reproduction Update. 2008;**14**:647-657

[62] Patrat C, Serres C, Jouannet P. The acrosome reaction in human spermatozoa. Biology of the Cell. 2000;**92**(3-4):255-266

[63] Bansal AK, Bilaspuri GS. Impacts of oxidative stress and antioxidants on semen functions. Veterinary Medicine International. 2011;**2011**:686137

[64] Calamera J, Buffone M, Ollero M, Alvarez J, Doncel GF. Superoxide dismutase content and fatty acid composition in subsets of human spermatozoa from normozoospermic, asthenozoospermic, and polyzoospermic semen samples. Molecular Reproduction and Development. 2003;**66**:422-430

[65] Khosrowbeygi A, Zarghami N. Fatty acid composition of human spermatozoa and seminal plasma levels of oxidative stress biomarkers in subfertile males. Prostaglandins, Leukotrienes, and Essential Fatty Acids. 2007;**77**:117-121

[66] Lampiao F. Free radicals generation in an in vitro fertilization setting and how to minimize them. World Journal of Obstetrics and Gynecology. 2012;**1**:29-34

[67] Sharma RK, Agarwal A. Role of reactive oxygen species in male infertility. Urology. 1996;**48**:835-850

[68] Hair WM, Gubbay O, Jabbour HN, Lincoln GA. Prolactin receptor expression in human testis and accessory tissues: Localization and function. Molecular Human Reproduction. 2002;**8**:606-611

[69] Palnitkar G, Phillips CL, Hoyos CM, Marren AJ, Bowman MC, Yee BJ. Linking sleep disturbance to idiopathic male infertility. Sleep Medicine Reviews. 2018

[70] Mitchell RN, Cotran RS. Acute and chronic inflammation. In: Kumar V, Cotran RS, Robbins SL, editors. Robbins Basic Pathology. Vol. 127. Philadelphia: Saunders Press; 2003. 33 p

[71] Purvis K, Christiansen E. Infection in the male reproductive tract. Impact, diagnosis and treatment in relation to male infertility. International Journal of Andrology. 1993;**16**(1):1-13

[72] Comhaire FH, Mahmoud AM, Depuydt CE, Zalata AA, Christophe AB. Mechanisms and effects of male genital tract infection on sperm quality and fertilizing potential: The andrologist's viewpoint. Human Reproduction Update. 1999;**5**(5):393-398

[73] Hales DB, Diemer T, Hales KH. Role of cytokines in testicular function. Endocrine. 1999;**10**(3):201-217

[74] Soder O, Sultana T, Jonsson C, Wahlgren A, Petersen C, Holst M. The interleukin-1 system in the testis. Andrologia. 2000;**32**(1):52-55

Chapter 3

Understanding the Epigenetic Modifications in Sperm Genome

Eswari Beeram

Abstract

Sperm genome condensation is mainly important as the genome expression should be repressed until it is fertilised with oocyte. In most of the mammals, protamines play an important role in genome condensation. In humans, histone variants were present in germ cells when compared with somatic cells. How successful replacement of histones by protamines occurs in most of the mammals is an interesting question. Little information is known about transition proteins that replace histones with protamines. Apart from condensation, which mechanisms prevent expression of X and Y chromosomes in sperm is to be studied. If exposed to genotoxic agents like Metosartan that damage testes should also be considered, in order for assisted reproductive technologies like in vitro fertilisation to succeed.

Keywords: assisted reproductive technology (ART), intra cytoplasmic sperm injection (ICSI), invitro fertilisation (IVF), stem cell factor (SCF), protein dependent kinase (PDK), glial cell derived neurotropic factor (GDNF), post translational modification (PTM), chromatin assembly factor (CAF), testes specific serine/threonine kinase 6 (TSSK6), nucleolar organising region (NOR), p- element induced wlmphy testes in drosophila (PIWI), a disintegrin and metalloprotease (ADAM)

1. Introduction

Spermiogenesis involves several steps and finally differentiate to A spermatogonia from stem cells [1]. Self renewal of stem cells was necessary for production of sperm cells throughout the life. C-Kit and SCF play an important role in determining the germ cell fate. Retinoic acid receptor plays a crucial role in proliferation of germ cells. Expression of Proteins like PP2A is reduced in later stages of the spermiogenesis and differentiation of A- spermatozoa in to B spermatozoa occurs through various intermediate stages like A_{pr}, A_{al}, A_{1-4} and finally to B- spermatozoa. Commitment to B- spermatozoa was followed by meiosis-I and ii leading to formation of round spermatids. During the separation of chromosomes, cohesins hold the sister chromatids and disassemble after the homologous recombination leading to separation of chromosomes, defects in which leads to stage IV arrest. The round spermatids undergo several morphological and cytological changes like elongation of sperm head, acrosome formation and shedding of the cytoplasm. During the process, several signalling mechanisms like PDK-Akt pathway, GDNF-GFR1 pathway, mTOR pathway, and MAP kinase pathways operate proceeding to spermiogenesis.

IntechOpen

2. Protamines are originated from histone H1

In humans and mammals histones was replaced by either protamines or histone variants in sperm cell. But recent discovery of protamine P1 show both N- terminal and C- terminal sequence similarity between each other, and where as histone variant precursor resembled to that of protamine P2. Histones are basic proteins rich in Arg and Lys residues where as protamines in Styela contain polyarginine tracts than compared with histones.

Sperm condensation is one of the important criteria to be considered during assisted reproductive technologies in order to prevent genetic defects in upcoming generation. Spermatid formation involves 12–14 steps, and finally elongation of nuclear material leads to elongated sperms with acrosome. In sperm, histones are replaced by protamines and in humans histone variants are present leading to sperm condensation. Disulfide bonds contribute additional stability to the condensation as it results in interlinking of protamines [2, 3]. Certain PTMs of histones was also one of the epigenetic modifications required for condensation. Decondensation of Sperm chromatin takes place after sperm penetration in to oocyte which leads to exposure of sperm DNA [4] to oocyte reducing agents like glutathione. As known, glutathione reduces disulfide bonds between the protamines and relaxing the sperm DNA. From the previous reports, agents like SDS, EDTA reduces the disulfide bonds in combined state. Glycosaminoglycans like heparin sulphate binds to receptors on sperm membrane and promotes decondensation instead with nonsulfated form heparin (**Figure 1**).

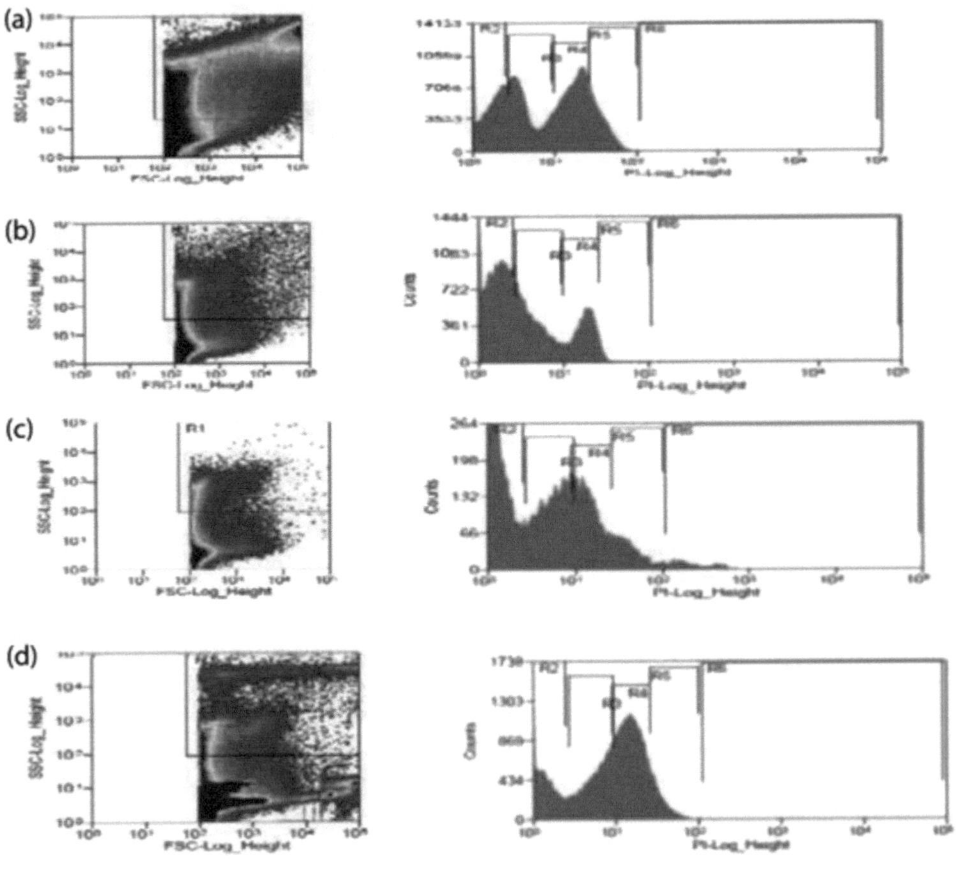

Figure 1.
Flow cytometry of spermatozoa showing DNA fragmentation. Where (a) is control, (b) is testes treated with Metosartan (c) with RNaseA +aspirin and (d) with RNaseA+metosartan.

Acrosome and mitochondrial sheath formation occurs at 6 and 16 steps of the sperm biogenesis. Acrosome vesicles are secreted from the Golgi vesicles and form acrosomes cap around the nucleus. Defect with vesicle fusion or vesicle proteins leads to abnormalities in sperm head. Mitochondria is the major energy reserve of the sperm and the movement of mitochondria occurs through IMT pathways. Finally the sperms shed their cytoplasm by forming a cytoplasmic droplet around the neck region and remains attached to Sertoli cells until they become mature. Apical epistatic interaction involves holding of sperms at Sertoli junctions through the help of adherens proteins like NECTIN, Integrin- laminin and cadherin-catenin. Loss of Protein leads to premature release of sperms from Sertoli cells into the lumen of seminiferous tubules and abnormalities leads to vice versa of the same.

3. Testes-specific histones

H1T1 was one of the variant of linker histone found during pachytene of the cell division. H1T2 was the other linker variant found in apical pole of spermatids and responsible for male fertility. In case of humans HilS1 is necessary for condensation in elongated spermatids. Certain Core histone variants like TH2A and TH2B are found to be elevated during elongation of spermatids and whereas the normal core histones show low amounts of expression. Gene knock outs of TH2A and TH2B induced male infertility but PTMs on core histones compensate the loss of these variants in the spermatids [5]. TH2A was found to be present at transcriptional start site [6] and where as TH2B is required during leptotene of the cell division.

Other histone variant is with core histone H3 which include H3.3, H3T and CenP. H3.3 is present at the stage of spermatids [7] and where as H3T was specifically expressed in testes and both differ by 5 amino acid residues from core histone H3.1. H3.3 represents actively transcripted regions where as H3.1 represents transcriptionally repressive regions and may be involved in replacement of Histones by protamines. H3.1 may be required for maintaining the repression of X and Y chromosomes where as H3.1 is involved in activating the genes required for transition protein and protamine synthesis.

Recently, humans contain histone variants instead of canonical histones which are subjected to acetylation at H_4K5, H4K8, H4K12 and H_4K16. In Drosophila H3 is also acetylated especially at H_3 K9 by Plant domain containing protein PYGO2 and responsible for open confirmation of chromatin. Presence of histone chaperones as identified recently in Drosophila named CAF1 (Chromatin Assembly Factor) and in humans was normal Heat shock protein variant namely HSPA2 (HSP 70.2). These chaperones acts as chromatin remodellers and responsible for exchange of transition proteins with protamines. ATP dependent remodeller proteins that act as histone chaperones was not known up to now, but above mentioned are some of the remodellers that help in chromatin remodelling in testes.

4. Various histone modifications during spermiogenesis

Histone modifications like phosphorylation, acetylation and ubiquitination play an important role in spermiogenesis [8]. Phosphorylation is found to be common on the four core histone proteins, and acetylation was mostly seen in H4, whereas ubiquitination was with respect to H2A and B. Phosphorylation and acetylation leads to neutralisation of charges on histones whereas ubiquitylation causes Rnf 8 mediated recruitment of transition proteins and found to be normal in gene knock out animals with respect to meiosis and repression of expression in germ cells.

Methylation is one of the main PTM to be considered during spermiogenesis. Lysine methylation is the most common methylation in histones during spermiogenesis. To some extent arginine methylation by type iii arginine methylases was also one of the common methylation that occurs in protamines like PRM2. Methylations like H2BK117 and H2BK121 is required for TH2B replacement in germ cells. Methylation in H3K9 was required for maintaining chromatin in repressed state [9], and it helps in maintaining some residual nucleosome core histones in paternal genome seen in sperm. Phosphorylation of H2A byTSSK6 is required for histone acetylation followed by condensation of chromatin [10, 11]. May be DNA double strand breaks activate TSSK6 in late spermatids forming ɤH2AX foci required for replacement of histones with protamines [12].

Poly ADP-ribosylation is one of the events involved in gene regulation and Cell proliferation. ADP-ribosylation was another important modification to be considered during meiotic programme and also during DNA condensation [13]. Both the steps requires ds break formation and as per recent reports poly ADP ribosylation was seen during stages of spermatocytes and spermatids but not in case of mature spermatids. Ds breaks activates enzyme Poly ADP ribosyl polymerase which was taken as a score of DNA damage that proceeds with ds break formation [14, 15].

Methylation, Ubiquitination, acetylation were some of the common modifications seen in sperm chromatin during late spermatid stages. However sumoylation is attributed to centromere and telomeric heterochromatin regions. Presence of canonical histones was necessary for the identification of the paternal genome by embryo. In late spermatid stage most of the genome mRNA is kept in repressed state where as Protamine and transition proteins synthesis occurs in early spermatocytes.

Phosphorylation is one of the PTM that protamine undergoes before its exchange with transition proteins. After loading on DNA dephosphorylation and disulfide bond formation of protamine occurs. Protamine P2 is synthesised as precursor and processed later on in order to get a functional protein. Disulfide bond formation mainly occurs during the transit of spermatozoa from caput to cauda. Thiol content has positive relation with tyrosine phosphorylation and infertility. Some of the residual Histones must be required in the sperm cells as it is necessary for gene expression and genetic imprinting of certain genes in paternal genome. Phosphorylation of protamines was effectively seen at some places and necessary for effective binding with DNA. Zinc stabilises the sperm chromatin mainly due to binding to protamines. Protamines interacts with toxic metals so pesticides used, damages DNA integrity by binding to protamines and some of them may also cause alkylation of protamines.

5. Nuclear basic proteins

Transition proteins TNP1 and TNP2 are involved in transition of histones to protamines. TNP2 was responsible for the condensation of DNA through interacting with PRM2 by methylating events. TNP1 and 2 are the basic proteins rich in lysine and arginine residues where as protamines consists of lysine and cysteines residues and loss of protein interactions between TNP2 and PRM2 results in prevention of histone replacement with protamines proved by spatiotemporal orientation of these genes on chromosome [16]. TNP1 is involved in decondensation of chromatin [17] at nucleosome core and relaxing DNA with the help of topoisomerase which removes positive supercoiling. TNP1 is also involved in repair of ss breaks of DNA generated during the chromatin remodelling. Histones are present as nucleosome core up to 11–12 step and replaced by TPs at 12–13 steps and by protamines in 13–15 steps. TNP1 and TNP2 are loaded on to DNA at apposition ends [18, 19] and the mutants of TNPs does not alter the expression of protamines PRM1 [20] and 2 (**Figure 2**).

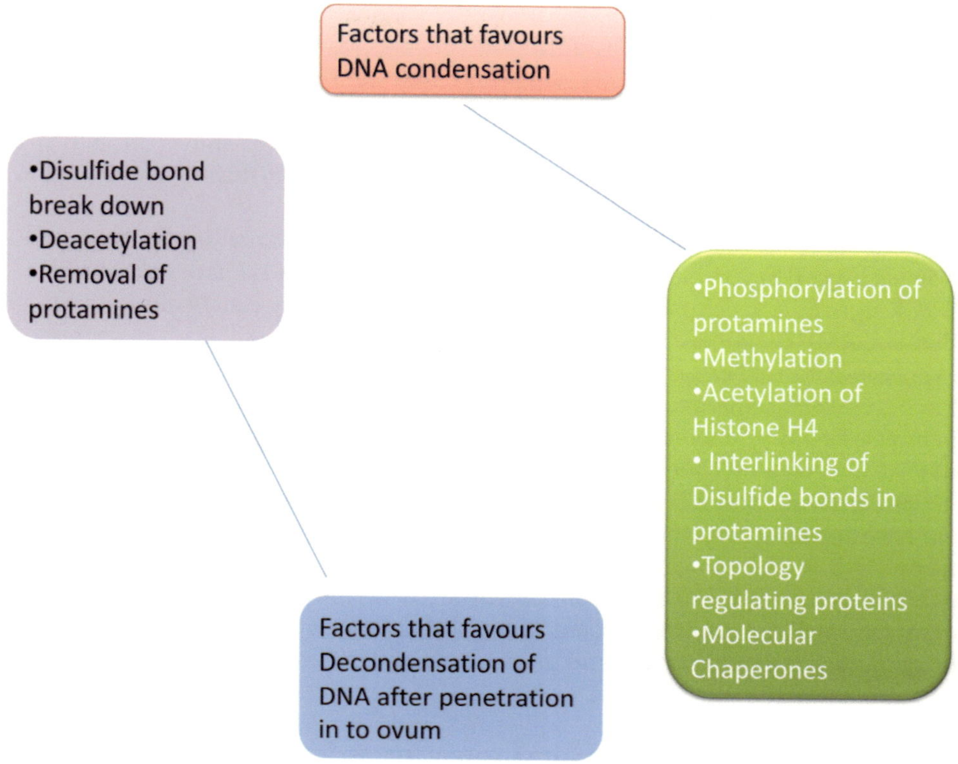

Figure 2.
Factors responsible for maintenance of genome integrity from parent to offspring.

Histone to protamine transition involves replacement of histones by protamines. From the previous reports, transition proteins play an important role in guiding this process. But recent report on male infertility has proved that ubiquitination of histones by RNF8 a ring domain containing proteins in the nucleus [21]. This protein mainly interacts with MIWI a PIWI protein and sequesters the protein RNF 8 in the cytoplasm. This interaction mainly prevents histone replacement by protamines even though the expression of protamines and transition proteins are normal. In this case not only the replacement of histones, but also the posttranslational modifications in protamines also play a major role in male fertility [22]. For example incorporation of Prm2 on chromatin requires phosphorylation of Prm2 to attain maturity of the protein so that it can interact with DNA. Phosphorylation of Prm2 is carried out by CAMK, loss of which leads to male infertility.

From the recent reports RNF8 is required for ubiquitination of H2A and H2B followed by H4 acetylation. Ubiquitinated H2 and H2B acts as platform for binding of MOF (Males absent of first) necessary for dosage compensation in drosophila fly and adds acetyl groups to H4 leading to free chromatin. The role of RNF8 is limited to spermatid stage and post meiotic, and plays an important role in male fertility. But how the ubiquitinated histones are protected from degradation by proteasome is a major question. But it is solved by spatial and temporal expression of proteasomal proteins especially in the late spermatid state.

Males defective in genes Tnp1 and Tnp2 does not effect the expression of proteins either protamines or Tnps. But abnormal retention of Tnp1 and 2 is the main reason for elevated levels in both Tnp−/− and as well as Tnp+/− mutants. The mutations would not affect the transition from histones to protamines. Histone to Protamine transition follows inter and intra disulfide bond formation in between cysteines of protamines there by centering the amino and carboxy terminal ends with DNA binding domain. Disulfide bonds are necessary for further compaction of DNA and four of seven cysteines in protamines were involved in disulfide bond formation. Reduction of disulfide bonds leads to decondensation of chromatin proved by X-ray crystallography. Intra and inter linking of protamines through disulfide bond formation occurs at spermatid stage especially during maturation in epididymis [23], before to 14 days of their release.

Inhibin B activates mainly five pathways namely GPCR signalling, calcium pathway [24], MAP kinase pathway, PI3 pathway, Phospholipase A2 pathway. In which GPCR signalling, calcium Pathway and MAP kinase pathway causes phosphorylation of CAMP Responsive Element Modulator (CREM). This will leads to decreased expression of Prm2 causing male infertility. As earlier discussed histone—Protamine replacement requires certain modifications in histones like acetylation. In mouse CHD5 promotes H4 acetylation and ablation of this gene leads to retention of H3 and decreased condensation of nuclear DNA in head. This gene is expressed in both brain and testes but with higher in testes. Haploid insufficiency of gene does not have any effect on male fertility but the DNA condensation is affected further from step 9 of spermiogenesis [25] with out affecting brain tissue. Abnormality of sperm was mainly due to defects in condensation of chromatin [26] but not due to other defects like cytoplasmic retention, apical epistatic specialisation, acrosomes biogenesis, flagella movement and mitochondrial sheath formation.

6. ABP as the main molecule for chromatin condensation and decondensation

Androgen Binding Protein (ABP) acts as carrier for steroid hormone [27] Dihydrotestosterone the potent form of testosterone which acts as acceptor of hydrogen atoms. It oxidises disulfide bonds in the nucleus of sperm at the time of

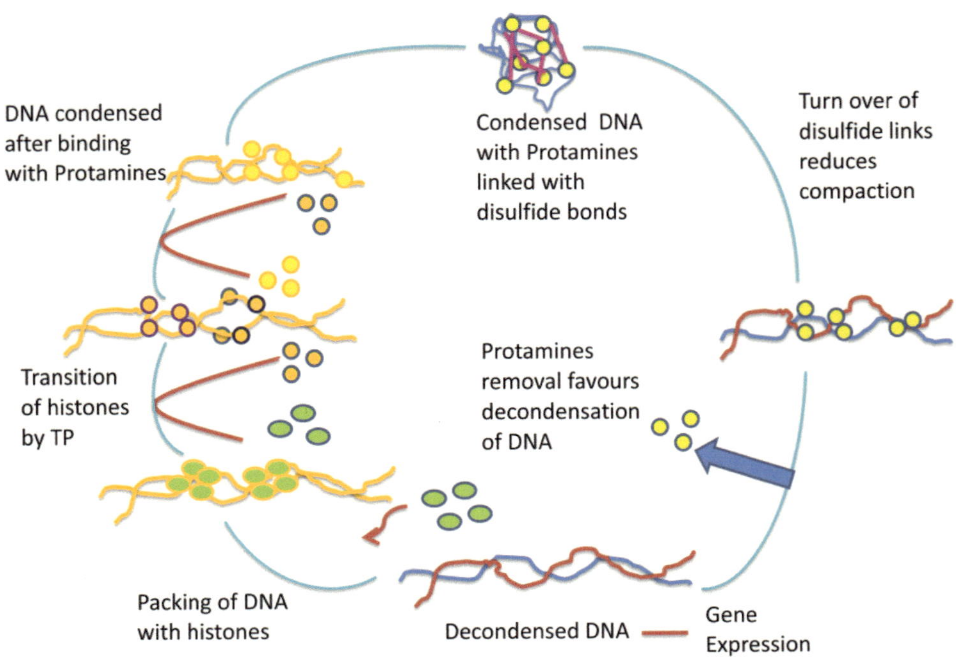

Figure 3.
Overall schematic representation of condensation and decondensation of sperm DNA.

maturation in caput epididymis. 3- Hydroxy steroid dehydrogenase is the enzyme that has both oxidase and reductase activities but oxidase activity requires activation by female sex hormones like oestrogens or Progesterone. The enzyme requires NADPH as reducing equivalent and later glutathione after oocyte penetration to induce decondensation [2]. The process requires 3- diol instead of dihydrotestosterone. The steps of condensation are ABP > ABP—Dihydrotestosterone > Nuclear Localisation > Release of Dihydrotestosterone > Condensation > Penetration in to oocyte by sperm > Decondensation > Decondensation further By Glutathione > Reducing disulfide bonds in DNA (**Figure 3**).

7. Cell cycle analysis in spermatozoa using aniline blue

In S phase the dye uptake is more compared to G1 phase, where as similar in M phase as that of the S phase because immature sperms are stained by aniline blue and in case of aneuploid and apoptotic cells the dye uptake is low. By aniline blue we cannot distinguish the dividing cells from the cells undergoing segregation of the nuclear content followed by cytokinesis. The maximum absorption spectrum of aniline blue is 234.5 nm which can be used to detect the dye by flow cytometry using detector at this wavelength. It is low cost effective compared to propidium iodide but it has yet to be used and by this, we can study the aneuploidy, sperm maturity and apoptosis of sperm cells by using ejaculated semen sample. Flow cytometry analysis of sperm suspension collected from epididymis can be performed after staining with aniline blue as protamines exclude aniline blue, only immature sperms takes aniline blue so, this property of dye can be used to study sperm maturity by flow cytometry.

8. Understanding the topology of spermatocytes

Spermatocyte recombination mainly occurs by double strand break formation and involves interactions between chromosome domains by forming nuclear territories. The telocentric chromosomes along with NORs form bouquet like structure at the periphery of the nucleus where as metacentric chromosomes at centre of the nucleus. If $2n = 24$, 8 bivalents are formed and attached to form bouquet structure. There was little exchange seen between the nonhomologous chromosomes in Mus species so evolutionary importance is less in these species. Heterochromatin surrounding the centromere form the basis for absence of recombination as it encodes proteins that keep the centromere integrity.

Constitutive heterochromatin in nucleolus makes the rDNA arrangement with difference in different species. Together with proximal arrangement with respect to telomere and metacentric chromosomes with NORs in long arms serve as excellent models for study of both NORs and bouquet formation, seen in maintenance of topology. Bouquet formation is necessary for interaction of chromosomal domains in nuclear territories. Two telocentric chromosome forms a single metacentric chromosome which forms the basis of recombination.

EtBr is normally used as intercalating dye to study DNA and also to stain DNA. Increased concentrations of EtBr causes decondensation of DNA as the bonds between the intercalated bases rearrange and results in loop formation. After certain concentration of dye, the decondensed DNA will be condensed again, i.e., biphasic kinetics was seen with the epididymal sperms. In late elongated spermatids histones are already replaced by protamines as cysteines present in protamines provide extra stability and these sperms are proven to resistant to DNase I digestion, up to shorter time periods.

9. Molecular chaperones are necessary for male fertility

Molecular chaperones are the proteins, which help in folding of proteins and prevent their aggregation. So after spermiogenesis, post testicular maturation in requires proteins like chaperones in addition to several other proteins in epididymis. Those are the proteins like HSP60, HSP70 family including HSPA2, HSPA5, and other than HSP 70 family include chaperonin containing t- complex protein and HSP90. HSP 70 plays an important role in maintaining proteins in partially folded state and facilitates in transport of those proteins in the membranes. HSPa2 is responsible for spermiogenesis and also aids in maturation of sperms. It binds to the plasma membrane of sperm along with its co chaperones and forms heterocomplex with CDC2 and cyclin B during G1- S phase and G2- M phase transitions. This protein is also present in ovial secretions along with HSPA5 and is necessary for capacitation of sperms.

As discussed previous the thiol content reflects the tyrosine phosphorylation. HSPa2 promotes condensation analogous to decondensation factor and terminates signalling by tyrosine phosphorylation. Chaperonin containing t- complex protein (CCT) binds to sperm plasma membrane and promotes ZP binding as it promotes binding to ZP receptors. CCT protein along with its co chaperones enters the sperm through endocytosis of receptor and ligand coated with caveolin protein in membrane rafts. This protein is mainly present in t-complex of sperm and prevents protein aggregation or misfolding. CCT is mainly composed of 8 subunits in which 3 subunits form the domains and substrate recognition was through electrostatic and hydrophobic interactions, and then transported to the central cavity of the protein.

HSP60 was the other molecular chaperone found in mitochondria and helps in transport of proteins in to mitochondria. HSPA5 also known as Bip aids in folding of proteins in endoplasmic reticulum and participates in ER stress signalling pathway. Like HSPA5 calcium binding protein Calmigen also express in ER and become arrested after late spermatid stage. HSPA8 the one of the member of HSP70 and was expressed ubiquitously and facilitates binding of sperm to ovum. So, injection of this protein with IVF may be useful as it is important for enhanced survival of sperm in vivo.

Calmigen and Calsporin were the variants of Calnexin and Calreticulin seen in testes and along with ADAM1A, ADAM2 and ADAM 3 were required for sperm capacitation by interacting with zona of oocyte and helps in sperm—oocyte interaction. Calreticulin is mainly necessary for calcium oscillations inside the sperm cells for hyper activation and capacitation. PDI (Protein Disulfide Isomerase) along with Calmigen is necessary for disulfide bond formation and remodelling in sperm.

10. Epigenetic modulations in sperm genome

Histone H3 undergoes demethylation at K9 due to loss of lysine demethylase in primordial germ cells after E7.5 days. In meiotic recombination histone mono, di tri methylations are responsible for DSBs and recombination. Methylation at pericentric regions [28] is responsible for preventing homologous recombination. Retrotransposons restrict methylating events and responsible for maintenance of genome imprinting. Reduced DNA methylation in retrotransposons leads to gene expression in LINE 1 transposons and proteins like PIWI and AUBERGINE undergoes methylation in repetitive elements of PGC and responsible for gene silencing mechanisms [29]. This pattern was found to be conserved in mice and in animals and mammals, in addition to mutational hotspots there are some recombination hotspots characterised by H3K4me3 and H3K9 acetylation.

Paternal genomes are hypomethylated compared to maternal genome and in Drosophila the protamine eviction was done by DHD (Dead Head) by reducing the disulfide bonds with the help of thioredoxin and NADPH. Protamines form oligomers by intrachain disulfide bonds. Molecular chaperone TAP/p32 acts on monomeric protamines and causes their eviction and found to be inactive on oligomers. DHD interacts physically with TAP/P32 to cause the eviction of protamines from DNA and TAP/P32 binds poorly to DNA. DHD normally found in sperm nucleus and was degraded after fertilisation. DHD domain was necessary for the reduction of disulfide bonds, DNA decondensation, and protamine eviction and also functions as chaperone. It shares some common properties with thioredoxins and also has unique properties necessary for the embryo formation. Mutation in DHD domain is non tolerant and results in haploid embryo formation with the absence of male pronucleus [30].

Proteomic profile of testes sperm was one of the important researches in progress nowadays. Normally in DNA condensing proteins the disulfide bonds are oxidised spontaneously and does not require any enzymatic source. There are certain proteins in sperm which require enzymes like thioredoxin/Glutathione reductase which acts on glutathione peroxidise and induces disulfide bond formation. Thioredoxin glutathione reductase catalyses isomerisation of disulfide bonds in these proteins and the protein was mainly localised at mid piece of mitochondrial sheath and was required for structural maintenance of mid piece and tail proteins. Those include proteins like mitochondrial capsule selenoprotein, two outer dense fibre (ODF) and glutathione-s-transferase M5. Differences in maternal and paternal chromosomes mainly occur at pericentric chromosomes, through which epigenetic message is conveyed to embryo.

11. Differentiation in meiotic events of sperm and oocyte in *C. elegans*

In oocyte, synaptonemal complex (SC) is formed along the lateral and central axis. In sperms condensation plate is formed after diplotene. Formation of karyosomes, [the aggregation of chromosomes] is characterised in both oocytes and sperms of *C. elegans* and other mammals and referred as karyosome stage in *C. elegans*. The meiotic process mainly differs in microtubule dynamics. In oocytes chromosome dependent spindle formation is necessary for chromosome segregation, where as in case of sperms centrioles are present. So, the spindle formation is mediated by centrioles.

There are some of the kinetochore differences observed in oocytes and sperms. In sperms, outer kinetochore proteins attract the inner proteins. CENP –c is present in spermatocytes and CENP- A is present in oocytes. Some of the kinases like AIR-2 is present in spermatocytes and PLK-1 is found in oocytes. SYP-1 is necessary protein of central element in SC and recruits AIR-2. Mutation in SYP-1 protein leads to random distribution of metaphase bivalents. Some of the kinases like AIR-2 phosphorylates Rec-8 protein which is required for cohesion of sister chromatids. Cytokinesis after meiosis –1 is incomplete in both sperms and oocyte without any necessity for re condensation of chromatin after diplotene.

12. Oxidative potential in testes and epididymis is required for spermiogenesis

GPRX 4 and PXRX4 are the two enzymes which are mainly required for compaction of chromatin in sperm mainly by sulfoxidation of protamines attached to

DNA. PXRX4 is necessary for condensation in testes where as GPRX4 is specifically in epididymis. Hydrogen peroxide acts as signalling molecule and causes phosphorylation of tyrosine molecules in the receptor, necessary for proliferation of sperm cells [31]. Abnormal signalling by hydrogen peroxide leads to sperm cancer which can be avoided by reduction of H2O2 by enzymes like SOD and catalase. Totally GPRX4 and PXRX4 is necessary for nuclear stability, condensation and spermiogenesis.

13. Factors responsible for condensation and decondensation of chromatin

Zinc is well known for maintenance of membrane stability and found to be present in seminal plasma. It is decreased during penetration of sperm in to the female reproductive tract and decrease of zinc causes premature decondensation of chromatin as it destabilises the sperm plasma membrane. Albumin also binds to zinc and accelerates decondensation. In humans heparin is involved in decondensation of chromatin. Zinc also binds to free thiols and increases stability of chromatin, necessary for reducing disulfide bonds and accelerating the reaction (**Figure 4**).

Few of the recent techniques used for measurement of DNA condensation and decondensation include using of TPM motions and energy. Condensation of DNA leads to decrease in length as protamines are organised as toroids. Where as decondensed chromatin is more in length as protamines are replaced by histones. Differences in motions of the DNA attached to the coverslip is captured and ultimately the difference in energy. Positive relation is seen between the persons with premature decondensation in DNA and infertility and DNA damage based on the studies in human subjects. Sperm fluorescent in situ hybridisation is other technique used to assess the relation between sperm DNA [32] condensation and abnormalities of head.

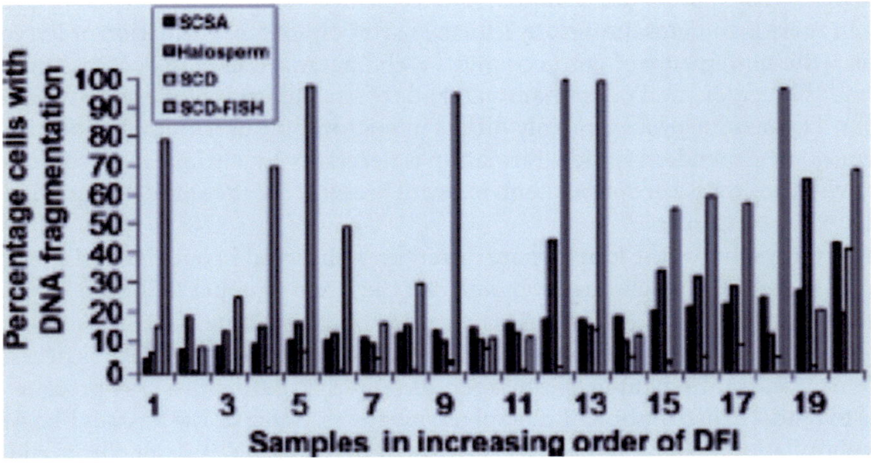

Figure 4.
Percentage of cells with DNA fragmentation using different techniques of assessment.

14. Assisted reproductive technologies required for success of reproductive outcome

ICSI and IVF are the techniques used in assisted reproductive technology, in which ICSI resulted in more percentage of PCC (pre mature condensation of chromatin) compared to IVF. It is mainly due to lack of activation of oocytes. and Pre mature condensation is due to the condensing factors released from the unactivated oocytes without affecting the sperms with intact plasma membrane. The main failure for ICSI is due to the injection of whole sperm in to oocytes. Fusion of oocytes and sperm membranes activates the oocytes lacking of which, was one of the main drawback seen in ICSI [33, 34]. Even damage to sperm membrane is another draw back seen with this technique.

Expression of decondensing factors like MPF is transient, as temporal expression is seen whereas in later stages sperm dependent factor SDF is mainly involved in activation of oocytes causing further decondensation of sperm chromatin. IVF does not include steps that cause damage to sperm DNA [35] and prevention of oocyte activation. The low rate of success is due to many reasons. One of the main reasons is DNA damage in spermatozoa. ART involves use of techniques which does not involve natural fertilisation. So, there may be chance of DNA damage. Sperm DNA lacks repair proteins that aids in protection against DNA damage. So, oocyte acts as source for repair proteins as it is active in gene expression. If the DNA damage overwhelms the oocyte capacity it leads to genetic aberrations in future generations. So, instead of choosing a single technique one has to get through the different techniques that help in selecting the single top spermatozoa.

When compared with high DNA damage the rate of pregnancy is more in case of IVF compared to ICSI. But in case of miss carriages rate it is more in ICSI compared to IVF. The reason is the post paternal factors play a pivotal role in repair of damage, and use of testicular sperm is helpful in ICSI if there is repeated miss carriages and low pregnancy rates. The assessment of sperm genome integrity is limited because different techniques used gives different outcomes. But SCSA is useful to assess testicular sperm for good outcome of results. Finally the outcome of ICSI cannot be predicted with respect to DNA condensation in both testicular sperm collected by biopsy and ejaculated spermatozoa in terms of pregnancy, cleavage and embryo formation.

15. Summary

Condensation of sperm genome was necessary for maintaining genome integrity by transition of histones by transition proteins which in turn by protamines. These proteins undergo some of PTM namely phosphorylation, Acetylation, poly ADP ribosylation and methylation. Further stability in interaction between DNA and protamine involves addition of disulfide bonds to form interlinking protamines. Dihydrotestosterone acts as hydrogen donor and acceptor in testes and necessary for maturation of sperms. Zinc acts as stabiliser of Genome through its interaction with protamines and toxicity due to metals responsible for male infertility [36] is due to interaction of these metal ions with protamines. So, safe ART is required to maintain genome integrity in offspring.

16. Metosartan acts as genotoxic agent of testes

Metosartan induces endometrial carcinoma in testes and causes changes in chromatin dynamics and causes prematurity in sperms. It causes competitive and non competitive inhibition of RNase present in male Wistar rats. It also decreases the sperm count, motility and induces abnormalities in sperm structure. It also causes apoptosis in both testes and sperm by increasing the permeability of mitochondria.

Abbreviations

ART	Assisted Reproductive Technology
ICSI	Intra Cytoplasmic Sperm Injection
IVF	In vitro Fertilisation
SCF	Stem Cell Factor
PDK	Protein Dependent Kinase
GDNF	Glial cell Derived Neurotropic Factor
PTM	Post Translational Modification
CAF	Chromatin Assembly Factor
TSSK6	Testes Specific Serine/Threonine Kinase 6
NOR	Nucleolar Organising Region
PIWI	P-element–induced wimpy testes in Drosophila
ADAM	A Disintegrin and Metalloprotease

Author details

Eswari Beeram
Sree Vidyanikethan Degree College, Andhra Pradesh, India

*Address all correspondence to: eshu.sonu@gmail.com

References

[1] Zhang Z, Shen X, Gude DR, Wilkinson BM, Justice MJ, Flickinger CJ, et al. MEIG1 is essential for spermiogenesis in mice. Proceedings of the National Academy of Sciences of the United States of America. 2009;**106**:17055-17060

[2] Thongkukiatkul A, Jungudomjaroen S, Ratanapahira C. Spermatogenesis and chromatin condensation in male germ cells of sea cucumber Holothuria leucospilota (Clark, 1920). Tissue & Cell. 2008;**40**(3):167-175

[3] Oliva R. Protamines and male infertility. Human Reproduction Update. 2006;**12**:417-435

[4] Meistrich ML, Reid BO, Barcellona WJ. Changes in sperm nuclei during spermatogenesis and epididymal maturation. Experimental Cell Research. 1976;**19**:72-78

[5] Goldberg RB, Geremia R, Bruce WR. Histone synthesis and replacement during spermatogenesis in the mouse. Differentiation. 1977;**7**:167-180

[6] Li B, Carey M, Workman JL. The role of chromatin during transcription. Cell. 2007;**128**:707-719

[7] Pradeepa MM, Rao MR. Chromatin remodeling during mammalian spermatogenesis: Role of testis specific histone variants and transition proteins. Society of Reproduction and Fertility Supplement. 2007;**63**:1-10

[8] Pivot-Pajot C, Caron C, Govin J, Vion A, Rousseaux S, Khochbin S. Acetylation dependent chromatin reorganization by BRDT, a testis-specific bromodomain containing protein. Molecular and Cellular Biology. 2003;**23**:5354-5365

[9] Bao J, Bedford MT. Epigenetic regulation of the histone-to-protamine transition during spermiogenesis. Reproduction. 2016;**151**:R55-R70

[10] Sosnik J, Miranda PV, Spiridonov NA, Yoon S-Y, Fissore RA, Johnson GR, et al. Tssk6 is required for relocalization and gamete fusion in the mouse. Journal of Cell Science. 2009;**122**:2741-2749

[11] Wang X, Wei Y, Fu G, Li H, Saiyin H, Lin G, et al. Tssk4 is essential for maintaining the structural integrity of sperm flagellum. Molecular Human Reproduction. 2015;**21**:136-145

[12] Marcon L, Boissonneault G. Transient DNA strand breaks during mouse and human spermiogenesis: New insights in stage specificity and link to chromatin remodeling. Biology of Reproduction. 2004;**70**:910-918

[13] Kashiwabara S, Noguchi J, Zhuang T, Ohmura K, Honda A, Sugiura S, et al. Regulation of spermatogenesis by testis specific, cytoplasmic poly(a) polymerase TPAP. Science. 2002;**298**:1999-2002

[14] Agarwal A, Said TM. Role of sperm chromatin abnormalities and DNA damage in male infertility. Human Reproduction Update. 2003;**9**:331-345

[15] Kodama H, Yamaguchi R, Fukuda J, Kasai H, Tanaka T. Increased oxidative deoxyribonucleic acid damage in the spermatozoa of infertile male patients. Fertility and Sterility. 1997;**68**:519-524

[16] Yu YE, Zhang Y, Unni E, Shirley CR, Deng JM, Russell LD, et al. Abnormal spermatogenesis and reduced fertility in transition nuclear protein 1-deficient mice. Proceedings of the National Academy of Sciences of the United States of America. 2000;**97**:4683-4688

[17] Brewer L, Corzett M, Balhorn R. Condensation of DNA by spermatid

basic nuclear proteins. The Journal of Biological Chemistry. 2002;**277**:38895-38900

[18] Balhorn R, Weston S, Thomas C, Wyrobek AJ. DNA packaging in mouse spermatids: Synthesis of protamine variants and four transition proteins. Experimental Cell Research. 1984;**150**:298-308

[19] Tanphaichitr N, Sobhon P, Taluppeth N, Chalermisarachai P. Basic nuclear proteins in testicular cells and ejaculated spermatozoa in man. Experimental Cell Research. 1978;**117**:347-356

[20] Lee K, Haugen HS, Clegg CH, Braun RE. Premature translation of protamine 1 mRNA causes precocious nuclear condensation and arrests spermatid differentiation in mice. Proceedings of the National Academy of Sciences of the United States of America. 1995;**92**:12451-12455

[21] Mailand N, Bekker-Jensen S, Faustrup H, Melander F, Bartek J, Lukas C, et al. RNF8 ubiquitylates histones at DNA double-strand breaks and promotes assembly of repair proteins. Cell. 2007;**131**:887-900

[22] Cho C, Willis WD, Goulding EH, Jung-Ha H, Choi YC, Hecht NB, et al. Haploinsufficiency of protamine-1 or −2 causes infertility in mice. Nature Genetics. 2001;**28**:82-86

[23] Hammadeh ME, Stieber M, Haidl G, Schmidt W. Association between sperm cell chromatin condensation, morphology based on strict criteria, and fertilization, cleavage and pregnancy rates in an IVF-program. Andrologia. 1998;**30**:29-35

[24] Taylor CT, Lawrence YM, Kingsland CR, et al. Oscillations in intracellular free calcium induced by spermatozoa in human oocytes at fertilization. Human Reproduction. 1993;**8**:2174-2179

[25] Kurtz K, Saperas N, Ausio J, Chiva M. Spermiogenic nuclear protein transitions and chromatin condensation. Proposal for an ancestral model of nuclear spermiogenesis. Journal of Experimental Zoology. Part B, Molecular and Developmental Evolution. 2009;**312B**:149-163

[26] Ward WS. Deoxyribonucleic acid loop domain tertiary structure in mammalian spermatozoa. Biology of Reproduction. 1993;**48**:1193-1201

[27] Schmidt WN, Taylor CA, Danzo BJ. The use of photoaffinity ligand to compare androgen-binding protein (ABP) present in rat Sertoli cell culture media with ABP present in epididymal cytosol. Endocrinology. 1981;**108**:786-794

[28] Martin C, Zhang Y. Mechanisms of epigenetic inheritance. Current Opinion in Cell Biology. 2007;**19**:266-272

[29] Yu Y, Gu J, Jin Y, Luo Y, Preall JB, Ma J, et al. Panoramix enforces piRNA-dependent cotranscriptional silencing. Science. 2015;**350**:339-342

[30] Kong A, Frigge ML, Stefansson K. Rate of de novo mutations and the importance of father's age to disease risk. Nature. 2012;**488**:471-475

[31] Gavriliouk D, Aitken RJ. Damage to sperm DNA mediated by reactive oxygen species: Its impact on human reproduction and the health trajectory of offspring. Advances in Experimental Medicine and Biology. 2014;**868**:23-47

[32] Silva PF, Gadella BM. Detection of damage in mammalian sperm cells. Theriogenology. 2006;**65**:958-978

[33] Schlegel PN, Girardi SK. Clinical review 87: in vitro fertilization for

male factor infertility. Clinics in Endocrinology and Metabolism. 1997;**82**:709-716

[34] Flaherty SP, Payne D, Swann NJ, Matthews CD. Assessment of fertilization failure and abnormal fertilization after intracytoplasmic sperm injection (ICSI). Reproduction, Fertility, and Development. 1995;**7**:197-210

[35] Simon L, Brunborg G, Stevenson M, Lutton D, McManus J, Lewis SEM. Clinical significance of sperm DNA damage in assisted reproduction outcome. Human Reproduction. 2010;**25**(7):1594-1608

[36] Wang XN, Li ZS, Ren Y, Jiang T, Wang YQ, Chen M, et al. The Wilms tumor gene, Wt1, is critical for mouse spermatogenesis via regulation of sertoli cell polarity and is associated with non-obstructive azoospermia in humans. PLoS Genetics. 2013;**9**:e1003645

Chapter 4

Ovarian Reserve

Nidhi Sharma and Sudakshina Chakrabarti

Abstract

The human ovary is a complex structure that is controlled by endocrine, paracrine, and autocrine mechanisms. The number of eggs retrieved after controlled ovarian stimulation in in vitro fertilization depends on the physiological follicular reserve pool of ovaries. Ovarian reserve is decided genetically and decreases with advancing age and gets affected by ovarian surgery, chemotherapy, radiotherapy, and autoimmune disorders. Environmental influences like chronic smoking, hyperglycemia, and conditions interfering ovarian vascularity also reduce the ovarian reserve. This chapter summarizes the methods to assess the ovarian reserve. This helps in deciding the initiating dose of gonadotropins for controlled ovarian hyper stimulation for optimal follicular response.

Keywords: ovary, controlled ovarian hyper stimulation, in vitro fertilization, ovarian reserve, ovulation

1. Introduction

Each natural ovulatory menstrual cycle has a 25% probability of spontaneous conception. Infertility is investigated when there is failure to conceive naturally following 1 year of unprotected intercourse in cases where the female is ≤35 years of age or following 6 months of unprotected intercourse for women >35 years of age. In 40% of the cases it can result due to female factor, in another 20% of cases it's the male factor, which is the cause, and combined factors can cause infertility in about 20% of cases. The causative female factors can be further classified into tubal factors (40%), ovulatory factors (40%), uterine factors (10%) and cervical factors (10%). The commonest etiology of female infertility is ovulation dysfunctions and fallopian tube anatomical and physiological obstruction. The cornerstone first line examinations and investigations for the subfertile couple should detect of ovulation and pituitary and ovarian secretion of hormones by hormonal assay (early follicular FSH and LH levels, mid-luteal progesterone) to assess the endogenous hypothalamo-pituitary-ovarian endometrial axis, and evaluation of tubal patency and function by diagnostic hysterolaparoscopy. GnRH hormone in hypothalamo-pituitary portal circulation cannot be detected in peripheral blood samples.

2. Physiology of folliculogenesis

Ovaries are almond-shaped organs located in the pelvis on either side of the uterus. In addition to production of ova the ovaries are also a distinct endocrine organ producing hormones primarily estrogen and progesterone that are very important for normal reproductive function. The adult ovary can be divided into

3 main regions superficial to deep. These are the a. Cortex that consists of tunica albuginea ovarian follicles (primordial, primary, secondary, small medium, large Graafian follicles, and corpus luteum, atretic follicles. The B. medulla consists of blood vessels and nerves in connective tissue. The innermost hilum contains large spiral arteries and Leydig cells.

Normally the ovary produces a single dominant follicle in each menstrual cycle that undergoes maturation and results in ovulation (**Figure 1**). The granulosa cells of the growing follicles produce estradiol during the first half of the menstrual cycle or the follicular phase. The folliculogenesis begins with recruitment of a primordial follicle into a pool of growing follicles and it is a long process almost a year for a primordial follicle ultimately resulting in ovulation of the follicle or death by atresia. The process of folliculogenesis can be divided into 2 phases. First phase is "preantral" or "gonadotrophin independent" phase, where there is growth and differentiation of oocyte. The preantral phase mainly controlled by local factors growths factors by autocrine and paracrine processes. The second phase is the "gonadotrophin dependent" phase or the "antral phase" when there is a fast growth in the size of the follicle itself and it is under the control of gonadotrophin. The Antral phase is regulated by FSH and LH and also by paracrine growth factors that cause intracellular signaling and multiplication of cells.

The process of this folliculogenesis goes through multiple sub phases too. These include: 1. primordial follicle recruitment; 2. preantral follicle development; 3. Selection and growth of antral follicle; and 4. follicle atresia. The primordial follicle is the reproductive unit of ovary. It gives rise to dominant follicle. In human female fetus, primordial follicles are formed 6 and 9 months of gestation and many of the primordial follicles undergo apoptosis. The number of primordial follicles decreases progressively due to recruitment and apoptosis and very few of them are present after menopause. Primordial follicle recruitment is completely dependent on paracrine mechanism largely controlled by growth factors especially TGF-beta superfamily.

A primary follicle is in the next sequence that has the presence of one or more cuboidal granulosa cells arranged in a single layer around the oocyte. The most important event at this stage is the FSH receptor expression and oocyte growth and

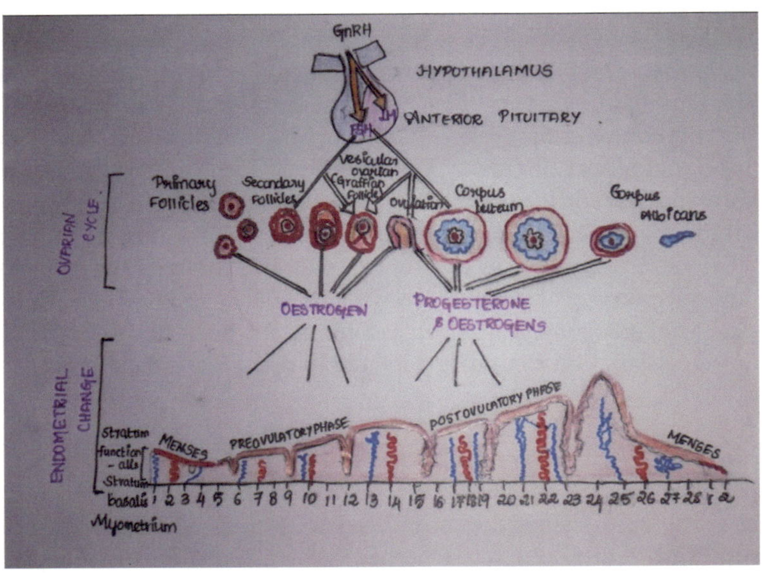

Figure 1.
Folliculogenesis, ovulation and corpus luteal formation.

maturation. Granulosa cells express receptors for FSH at this stage and the stimulus for this is FSH itself. Further development of primary follicle into preantral follicle is FSH dependent. The development of primary follicle is associated with striking change in oocyte too. Even there is a development of intimate connections between oocyte and granulose cells through the transzonal oocyte processes and gap junctions (cumulus oophorus complex). FSH is an important factor in supporting follicle growth after antrum formation and in also preventing apoptosis thus it is a survival factor for antral follicles. Thus FSH plays a very important role in selection and dominant follicle development. The proliferation of granulosa cells is a very important feature for development of dominant follicles. FSH is the most important factor for granulosa cell proliferation.

As the granulosa cells proliferate and a dominant follicle develops it acquires the capacity to produce estradiol. FSH mediates the granulosa cells to acquire the above potential. The progressive increase in estradiol production by the dominant follicle from Day 7-Day 12 of menstrual cycle is only possible due to increased levels in P450AROM gene expression by FSH in granulosa cells.

The physiologic mechanism by which dominant follicle produces estradiol is the two cells two-gonadotrophin concept. When FSH recruits follicles to preovulatory development, their granulosa cells develop LH receptors, start undertaking aromatization and also inhibin production. Inhibin has the capability to increase LH stimulated thecal androgen production. LH receptors are present on theca cells throughout the menstrual cycle. LH acts on theca cells to produce primarily androstenedione and to a lesser extent testosterone. Theca cell synthesized androstenedione is transported by paracrine circulation into the granulosa cells. In granulosa cells androstenedione and testosterone are aromatized to estrone and finally into estradiol by 17-β-hydroxysteroid dehydrogenase type I. This is known as the two-cell, i.e., theca cell and follicular cell, two-gonadotropin, i.e., FSH and LH and two hormone, i.e., estradiol and progesterone theory of regulation of estrogen synthesis in the human ovary as shown in **Figure 2**. Granulosa cell derived inhibin takes part in a paracrine mechanism communicating with theca cells and thus amplifying androgen synthesis. This theca cell derived androgen is converted to estradiol in granulosa cells of preovulatory follicles. Inhibin B has an early follicular phase elevation and lower values after ovulation. Thus it suggests Inhibin B is a granulosa cell product and can be a marker for follicular function, oocyte number and thus plays a role in follicular development in early part of the cycle.

2.1 Follicular phase

The follicular phase starts from the first day of menstrual cycle D1 until ovulation. Basal body temperature chart normally shows lower values during this phase. Development growth trajectories of the ovarian follicles characterize this first phase of the cycle. Folliculogenesis starts during the last few days of the preceding menstrual cycle and continues till the release of the mature follicle at the time of ovulation. The primary development of the follicle to the preantral follicle is not gonadotropin dependent, and further follicular growth beyond this point requires gonadotropin action.

The secretion of gonadotropins from anterior pituitary is regulated by gonadotropin releasing hormone (GnRH), steroid hormones, and various peptides released by the dominant follicle. The growth of follicular size and number of granulosa cells in each follicle leads to an increase in estradiol serum concentrations in the early follicular phase. FSH receptors exist only on the granulosa cell membrane. There is increase in the number of FSH receptors with the gradual rise in serum FSH levels during the late follicular phase. The rise in serum FSH along with the rise in FSH

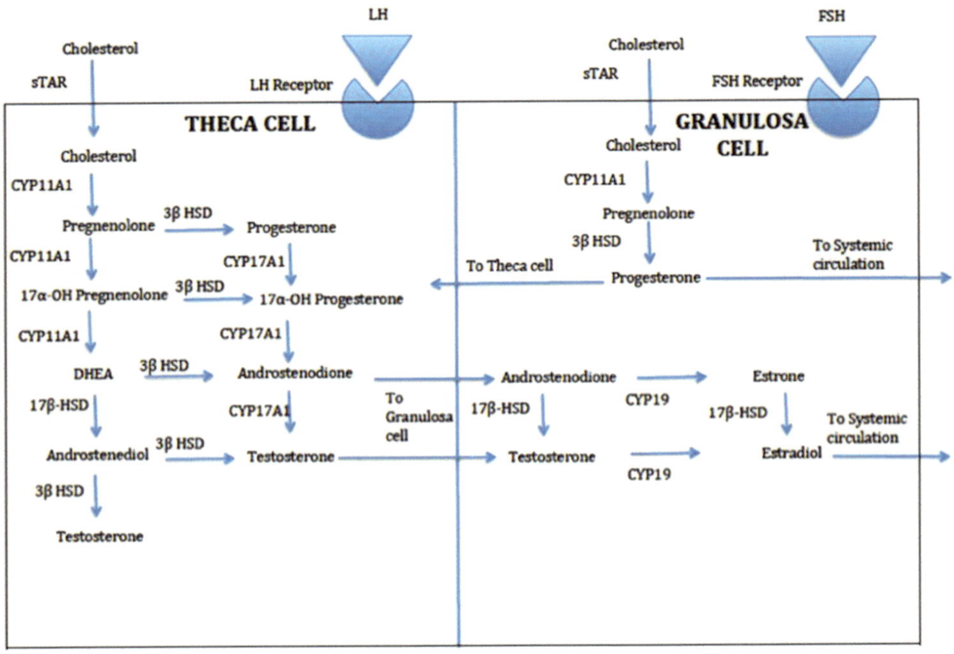

Figure 2.
Theca and granulosa cells (two cells) respond to luteinizing hormone and follicle stimulating hormone (two gonadotropins) to produce 17-OH progesterone and estradiol (two hormones).

receptors leads to an increase in estradiol secretion by granulosa cells. It has to be noted at this point clearly that the increase in FSH receptor numbers is due to an increase in the population of granulosa cells and not an increase in the concentration of FSH receptors per granulosa cell. FSH has a positive stimulating effect for the formation of LH receptors on granulosa cells thus allowing the production of small quantities of progesterone and 17-hydroxyprogesterone (17-OHP) that exert a positive feedback on the estrogen-primed pituitary to augment luteinizing hormone (LH) release. Without LH, the increased progesterone synthesis from granulosa cells under the influence of FSH advances the endometrium and the resulting asynchronous development reduces the chances of embryo implantation (**Figure 2**). This phenomenon is also called as ENLOP or Elevated Non Luteinised Origin of Progesterone leading to displaced window of implantation. The addition of LH in follicular phase reduces premature progesterone increase and improves the likelihood of implantation and clinical pregnancy.

FSH is elevated during the early follicular phase, declines as estradiol secretion increases from the granulosa cells, has a second rise before ovulation and then begins to decline until ovulation. FSH also stimulates several steroidogenic enzymes including aromatase, and 3β-hydroxysteroid dehydrogenase (3β-HSD). The secondary rise of FSH is important for inducing LH receptors on theca cells and granulosa cells and thereby preparing for the action of LH surge.

2.2 Luteal phase

The positive feedback from the rising estrogen levels during the follicular phase results in gradual increase in LH level by mid follicular phase that is low to start with during the early follicular phase. Estradiol levels must be greater than 200 pg/mL for approximately 50 hours in duration for the positive feedback effect of LH release to occur. During the early follicular phase, LH secretion occurs at a pulse frequency of

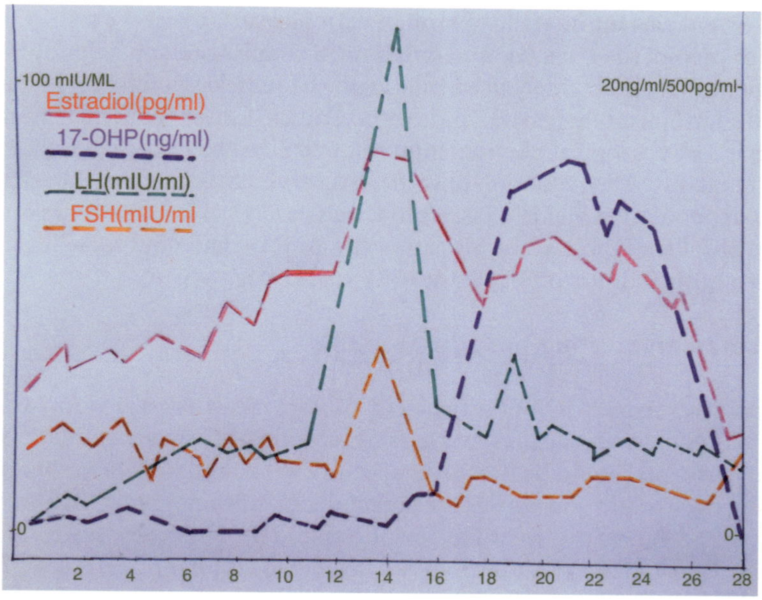

Figure 3.
The cyclical harmonious balance of gonadotropin secretion from pituitary and estrogen and progesterone secretion from ovary results in LH surge resulting in final maturation of oocyte and ovulation.

60 to 90 minutes with relatively constant pulse amplitude. During the late follicular phase prior to ovulation, the pulse frequency and may be amplitude of LH secretion increases. LH pulse amplitude increase results in ovulation [1, 2]. After ovulation corpus luteum is formed and theca cells continue to secrete progesterone.

The reduction of steroid production by the corpus luteum and the sudden fall of inhibin A allow the follicle stimulating hormone (FSH) to increase during the last few days of the menstrual cycle. In the late luteal phase, as corpus luteum lso degenerates there is no the estrogen and progesterone secretion from the ovary resulting in FSH rise because of increased GnRH pulsatile secretion. This elevation in FSH is very crucial for the recruitment of a cohort of ovarian follicles in each ovary out of that one follicle will be destined to ovulate during the next menstrual cycle. As menstruation starts the FSH levels begin to decline due to the negative feedback of estrogen and the negative effects of inhibin B produced by the developing follicle [1, 2]. The cyclical hormone changes are depicted in **Figure 3**.

3. Ovarian reserve

Ovarian reserve plays an important role in achieving pregnancy following any treatment in infertile and sub fertile women. The main function of the ovary in a woman is the production of a mature and viable oocyte that is capable of fertilization and subsequently leads to an embryo development and implantation. At birth, each ovary has a fixed number of oocytes available for folliculogenesis during the later life. This fixed number of available oocytes is termed as "the ovarian reserve" of the woman. Delayed childbearing, voluntary or involuntary, is a common feature in couples visiting fertility clinics nowadays as they are career oriented and mostly working. The estimation of ovarian reserve is routinely performed prior to interventions through various ovarian reserve tests (ORTs) in an effort to predict the response and outcome in couples in vitro fertilization techniques and to even counsel them. The ovarian reserve estimation has to be routinely performed prior to any interventions for infertility through various ovarian reserve tests (ORTs) in an effort to predict the response and outcome in couples seeking help for infertility treatment such. The widely used tests are basal follicle stimulating hormone, Anti-Mullerian Hormone (AMH) and Antral Follicle Count (AFC). Ovarian reserve reduction is a physiological phenomenon characterized by declining follicular pool and oocyte quality. The reduction of ovarian reserve starts at about 30 years in south Asian population and at 35 years in Caucasians [3].This rate of age-related reduction of follicle count in the human ovary is more than doubles when numbers fall below a critical figure of 25,000 at ~37.5 years of age [4].

3.1 Ovarian reserve testing

Ovarian reserve tests (ORT) serve as an indirect measures of a woman's remaining follicular pool when she presents herself for infertility treatment. ORT should be easy to perform, should be sensitive, specific, valid, and help to individualize the starting dose of gonadotropins for multifollicular development. The ovarian reserve testing helps to differentiate normoresponders, hyporesponders, and hyper-responders. Ovarian reserve is deciphered through a number of markers. These markers also help to prognosticate poor responders. Ovarian reserve is predicted clinically using a combination of clinical, biochemical and biophysical tests.

The tests are being used all over the world but the sensitivity and specificity of these test to detect the oocyte number, quality, and fecundity has to be still ascertained with further research [5]. More recently, their value in predicting hyper-response and hypo response and thus using safe stimulation regimes to prevent OHSS is also explored [2]. The interpretation of the results of the ovarian reserve test is complicated by the lack of uniform definitions for hypo or hyper-responders and uniform threshold values to identify abnormal results. Several static and dynamic ovarian functional markers like biological (age), biochemical, biophysical, and histological tests have been used to identify ovarian reserve [1, 2].

In most cases of decreased ovarian reserve, the cause remains undetected. In specific cases like exposure to chemotherapy, pelvic irradiation, and genetic abnormalities there is a premature decrease in ovarian pool of oocytes. Cigarette smoking has been associated with a decrease in ovarian reserve. With diminished ovarian reserve a reproductive age woman has regular periods with normal or shortened duration of menstrual cycles but there is a decrease in response to ovarian stimulation and fecundity. Thus women of same age can differ in their response to ovarian stimulation and thus the fecundity can vary.

3.1.1 Age

It is long established that ovarian reserve reduces progressively with age. This is due to a combination of two factors the body 'spending' the eggs through routine ovulation and the ovaries aging and preparing for menopause. Individual variation of the ovarian reserve can be explained by the two instances given as- a young woman with certain reproductive health problems may start out with smaller than the normal reserve of healthy eggs, and some women's reserves decrease more quickly than others with age. Fecundity in both natural and stimulated ovarian cycles declines with maternal age, beginning in the late 20s and becoming more abrupt in the late 30s. The fall in ovarian reserve with age in is a universal phenomenon in all ethinic groups. The initiation and rate of this decline varies considerably with ethinicity. Calender Age *per se* cannot determine ovarian responses. Ovarian reserve can also be traced indirectly by other biochemical and biophysical markers of ovarian function [6–11].

3.1.2 Basal follicle stimulating hormone

One of the most classically used biochemical levels to measure ovarian reserve is the Basal follicle stimulating hormone (FSH) levels measured on day 3 of the menstrual cycle. An increase in FSH levels occurs due to follicle depletion as the age of the woman progresses [9, 10]. The measurement of FSH is easy, and inexpensive reproducible and its specific. FSH levels are known to have diurnal, intra- and intercycle variations that have to be kept in mind. There is definite precise parameter value to detect a woman with poor ovarian reserve. A vague demarking values more than 25 IU/L was used arbitrarily in some studies to detect high basal FSH. Several subsequent reviews did not identify values to satisfy the specificity and sensitivity for basal FSH as a test for poor ovarian response to stimulation or prediction of non-pregnancy. In women with regular menstrual cycles, FSH can predict a poor response adequately only at very high levels, and hence will be helpful only to a small number of women as a screening test for ovarian reserve testing and further counseling. It is thus clear that the ovarian aging begins several years prior to any elevation in FSH levels is noted and thus a normal test cannot rule out a poor ovarian response in some women. When FSH level is combined with other markers it can be used to counsel couples and planning treatment option regarding a poor response but it should not be used to exclude regularly cycling women from ART. The specificity of basal FSH testing in a general sub-fertile population or elevated levels in young, regularly cycling women is thus unclear and needs further studies [11–13]. Additionally the reliability of FSH is challengeable because of its pulsatile and circadian release and its isoforms. There are no cut off values available to predict poor responders.

3.1.3 Anti-Mullerian hormone

Anti-Mullerian hormone (AMH) is a dimeric glycoprotein exclusively produced by granulosa cells of preantral (primary and secondary) and very small and small antral follicles (2–6 mm) in the ovary. The serum levels of AMH reflect the number of follicles that have made the transition from primordial pool into the growing pool but still it is not under gonadotrophin control. The secretion of AMH starts once there is a follicular transition from the primordial to the primary stage, and it continues until the follicles reach till the follicles attain antral stages of diameters 2–6 mm. The number of the small Antral Follicles indirectly reflects size of the primordial follicle pool. With the decrease in the number of the antral follicles with age, AMH production seems to reduce and become undetectable at and after menopause. The physiological function of AMH is to modulate primordial follicle recruitment. It inhibits the action of FSH on follicular growth and selection. AMH is considered to be reflective of FSH independent follicular growth, so it is a direct measure of ovarian reserve. AMH reflects qualitative and quantitative assessment of ovarian reserve. AMH levels also strongly correlate with basal antral follicle count (AFC) measured by transvaginal ultrasonography. Serum AMH levels correlate inversely with age from 25 years onwards and reaches undetectable levels after menopause, thus AMH levels is an important ovarian reserve marker. Serum AMH levels can be measured on any day of the cycle and does not exhibit inter-cycle variability unlike other biochemical markers. Threshold values of 0.2–1.26 ng/ml, have been used to identify poor responders with 80–87% sensitivity and 64–93% specificity. Thus by understanding of its clinical implications, AMH too has the potential to predict a hyper-response during treatment as well. The nomograms of the values of AMH can predict and identify the age-related physiological decline in the AMH levels and thus ovarian reserve, and abnormal deviation in the levels of AMH can be used for counseling couples wishing to delay childbirth. Still the available evidence is not sufficient enough to suggest that serum AMH can be used as a single marker to predict pregnancy. Furthermore, studies of the levels of follicular fluid AMH has shown that oocytes obtained from follicles with higher levels of AMH have a better fertility potential compared to those with lower AMH levels [14–16]. Serum AMH estimations have also been useful to diagnose "Transitional Ovarian Failure" and "Insipient Ovarian Failure."

Studies conducted longitudinally in fertile women have clearly shown a decline in serum AMH levels with progressing age. AMH is one of the earliest markers to show a decline progressively in young women with aging thus offering the probability of a screening test for women to counsel against delay in childbirth. Levels of 0.5–1.26 ng/ml of AMH suggests impending menopause in next 3–5 years [17, 18]. AMH is also a most promising marker for predicting age of natural menopause too. The serum levels of AMH are not controlled by hypothalamus pituitary axis that makes it important marker in diagnosing conditions such as PCOS and premature ovarian failure.

3.1.4 Inhibin B

Inhibin B is a glycoprotein hormone produced by small ovarian follicular granulosa cells and thereby it is an indirect indicator of the follicular pool. Inhibin B is not a reliable parameter for measuring ovarian reserve though serum levels <45 pg/ml have been associated with poor response to controlled ovarian stimulation since it is not a reliable predictor of pregnancy. Inhibin B levels are lower in poor responders than in women with normal ovarian reserve. Inhibin B levels if exaggerated in stimulated cycle is an indicator of hyper response thus it can be used to monitor the response to exogenous FSH. Use of Inhibin B as a sole predictor of ovarian response is not recommended [19].

3.1.5 Basal estradiol

Estradiol is a steroid hormone secreted by the granulosa cells of the growing ovarian follicles. Day 2 or Day 3 basal estradiol is commonly assessed for observing the early oocyte development. Estradiol also exerts a negative feedback on the secretion of FSH from the pituitary thus high basal estradiol can reduce the FSH levels. Thus it is a helpful parameter in combination with FSH to establish the baseline ovarian reserve. Elevated basal estradiol has been associated with a poor response to ovarian stimulation. An early rise in serum estradiol is a characteristic sign of reproductive aging and can lower the elevated basal FSH into normal range thus resulting in misinterpretation of the test.

4. Clomiphene citrate challenge test

This is a dynamic test of ovarian function. This basically involves the Day 3 testing of basal FSH levels and serum estradiol. Administering 100 mg of Clomiphene citrate tablets per day for 5 days from Day 5 to Day 9 of the cycle follows this. The FSH level is measured on Day 10 of the cycle. In cases of low reserve FSH is elevated on Day 10. FSH is the primary stimulus for final follicular maturation. It is under negative feedback from estradiol and inhibin B. Basal FSH levels are elevated it indicates a diminished follicular pool. Clomiphene citrate challenge test is a good predictor of ovarian reserve but not an absolute indicator of ovarian hypofunction. Thus the clinical value of CCCT is not clearly better than basal FSH and AFC in combination. The Day 3 or Day10 FSH levels more than 10 mIU/ml is considered abnormal by most studies. Though there are different opinions still CCCT remains a gold standard in testing ovarian reserve. The justification of this test is that as the ovarian follicle develops in patients with normal ovarian function and will produce levels of inhibin and estradiol sufficient enough to suppress FSH production by Day 10 of the cycle concerned [20].Other dynamic tests used are GAST (GnRH Analogue Stimulation Test) and EFFORT (Exogenous FSH Ovarian Reserve Test).

5. Ultrasound parameters

5.1 Antral follicle count

After menarche, gradually a regular bi-fortnight ovulation is established. The immature oocyte covered with granulosa and theca cells rests in a small fluid filled cavity called as the antral follicle. These small fluid filled cavities are visualized sonologically in early follicular phase. These reflect follicles that were selected from the primordial follicle in this wave (wave theory of folliculogenensis) and so the antral follicle counts may vary in various mentstral cycles. There is no clear-cut consensus on the criteria to identify antral follicles. Various litreture reviews suggest that the follicles with a diameter of 2 to 10 mm can be considered as AFa [5, 21]. Thus, the antral follicle count (AFC) is the number of follicles with cavity less than 10 mm in diameter with Transvaginal Ultrasound (TVUS) imaging in the early follicular phase of the cycle (**Figure 4a–c**). Antral follicle count is a quantitative aspect of ovarian aging. As a direct marker of the cohort of growing follicles

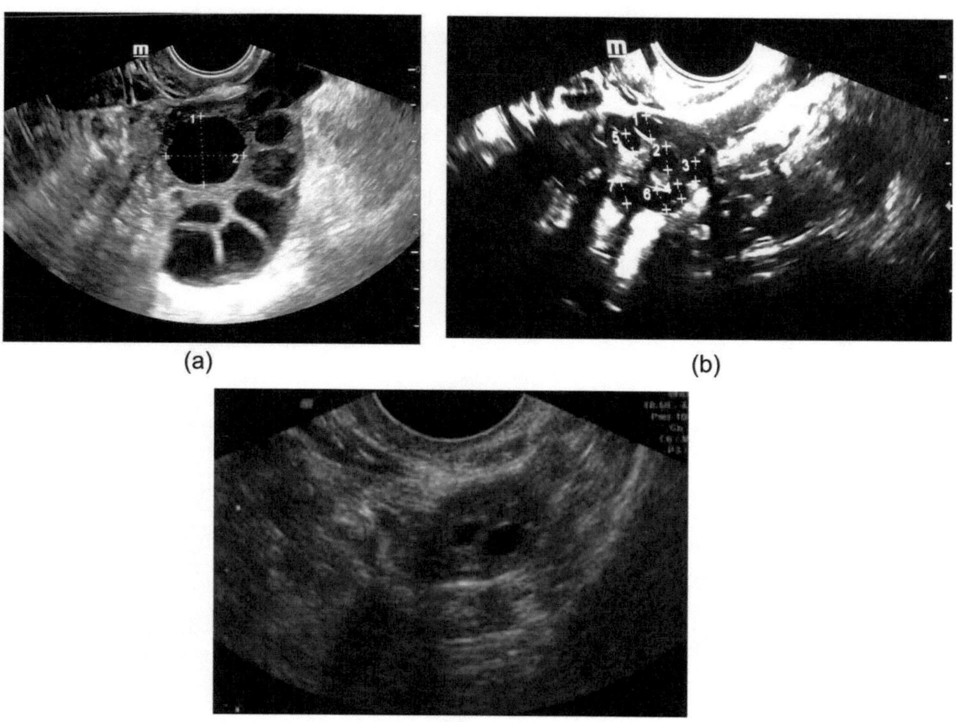

Figure 4.
(a) Ovarian antral follicular count in hypo responders; (b) ovarian antral follicular count in normal responders; and (c) ovarian antral follicular count in hyper responders.

in the early menstrual cycle, the AFC is believed to correlate strongly with the number of primordial follicles present in the ovary and, thus, the ovarian reserve. Antral Follicles are routinely measured by 2 D transvaginal ultrasonography in the early follicular phase, by taking the mean of two perpendicular measurements. Inversion made is useful for counting multiple follicles. The numbers of follicles in both ovaries are added for the total Antral Follicle count. (AFC). AFC has been predominantly used as a marker of ovarian reserve over a period of time. A count of 8–10 is taken as a normal response of ovaries. Different diameters are used to define antral follicles of varying sizes as those measuring 2–6 and 7–10 mm. There is no clear consensus regarding the size of antral follicles, which truly represent ovarian reserve. The number of small antral follicles (2–6 mm) is significantly related to age and also to all endocrine ORTs tested, suggesting the number of small antral follicles represents the functional ovarian reserve. It is seen that the number of antral follicles of 2–6 mm in size decreases with age and correlates with other markers such as serum basal FSH and CCCT whereas follicles of size 7–10 mm remains constant and thus, the former appears to be a more reliable marker of ovarian reserve. Measurements taken repeatedly of the antral follicles have shown that there is only a limited intercycle variability. 3D ultrasound imaging also does not carry any better advantage in comparison to 2D ultrasound for the detection of functional ovarian reserve [22–25]. Meta-analyses showed that women with AFC less than four were 8.7 times more likely not to get pregnant after IVF (two studies; 95% CI,) than women with AFC four or more. The sensitivity and specificity of AFC to predict cycle cancelation was 66.7 and 94.7%, respectively [21].

5.2 Ovarian volume

The volume of the ovaries is calculated by imaging and callipering the ovary in three perpendicular planes with using the formula of ellipsoid volume as ($L1 \times L2 \times L3 \times \pi/6$). An alternative automatic method is calculation of Ovarian volume through "virtual organ computer-aided analysis" or VOCAL. The predictive performance of ovarian volume toward poor response is clearly inferior compared with that of AFC. Therefore, the AFC may be considered the test of first choice when estimating quantitative ovarian reserve before IVF. Total Basal Ovarian Volume (BOV) is obtained by adding the volumes of both. The ovarian volume is constant till the perimenopausal period and the measurement does not increase the

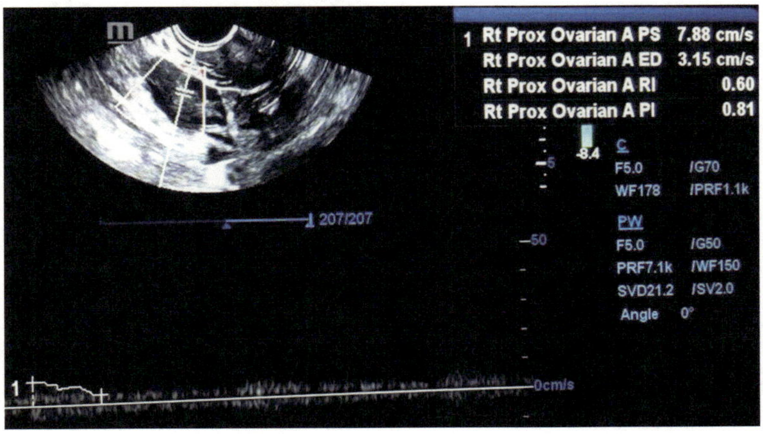

Figure 5.
Doppler ovarian stromal vascularity measurements with 2D doppler calculation of pulsatility index and resistivity index.

positive predictive value of AFC. Furthermore, the decrease in the Basal Ovarian Volume is a very late phenomenon women >40 years [25, 26]. Ovarian volume measurement, at a cut off value of 3 cm^3, showed specificity for prediction of cycle cancelation and non-pregnancy of 92% (three studies, 95% CI, 89–94) and 93% (three studies, 95% CI), respectively [21].

5.3 Ovarian stromal vascularity

The observation of the ovarian stromal Doppler flow during ovarian stimulation has been studied in IVF cycles. Poor ovarian stromal vascularization impairs the access of gonadotropins to the ovarian follicles. Power Doppler US in combination with 3D VOCAL is an appropriate approach for correlating the ovarian vascular network with the ovarian response to ART. The gradual increase in the Doppler flow noted during stimulation may provide additional information to AFC (**Figure 5**) [27–36].

6. Conclusion

Ovarian pathophysiology is complex. Ovarian folliculogenesis follicular rupture and luteal transition should be studied elaborately. Endometrial evaluation should be also done in a nonstimulated cycle. Serum hormone values should be measured in normal non-induced menstrual cycle to study the ovarian reserve and detect any undiagnosed synchronizing defects in embryo invasion and endometrial implantation window. Sonoendocrinology is a new imaging science deciphers the hormonal action on target organs. Antral follicle count, at a cut off value of less than four, had high specificity for the prediction of cycle cancelation in assisted reproduction. Ovarian volume, at a cut-off value 3 mL^3, had high specificity for the prediction of non-pregnancy and cycle cancelation in assisted reproduction. Doppler studies of ovarian stromal blood flow are promising, but more research is needed. AFC and ovarian volume provide direct measurements of ovarian response, while AMH, Inhibin B and estradiol are released from the growing follicles and so they reflect the follicular cohort that has been selected from the follicular pool.

Author details

Nidhi Sharma* and Sudakshina Chakrabarti
Saveetha Medical college and hospital Chennai, India

*Address all correspondence to: drbonuramkumar@yahoo.co.in

References

[1] Groome NP et al. Measurement of dimeric inhibin B throughout the human menstrual cycle. The Journal of Clinical Endocrinology and Metabolism. 1996;**81**(4):1401-1405

[2] Welt CK et al. Control of follicle-stimulating hormone by estradiol and the inhibins: Critical role of estradiol at the hypothalamus during the luteal-follicular transition. The Journal of Clinical Endocrinology and Metabolism. 2003;**88**(4):1766-1771

[3] Williams CJ, Erickson GF. Morphology and physiology of the ovary. (updated 2012 Jan) In : Feingold KR Anawalt B, Boyce A,et.al. editors. Endotext (Internet). South Dartmouth (MA): MD Text.com, Inc,Inc; 2000

[4] Faddy MJ, Gosden RG, Gougeon A, Richardson SJ, Nelson JF. Accelerated disappearance of ovarian follicles in mid-life: Implications for forecasting menopause. Human Reproduction. 1992;**7**:1342-1346

[5] Frattarelli JL, Levi AJ, Miller BT, Segars JH. A prospective assessment of the predictive value of basal antral follicles in in vitro fertilization cycles. Fertility and Sterility. 2003;**80**(2):350-355

[6] Wood JW. Fecundity and natural fertility in humans. Oxford Reviews of Reproductive Biology. 1989;**11**:61-109

[7] Piette C, de Mouzon J, Bachelot A, Spira A. *In-vitro* fertilization (influence of woman's age on pregnancy rates). Human Reproduction. 1990;**5**:56-59

[8] Padilla SL, Garcia JE. Effect of maternal age and number of *in vitro* fertilization procedures on pregnancy outcome. Fertility and Sterility. 1989;**52**:270-273

[9] Scott RT, Toner JP, Muasher SJ, Oehninger S, Robinson S, Rosenwaks Z. Follicle-stimulating hormone levels on cycle day 3 are predictive of *in vitro* fertilization outcome. Fertility and Sterility. 1989;**51**:651-654

[10] Toner JP, Philput CB, Jones GS, Muasher SJ. Basal follicle stimulating hormone level is a better predictor of *in vitro* fertilization performance than age. Fertility and Sterility. 1991;**55**:784-791

[11] Sharif K, Elgendy M, Lashen H, Afnan M. Age and basal follicle stimulating hormone as predictors of *in vitro* fertilization outcome. British Journal of Obstetrics and Gynaecology. 1998;**105**:107-112

[12] Erdem M, Erdem A, Gursoy R, Biberoglu K. Comparison of basal and clomiphene citrate induced FSH and inhibin B, ovarian volume and antral follicle counts as ovarian reserve tests and predictors of poor ovarian response in IVF. Journal of Assisted Reproduction and Genetics. 2004;**21**:37-45

[13] Scott RT Jr, Hofmann GE, Oehninger S, Muasher SJ. Intercycle variability of day 3 follicle-stimulating hormone levels and its effect on stimulation quality in *in vitro* fertilization. Fertility and Sterility. 1990;**54**:297-302

[14] Muttukrishna S, McGarrigle H, Wakim R, Khadum I, Ranieri DM, Serhal P. Antral follicle count, anti-Mullerian hormone and inhibin B: Predictors of ovarian response in assisted reproductive technology? BJOG : An International Journal of Obstetrics and Gynaecology. 2005;**112**:1384-1390

[15] Tremellen KP, Kolo M, Gilmore A, Lekamge DN. Anti-Mullerian hormone as a marker of ovarian reserve. Australian and New Zealand Journal

of Obstetrics and Gynaecology. 2005;**45**:20-24

[16] La Marca A, Giulini S, Tirelli A, Bertucci E, Marsella T, Xella S, et al. Anti-Müllerian hormone measurement on any day of the menstrual cycle strongly predicts ovarian response in assisted reproductive technology. Human Reproduction. 2007;**22**:766-771

[17] Nelson SM, Yates RW, Lyall H, Jamieson M, Traynor I, Gaudoin M, et al. Anti-Müllerian hormone-based approach to controlled ovarian stimulation for assisted conception. Human Reproduction. 2009;**24**:867-867

[18] Nelson SM, Messow MC, McConnachie A, Wallace H, Kelsey T, Fleming R, et al. External validation of nomogram for the decline in serum anti-Müllerian hormone in women: A population study of 15,834 infertility patients. Reproductive Biomedicine Online. 2011;**23**:204-206

[19] Jirge PR. Ovarian reserve tests. Journal of Human Reproductive Sciences. 2011;**4**(3):108-113

[20] Mukta A et al. Assessment of ovarian reserve in infertility. The Journal of Obstetrics and Gynecology of India. 2009;**59**(6):569-572

[21] Jayaprakasan K, Deb S, Batcha M, et al. The cohort of antral follicles measuring 2-6 mm reflects the quantitative status of ovarian reserve as assessed by serum levels of anti-Mullerian hormone and response to controlled ovarian stimulation. Fertility and Sterility. 2010;**94**(5):1775-1781

[22] Hendriks DJ, Broekmans FJ, Bancsi LF, Looman CW, de Jong FH, te Velde ER. Single and repeated GnRH agonist stimulation tests compared with basal markers of ovarian reserve in the prediction of outcome in IVF. Journal of Assisted Reproduction and Genetics. 2005;Feb **22**(2):65-73

[23] Haadsma MA, Bukman A, Groen H, Roeloffzen EM, Groenewoud ER, Heineman MJ, et al. The number of small antral follicles (2-6 mm) determines the outcome of endocrine ovarian reserve tests in a subfertile population. Human Reproduction. 2007;**22**:1932-1941

[24] Bancsi LF, Broekmans FJ, Looman CW, Habbema JD, Velde ER. Impact of repeated antral follicle counts on the prediction of poor ovarian response in women undergoing *in vitro* fertilization. Fertility and Sterility. 2004;**81**:35-41

[25] Hendriks DJ, Kwee J, Mol BW, te VeldeER,BroekmansFJ.Ultrasonography as a tool for the prediction of outcome in IVF patients: A comparative meta-analysis of ovarian volume and antral follicle count. Fertility and Sterility. 2007;**87**:764-767

[26] Kwee J, Elting ME, Schats R, McDonnell J, Lambalk CB. Ovarian volume and antral follicle count for the prediction of low and hyper responders with *in vitro* fertilization. Reproductive Biology and Endocrinology. 2007;**5**:9

[27] Jayaprakasan K, Hilwah N, Kendall NR, Hopkisson JF, Campbell BK, JohnsonI R, et al. Does 3D ultrasound offer any advantage in the pretreatment assessment of ovarian reserve and prediction of outcome after assisted reproduction treatment? Human Reproduction. 2007;**22**:1925-1931

[28] Kwee J, Schats R, McDonnell J, Schoemaker J, Lambalk CB. The clomiphene citrate challenge test versus the exogenous follicle-stimulating hormone ovarian reserve test as a single test for identification of low responders and hyper responders to in vitro fertilization. Fertility and Sterility. 2006;**85**:1714-1722

[29] Broer SL, Dólleman M, Opmeer BC, Fauser BC, Mol BW, Broekmans FJ.

AMH and AFC as predictors of excessive response in controlled ovarian hyperstimulation: A meta-analysis. Human Reproduction Update. 2011;**17**:46-54

[30] Kahraman S, Vicdan K, Işik AZ, Ozgün OD, Alaybeyoğlu L, Polat G, et al. Clomiphene citrate challenge test in the assessment of ovarian reserve before controlled ovarian hyperstimulation for intracytoplasmic sperm injection. European Journal of Obstetrics & Gynecology and Reproductive Biology. 1997;**73**:177-182

[31] Chuang CC, Chen CD, Chao KH, Chen SU, Ho HN, Yang Y. Age is a better predictor of pregnancy potential than basal follicle-stimulating hormone levels in women undergoing *in vitro* fertilization. Fertility and Sterility. 2003;**79**:63-68

[32] de Bruin JP, te Velde ER. Female reproductive ageing: Concepts and consequences. In: Tulandi T, Gosden RG, editors. Preservation of Fertility. London UK: Taylor and Francis; 2004

[33] Fanchin R, Taieb J, Lozano DH, Ducot B, Frydman R, Bouyer J. High reproducibility of serum anti-Mullerian hormone measurements suggests a multi-staged follicular secretion and strengthens its role in the assessment of ovarian follicular status. Human Reproduction. 2005;**20**:923-927

[34] Higgins RV, van Nagell JR, Woods CH, Thompson EA, Kryscio RJ. Interobserver variation in ovarian measurements using transvaginal sonography. Gynecologic Oncology. 1990;**39**:69-71

[35] Järvelä IY, Sladkevicius P, Kelly S, Ojha K, Campbell S, Nargund G. Quantification of ovarian power doppler signal with three-dimensional ultrasonography to predict response during *in vitro* fertilization. Obstetrics and Gynecology. 2003;**102**:816-822

[36] Gibreel A, Maheshwari A, Bhattacharya S, Johnson NP. Ultrasound tests of ovarian reserve; a systematic review of accuracy in predicting fertility outcomes. Human Fertility. 2009;**12**(2):95-106

Chapter 5

Paternal Effects on Embryonic, Fetal and Offspring Health: The Role of Epigenetics in the ICSI and ROSI Era

Jan Tesarik

Abstract

Paternal effects on the developmental potential of human embryos have been studied since the early 1990s, particularly with respect to newly emerging assisted reproduction technologies. Both genetic and epigenetic paternal effects can influence postfertilization development and cause implantation failure or miscarriage. However, it is only over the last few years that issues related to paternal effects associated with different assisted reproduction techniques on the health status of newborn and adult progeny have been focused. At the same time, new findings point out different, yet unexplored, areas of research into the potentially responsible factors, including the activity of the sperm-derived oocyte-activating factor and the oocyte signaling pathways mediating its action, the methylation status of both imprinted and non-imprinted genes, correct replacement of sperm nuclear protamines with oocyte-derived histones, the histone acetylation status, and the function of sperm-borne small RNAs. It is increasingly important to know how these developmentally important epigenetic regulators can be altered in the context of the current micromanipulation-assisted fertilization techniques, intracytoplasmic sperm injection (ICSI) and round spermatid injection (ROSI). Last but not least, transgenerational transmission of acquired, environmentally conditioned disorders from fathers to offspring is a newly emerging issue which warrants further research.

Keywords: paternal effects, embryonic health, fetal health, offspring health, epigenetics, ICSI, ROSI, assisted reproduction, epigenetic inheritance

1. Introduction

There are two types of paternal factors involved in problems of embryonic, fetal and offspring health: the genetic ones and the epigenetic ones. The terms "hard" and "soft" inheritance, first introduced in 1980 [1], are increasingly used to refer to the genetic and epigenetic inheritance, respectively [2, 3]. These terms reflect very nicely the nature of the two kinds of inheritance. The genetic inheritance, the hard one, is based on transmission of DNA sequences, and it is this type of inheritance which has been the main subject of human genetic studies for the past 60 years. On the other hand, a number of studies carried out over the past 20 years have revealed that phenotypes are affected by more complex layers of information besides DNA

IntechOpen

sequences. These factors, interposed between the DNA sequence of a gene and its phenotypic expression, are termed epigenetic marks and can be modified by environmental exposures [4].

This chapter reviews the current knowledge about the factors affecting epigenetic marks in human gametes and embryos and about the ways how improper function of the male gametes during the process of fertilization can influence further embryonic and fetal development, with particular attention to possible adverse epigenetic effects related to the new micromanipulation-assisted fertilization technologies, intracytoplasmic sperm injection (ICSI) and round spermatid injection (ROSI).

2. Hard and soft hereditary elements

Hard hereditary elements are stable DNA sequences constituting specific genes that can only be modified by mutations or deletions. The system of soft hereditary elements is made up by a variety of molecules (epigenetic factors) that interact with each other and determine if, and to what extent, individual genes will be expressed at any given time of life. Early studies into epigenetic regulations in mammals largely focused on two constitutive events: genomic imprinting [5, 6] and X chromosome inactivation [7, 8]. However, later studies have pointed out that epigenetic regulation is a much more ample phenomenon than thought previously, involving a number of both imprinted and non-imprinted genes, and their role is particularly important in developmental processes, such as embryogenesis and organogenesis [9].

DNA methylation at the 5′ position of cytosin in CpG dinucleotides [2, 10] and histone acetylation are the two most widely known processes involved in epigenetic regulations. However, more recent studies have revealed other players in these complex processes, especially non-coding RNAs (siRNAs, microRNAs, and piRNAs) [11–18], some of which have been detected in the germline [14, 15, 17, 18], as well as factors regulating higher-level organization of chromatin [19, 20]. Some of these elements can be modified by environmental factors leading to alternate gene expression [18–20].

3. Gamete and embryo epigenetics

In spite of the ample knowledge about epigenetic mechanisms involved in gene expression control during the early embryogenesis fetal development and adult life [9], the environmental epigenetic inheritance through gametes was initially thought impossible because of the belief that all epigenetic marks, including DNA methylation, histone acetylation status and small RNAs, are completely erased and subsequently reset during germline reprogramming [21]. In mammals, these events take place both in the germline and in zygote immediately after fertilization [21, 22]. However, it is now known that this reset is not complete, and some parental imprinted loci can resist the global demethylation after fertilization, owing to the action of different mechanisms [23–26]. These findings explain previous observations on transgenerational transmission of environmentally conditioned disorders. For instance, the incidence of effects of parental ionizing irradiation on genomic instability in the offspring is too high to be explained by radiation-induced mutations which occur at a substantially lower rate [27]. Epigenetic inheritance through gametes can also explain transgenerational transmission of obesity [28, 29], diabetes [30, 31], and some types of cancer [32, 33].

All these data converge to suggest that epigenetic marks carried by the fertilizing spermatozoon are important for a variety of physiological and pathological processes that can affect offspring throughout life.

4. Potential sources of paternal epigenetic issues

It has been known since the early 2000 that human embryonic development is subject to paternal effects that can affect not only the early postfertilization events but also later phases of preimplantation and postimplantaion development [34–36]. Two types of paternal effects were distinguished: the early paternal effect and the late paternal effect [35]. The early paternal effect was reflected by an impairment of postfertilization development as early as the 1-cell zygote stage and subsequently was often associated with irregular cleavage divisions and blastomere fragmentation [34]. The late paternal effect was not detectable during the early cleavage stages, but became manifest after the 8-cell stage [35, 36]. Unlike the early paternal effect, the late paternal effect was often, though not always, associated with abnormally increased levels of DNA fragmentation in the father's sperm [35]. Both types of paternal effect reduced the chance of pregnancy [36].

In view of more recent data about sperm epigenetics, the meaning of these early observations can now be extended and reinterpreted. Since both the early and the late paternal effect were evaluated only in patients treated by intracytoplasmic sperm injection (ICSI), facilitating fertilization with spermatozoa carrying different morphological and functional abnormalities, which would not be capable of fertilizing oocytes by their proper means, the analysis of the resulting embryos can yield valuable information about the impact of sperm abnormalities and immaturity on fertilization and early development.

4.1 Fertilization with abnormal spermatozoa

ICSI has made it possible to achieve fertilization, embryonic and fetal development and childbirth by using spermatozoa with severe morphological and functional abnormalities. However, these abnormalities cannot be blamed for most of the negative paternal effects observed in ICSI-derived embryos. In fact, data have shown that fertilization with spermatozoa from certain individuals consistently leads to the formation of embryos with developmental abnormalities detectable as early as the 1-cell zygote stage [34]. Interestingly, these abnormalities almost always included abnormal pattern of the formation of nucleolar precursor bodies (NPBs) in the zygote pronuclei [34], as characterized previously [37]. The process of NPB assembly in human zygotes requires an early onset of RNA synthesis activity in the adjacent chromatin regions [38, 39]. The nature of the RNA molecules synthesized at this stage is unknown, but they are likely to be non-coding ones, since the first signs of embryonic gene expression can only be detected between the 4-cell and the 8-cell stage of the human preimplantation development [40–42]. These non-coding RNA species may be involved in the early epigenetic events that condition further embryonic development. Interestingly, the assembly of NPBs and the accompanying pronuclear RNA synthesis coincide with the assembly of microtubule organizing centers in human zygotes [43], and abnormalities of NPB assembly are associated with abnormal development of human preimplantation embryos [37, 44] and an increased risk of embryo aneuploidy [45].

Some conditions potentially responsible for sperm epigenetic abnormalities, such as advanced paternal age [46], tobacco smoking [47], and various lifestyle factors including dietary habits, physical activity or alcohol consumption [48], have been pointed out. However, a more comprehensive analysis of factors involved in these phenomena remains a big challenge for future research.

4.2 Fertilization with immature male germ cells

The final stage of sperm maturation is achieved during sperm passage through the epididymis. However, spermatozoa recovered directly from the testis [49, 50] and even round spermatids [51–55] are able to fertilize human oocytes and generate normal offspring when incorporated into oocytes via ICSI and ROSI, respectively. Moreover, live offspring was born in mice after fertilization with secondary spermatocytes [56], and in humans after fertilization with round spermatids developed in vitro from germ cells of men with spermatogenic arrest at the primary spermatocyte stage [57, 58].

Recent reports on the postnatal development of 108 babies born after fertilization of oocytes by round spermatid injection (ROSI), 90 of them in Japan and 18 in Spain [59], did not show any significant differences as compared with naturally conceived babies in either physical or cognitive development during the first 2 years after birth, and none of them developed any of the syndromes associated with genomic imprinting defects [59]. Thus, the use of immature male germ cells for fertilization, in spite of the still relatively low success rates, does not appear to be associated with an increased risk of epigenetic abnormalities in the offspring.

4.3 Disorders of paternally induced oocyte activation

As discussed in the previous sections, human embryonic development appears to be particularly sensitive to epigenetic events taking place during an early phase of the fertilization process, referred to as oocyte activation. Oocyte activation has been extensively studied since the mid-1990s, especially in relation with the new technologies. Both ICSI and ROSI avoid the initial contact between the surfaces of the fertilizing spermatozoon and the oocyte preceding their fusion during natural fertilization. Yet, this contact activates a series of signal transduction events that participate in physiological oocyte activation [60, 61].

These early signal transduction events are obviously by-passed when oocytes are fertilized by ICSI. This shortcut, however, does not prevent fertilization in most mammalian species. In fact, sperm-induced oocyte activation is driven by repeated rises of free cytosolic Ca^{2+} ions, referred to as calcium oscillations, mediated by periodic release and uptake of calcium by two types of calcium stores (basically endoplasmic reticulum), one opened by inositol trisphosphate (IP3) and the other by the very increase in free cytosolic calcium in its vicinity [62, 63]. In order to sustain the periodic calcium oscillations, the oocyte's calcium stores have to be sensitized by a soluble factor released from the fertilizing spermatozoon, initially called "oscillin" and later identified as a special form of phospholipase C (PLC) referred to as PLCζ [64]. Even in the absence of the initial contact between the sperm and oocyte surfaces, the release of PLCζ from the injected spermatozoon to the oocyte cytoplasm, together with an early extracellular calcium influx produced by the ICSI procedure itself, is sufficient to sustain calcium oscillations needed for proper oocyte activation [65]. However, the temporal pattern of the oscillations after ICSI (**Figure 1**) is slightly different from that following sperm-oocyte fusion (**Figure 2**). The release of PLCζ from the spermatozoon to the oocyte cytoplasm marks the spatial pattern of the first calcium rise, which propagates in a wave-like manner from the sperm position site across the oocyte (**Figure 3**).

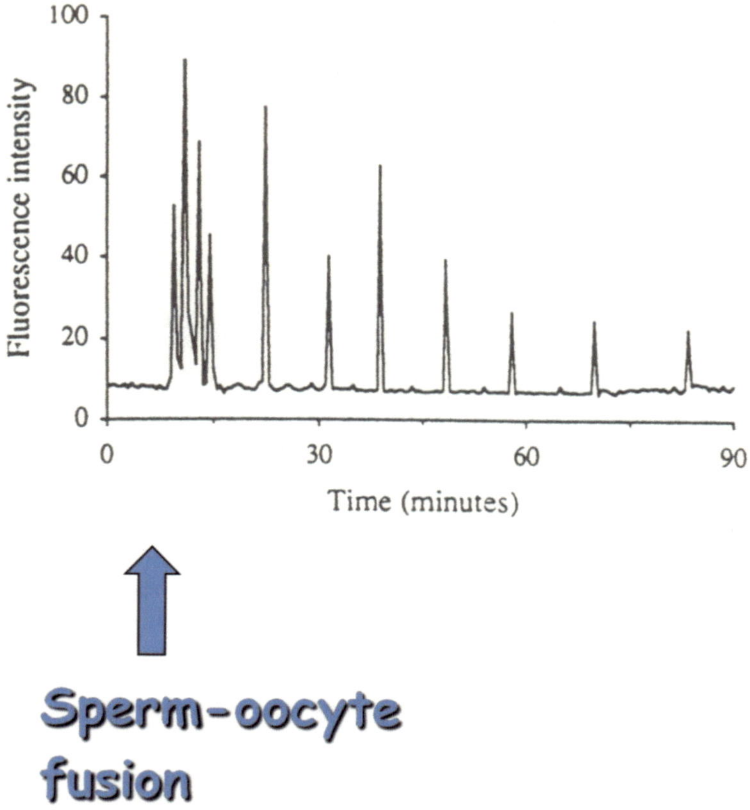

Figure 1.
Oscillations of free cytosolic Ca^{2+} concentration induced by sperm-oocyte fusion, recorded by confocal microscopy in a living human oocyte loaded with fluorescent calcium indicator Fluo-3 as described [65].

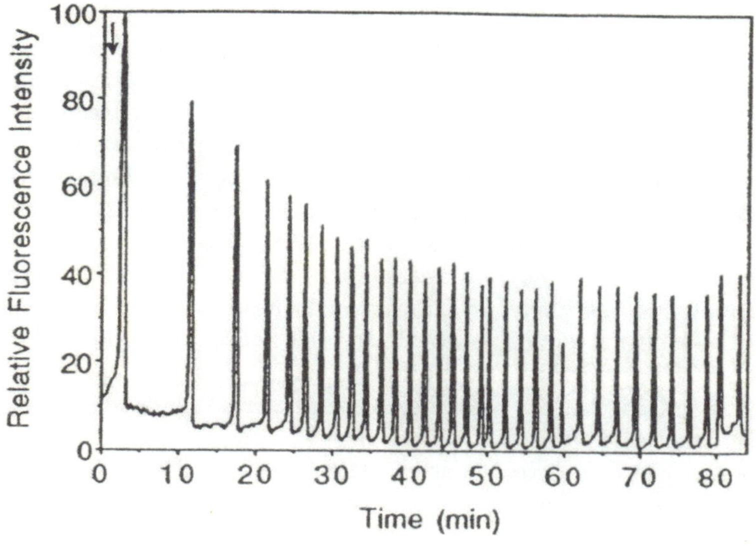

Figure 2.
Oscillations of free cytosolic Ca^{2+} concentration after ICSI (arrow), recorded by confocal microscopy in a living human oocyte loaded with fluorescent calcium indicator Fluo-3 as described [65].

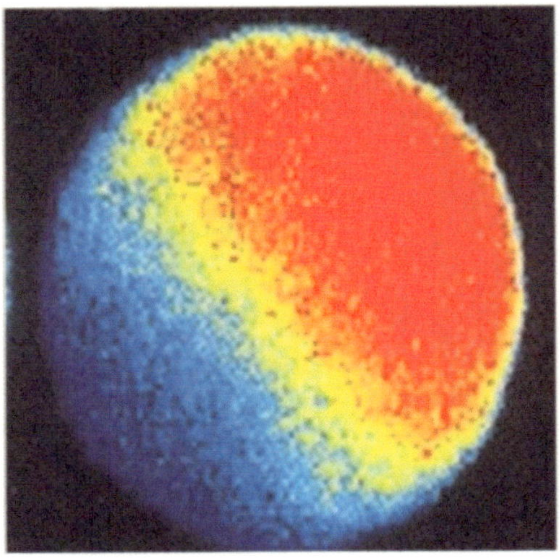

Figure 3.
Spatial propagation of the first sperm-induced increase in free cytosolic Ca^{2+} concentration, recorded by confocal microscopy in a living human oocyte loaded with fluorescent calcium indicator Fluo-3 as described [65].

In spite of the fact that the slight difference in the temporal pattern of the first sperm-induced calcium rise does not appear to have any impact on zygote and embryo development, the frequency and duration of the ongoing calcium rises have been shown to affect embryo development in different mammalian species [66–68] including the human [69]. Recent findings have pointed out the possibility that inherent abnormalities of the sperm-born PLCζ, but also in the oocyte response mechanisms, including steps downstream of the calcium releasing machinery, may influence mitotic divisions and gene expression during subsequent development and have to be considered an additional epigenetic risk factors to be taken into consideration in relation with the current-assisted fertilization technologies [70].

5. Current clinical experience

Several studies have suggested that both IVF and ICSI may increase the risk of certain types of birth defects in general [71–73] and heart defects in particular [74, 75]. However, there does not appear to exist a significant difference between the children conceived by conventional IVF and by ICSI [76, 77]. During the early years of its use, ICSI was preferentially employed in cases of poor sperm quality, while conventional IVF was used in cases with normal or nearly normal sperm, and the lack of significant differences between the outcomes of conventional IVF and ICSI suggests that sperm quality, as reflected by spermogram, spermocytogram and other standard sperm evaluation methods, has little, if any, impact on the health of offspring. Hence, the trend toward a higher risk of birth defects after IVF and ICSI as compared with natural conception is likely to be related to different, largely sperm-independent factors, such as the underlying cause of infertility, higher maternal age or a higher incidence of twin pregnancies [75, 78].

Even though there is no strong correlation between the conventional sperm parameters and ICSI outcome, sperm abnormalities, especially morphological ones, were shown to be associated with different genetic and epigenetic abnormalities [79], such as increased sperm DNA fragmentation [80] or abnormal patterns of DNA methylation [81]. Morphological abnormalities of the human sperm head have been shown to be associated with different types of genetic abnormalities [79], increased sperm DNA fragmentation [80] and different potentially harmful epigenetic factors, such as abnormal patterns of DNA methylation [81] and the absence or defective function of the sperm-derived oocyte-activating factor [82]. These observations explain the findings of increased implantation and pregnancy rate and decreased miscarriage rate [83–85], as well as a significantly decreased risk of major birth defects [86, 87], with the use of high-magnification ICSI (IMSI) as compared with conventional ICSI, although some studies failed to confirm these differences [88, 89].

As to fertilization by ICSI with immature (testicular) spermatozoa and by round spermatid injection (ROSI), the initial fears that incomplete or defective DNA methylation and chromatin configuration of these immature germ cells might cause syndromes related to genomic imprinting abnormalities [90] were not confirmed. In fact, no increase in the frequency of health problems caused by genomic imprinting abnormalities, such as Beckwith-Wiedemann, Prader-Willi, and Angelman syndromes, has been detected in children born after ICSI with testicular spermatozoa [91] and ROSI [59]. A recent study [92] has suggested that the supposed increase of imprinting errors, present in the sperm of infertile patients, does not have an obvious influence on assisted reproduction outcome or the imprinting of offspring, probably because the imprinting errors in sperm are selectively discarded or corrected during development [20, 93].

In contrast to the reassuring clinical data concerning the potential epigenetic risk of using abnormal and immature male germ cells for fertilization, there is increasing concern about the possible transmission of epigenetic abnormalities and diseases acquired during the father's life via his spermatozoa. This risk is difficult to evaluate with the use of currently available diagnostic methods because it is not necessarily associated either with sperm morphology or with its DNA integrity. It was actually demonstrated in humans that nutritional status and physical activity levels were associated with dynamic epigenetic changes in spermatozoa, including DNA methylation patterns and small RNA expression [94–97]. This kind of acquired epigenetic changes in spermatozoa is suspected to mediate transgenerational epigenetic inheritance of neurological disorders [95] and susceptibility to diabetes [31] and obesity [96, 97], and this list does not appear to be definitive, since new evidence of environmentally driven sperm-borne epigenetic factors, which are capable of altering the phenotype of the next generation, is emerging on a large scale. Paternal aging [46] and smoking [47] were also shown to affect sperm DNA methylation patterns, with still ill-defined developmental and health consequences for the offspring.

6. Future prospects for paternal epigenetic diagnosis and treatment

Abnormal patterns of sperm DNA methylation, small RNA expression, and chromatin configuration can now be detected with a relative ease. However, many of these abnormalities lack clinical significance because they might be corrected during fertilization and postfertilization development. The mechanisms responsible for this repair are still largely hypothetical and poorly understood. However, they are very likely to exist because a recent publication, based on the analysis of 1280 IVF-related treatment cycles, did not show any influence of either male age or sperm parameters on clinical pregnancy and live birth outcomes [92], in spite of the existence of data suggesting that there are very clear consequences of aging in the sperm epigenome that can be directly detected in DNA methylation patterns [46].

Obviously, further studies are needed to assess whether any effects of male age and sperm parameters on the offspring health status can be detected later in life.

In order to be able to distinguish between "benign" paternal epigenetic alterations that can be repaired spontaneously, on the one hand, and clinically relevant alterations that can cause negative effects on the embryonic, fetal and offspring health, studies are needed to relate DNA methylation status of specific genes and the expression pattern of specific small RNAs with specific developmental abnormalities. This work can be done by analyzing nucleic acids extracted directly from sperm cells or by using the "liquid biopsy" approach, based on the use of soluble nucleic acids isolated from blood plasma or seminal fluid. This latter approach is particularly interesting in azoospermic men so as to avoid the need for testicular biopsy to obtain a sample.

The identification of the developmentally relevant sperm epigenetic abnormalities is a necessary pre-requisite to design possible therapeutic interventions. These may go from relatively simple to more complex ones. It has been shown in the mouse that several waves of microRNAs and tRNA fragments are shipped to sperm during post-testicular maturation in the epididymis [98]. If some pathogenic paternal epigenetic signals are conveyed to sperm essentially during epididymal passage, ICSI with spermatozoa retrieved surgically from the testis, the technique already used with success in men with elevated levels of sperm DNA fragmentation [99, 100], might be a relatively simple and immediately available solution. If this approach is not possible, other, more sophisticated technologies, such as injecting specific microRNA molecules, capable of repairing specific epigenetic defects, into the early zygote [98] or induction of DNA methylation of the genes of interest by a Dnmt3-type *de novo* DNA methyltransferase targeted to the corresponding sperm DNA sequence by a nuclease-inactivated CRISPR variant (dCas9) [101], may be explored.

7. Conclusions

Since the availability of cell micromanipulation technologies enabling fertilization of human oocytes by ICSI with immature (testicular) spermatozoa and by round spermatid injection (ROSI), the role of paternal factors on embryonic, fetal, and offspring health needed a profound revision. While genetic abnormalities contributed by injected spermatozoa or spermatids can be controlled by preimplantation genetic testing and usually lead to a miscarriage, sperm-borne epigenetic abnormalities are much more difficult to detect and may be at the origin of different health problems throughout the offspring life. The current knowledge of the origin, nature, and mechanism of action of these sperm-borne epigenetic factors is outlined in this chapter. Surprisingly, in spite of multiple types of sperm epigenetic abnormalities associated with defective spermatogenesis and male aging, the current clinical experience is reassuring. In fact, no significant increase in the prevalence of diseases attributable to abnormal genomic imprinting was detected in children conceived by testicular spermatozoa or spermatids, probably because of the existence of efficient repair mechanisms acting in postfertilization stages of development.

By contrast, there is increasing evidence suggesting that transgenerational inheritance of paternally acquired epigenetic abnormalities via spermatozoa is more frequent than previously thought and can occur even in cases with normal conventional sperm parameters and during natural conception. The known pathologies transmitted in this way include neurological disorders, obesity, and diabetes, and their list is in continuous expansion. Future diagnostic and therapeutic possibilities applicable in these cases are discussed.

Conflict of interest

The author declares no conflict of interest related to this chapter.

Author details

Jan Tesarik
MARGen Clinic, Granada, Spain

*Address all correspondence to: jtesarik@clinicamargen.com

References

[1] Mayr E, Provine WB. The Evolutionary Synthesis: Perspectives on the Unification of Biology. Cambridge, MA: Harvard University Press; 1980

[2] Richards EJ. Inherited epigenetic variation—revisiting soft inheritance. Nature Reviews. Genetics. 2006;**7**: 395-401. DOI: 10.1038/nrg1834

[3] Wei Y, Schatten H, Sun Q-Y. Environmental epigenetic inheritance through gametes and implications for human reproduction. Human Reproduction Update. 2015;**21**:194-208. DOI: 10.1093/humupd/dmu061

[4] Duffie R, Ajjan S, Greenberg MV, Zamudio N, Escamilla del Arenal M, Iranzo J, et al. The Gpr1/Zdbf2 locus provides new paradigms for transient and dynamic genomic imprinting in mammals. Genes & Development. 2014;**28**:463-478. DOI: 10.1101/gad.232058.113

[5] Falls JG, Pulford DJ, Wylie AA, Jirtle RL. Genomic imprinting: Implications for human disease. The American Journal of Pathology. 1999;**154**:635-647

[6] Reik W, Walter J. Genomic imprinting: Parental influence on the genome. Nature Reviews. Genetics. 2001;**2**:21-32. DOI: 10.1038/35047554

[7] Huynh KD, Lee JT. X-chromosome inactivation: A hypothesis linking ontogeny and phylogeny. Nature Reviews. Genetics. 2005;**6**:410-418. DOI: 10.1038/nrg1604

[8] Thorvaldsen JL, Verona RI, Bartolomei MS. X-tra! X-tra! News from the mouse X chromosome. Developmental Biology. 2006;**298**:344-353. DOI: 10.1016/j.ydbio.2006.07.011

[9] Christophersen NS, Helin K. Epigenetic control of embryonic stem cell fate. The Journal of Experimental Medicine. 2010;**207**:2287-2295. DOI: 10.1084/jem.20101438

[10] Klose RJ, Bird AP. Genomic DNA methylation: The mark and its mediators. Trends in Biochemical Sciences. 2006;**31**:89-97. DOI: 10.1016/j.tibs.2005.12.008

[11] Fire A, Xu S, Montgomery MK, Kostas SA, Driver SE, Mello CC. Potent and specific genetic interference by double-stranded RNA in *Caenorhabditis elegans*. Nature. 1998;**391**:806-811. DOI: 10.1038/35888

[12] Rassoulzadegan M, Grandjean V, Gounon P, Vincent S, Gillot I, Cuzin F. RNA-mediated non-mendelian inheritance of an epigenetic change in the mouse. Nature. 2006;**441**:469-474. DOI: 10.1038/nature04674

[13] Grandjean V, Gounon P, Wagner N, Martin L, Wagner KD, Bernex F, et al. The miR-124-Sox9 paramutation: RNA-mediated epigenetic control of embryonic and adult growth. Development. 2009;**136**:3647-3655. DOI: 10.1242/dev.041061

[14] Watanabe T, Takeda A, Tsukiyama T, Mise K, Okuno T, Sasaki H, et al. Identification and characterization of two novel classes of small RNAs in the mouse germline: Retrotransposon-derived siRNAs in oocytes and germline small RNAs in testes. Genes & Development. 2006;**20**:1732-1743. DOI: 10.1101/gad.1425706

[15] Ashe A, Sapetschnig A, Weick EM, Mitchell J, Bagijn MP, Cording AC, et al. piRNAs can trigger a multigenerational epigenetic memory in the germline of *C. elegans*. Cell. 2012;**150**:88-99. DOI: 10.1016/j.cell.2012.06.018

[16] Bagijn MP, Goldstein LD, Sapetschnig A, Weick EM, Bouasker S,

Lehrbach NJ, et al. Function, targets, and evolution of *Caenorhabditis elegans* piRNAs. Science. 2012;**337**:574-578. DOI: 10.1126/science.1220952

[17] Lee HC, Gu W, Shirayama M, Youngman E, Conte D Jr, Mello CC. *C. elegans* piRNAs mediate the genome-wide surveillance of germline transcripts. Cell. 2012;**150**:78-87. DOI: 10.1016/j.cell.2012.06.016

[18] Shirayama M, Seth M, Lee HC, Gu W, Ishidate T, Conte D Jr, et al. piRNAs initiate an epigenetic memory of nonself RNA in the *C. elegans* germline. Cell. 2012;**150**:65-77. DOI: 10.1016/j.cell.2012.06015

[19] Becker JS, McCarthy RL, Sidoli S, Donahue G, Kaeding KE, He Z, et al. Genomic and proteomic resolution of heterochromatin and its restriction of alternate fate genes. Molecular Cell. 2017;**68**:1023-1037.e15. DOI: 10.1016/j.molcel.2017.11.030

[20] Wang C, Liu X, Gao Y, Yang L, Li C, Liu W, et al. Reprogramming of H3K9me3-dependent heterochromatin during mammalian embryo development. Nature Cell Biology. 2018;**20**:620-631. DOI: 10.1038/s41556-018-0093-4

[21] Hackett JA, Surani MA. Beyond DNA: Programming and inheritance of parental methylomes. Cell. 2013;**153**:737-739. DOI: 10.1016/j.cell.2013.04.044

[22] Hackett JA, Sengupta R, Zylicz JJ, Murakami K, Lee C, Down TA, et al. Germline DNA demethylation dynamics and imprint erasure through 5-hydroxymethylcytosine. Science. 2013;**339**:448-452. DOI: 10.1126/science.1229277

[23] Nakamura T, Liu YJ, Nakashima H, Umehara H, Inoue K, Matoba S, et al. PGC7 binds histone H3K9me2 to protect against conversion of 5mC to 5hmC in early embryos. Nature. 2012;**486**:415-419. DOI: 10.1038/nature11093

[24] Messerschmidt DM. Should I stay or should I go: Protection and maintenance of DNA methylation at imprinted genes. Epigenetics. 2012;7:969-975. DOI: 10.4161/epi.21337

[25] Messerschmidt DM, de Vries W, Ito M, Solter D, Ferguson-Smith A, Knowles BB. Trim28 is required for epigenetic stability during mouse oocyte to embryo transition. Science. 2012;**335**:1499-1502. DOI: 10.1126/science.1216154

[26] Jiang L, Zhang J, Wang JJ, Wang L, Zhang L, Li G, et al. Sperm, but not oocyte, DNA methylome is inherited by zebrafish early embryos. Cell. 2013;**153**:773-784. DOI: 10.1016/j.cell.2013.04.041

[27] Dubrova YE. Radiation-induced transgenerational instability. Oncogene. 2003;**22**:7087-7093. DOI: 10.1038/sj.onc.1206993

[28] Gluckman PD, Hanson MA, Bateson P, Beedle AS, Law CM, Bhutta ZA, et al. Towards a new developmental synthesis: Adaptive developmental plasticity and human disease. Lancet. 2009;**373**:1654-1657. DOI: 10.1016/S0140-6736(09)60234-8

[29] Li L, Law C, Lo Conte R, Power C. Intergenerational influences on childhood body mass index: The effect of parental body mass index trajectories. The American Journal of Clinical Nutrition. 2009;**89**:551-557. DOI: 10.3945/ajcn.2008.26759

[30] Whitaker RC, Wright JA, Pepe MS, Seidel KD, Dietz WH. Predicting obesity in young adulthood from childhood and parental obesity. The New England Journal of Medicine. 1997;**337**:869-873. DOI: 10.1056/NEJM199709253371301

[31] Wei Y, Yang CR, Wei YP, Zhao ZA, Hou Y, Schatten H, et al. Paternally induced transgerenational inheritance of susceptibility to diabetes in mammals. Proceedings of the National Academy of Sciences of the United States of America. 2014;**111**:1873-1878. DOI: 10.1073/pnas.1321195111

[32] Suter CM, Martin DL, Ward RL. Germline epimutation of MLH1 in individuals with multiple cancers. Nature Genetics. 2004;**36**:497-501. DOI: 10.1038/ng1342

[33] Chan TL, Yuen ST, Kong CK, Chan YW, Chan YS, NG WF, et al. Heritable gernline epimutation of MSH2 in a family with hereditary nonpolyposis colorectal cancer. Nature Genetics. 2006;**37**:1178-1183. DOI: 10.1038/ng1866

[34] Tesarik J, Mendoza C, Greco E. Paternal effects acting during the first cell cycle of human preimplantation development after ICSI. Human Reproduction. 2002;**17**:184-189. DOI: 10.1093/humrep/17.1.184

[35] Tesarik J, Greco E, Mendoza C. Late, but not early, paternal effect on human embryo development is related to sperm DNA fragmentation. Human Reproduction. 2004;**19**:611-615. DOI: 10.1093/humrep/deh127

[36] Tesarik J. Paternal effects on cell division in the preimplantation embryo. Reproductive Biomedicine Online. 2005;**10**:370-375. DOI: 10.1016/S1472-6483(10)61798-1

[37] Tesarik J, Greco E. The probability of abnormal preimplantation development can be predicted by a single static observation on pronuclear stage morphology. Human Reproduction. 1999;**14**:1318-1323. DOI: 10.1093/humrep/14.5.1318

[38] Tesarik J, Kopecny V. Nucleic acid synthesis and development of human male pronucleus. Journal of Reproduction and Fertility. 1989;**86**:549-558. DOI: 10.1530/jrf.0.0860549

[39] Tesarik J, Kopecny V. Assembly of the nucleolar precursor bodies in human male pronuclei is correlated with an early RNA synthetic activity. Experimental Cell Research. 1990;**191**:153-156. DOI: 10.1016/0014-4827(90)90050-K

[40] Tesarik J, Kopecny V, Plachot M, Mandelbaum J. Activation of nucleolar and extranucleolar RNA synthesis and changes in the ribosomal content of human embryos developing in vitro. Journal of Reproduction and Fertility. 1986;**78**:463-470. DOI: 10.1530/jrf.0.0780463

[41] Braude P, Bolton V, Moore S. Human gene expression first occurs between the four- and eight-cell stages of preimplntation development. Nature. 1988;**332**:459-461. DOI: 10.1038/332459a0

[42] Tesarik J, Kopecny V, Plachot M, Mandelbaum J. Early morphological signs of embryonic genome expression in human preimplantation development as revealed by quantitative electron microscopy. Developmental Biology. 1988;**128**:15-20. DOI: 10.1016/0012-1606(88)90261-8

[43] Sathananthan AH, Ratnam SS, Ng SC, Tarín JJ, Gianaroli L, Trounson A. The sperm centriole: Its inheritance, replication and perpetuation in early human embryos. Human Reproduction. 1996;**11**:345-356

[44] Balaban B, Urman B, Isiklar A, Alatas C, Aksoy S, Mercan R, et al. The effect of pronuclear morphology on embryo quality parameters and blastocyst transfer outcome. Human Reproduction. 2001;**16**:2357-2361. DOI: 10.1093/humrep/16.11.2357

[45] Balaban B, Yakin K, Urman B, Isiklar A, Tesarik J. Pronuclear morphology predicts embryo development and chromosome constitution. Reproductive Biomedicine Online. 2004;**8**:695-700. DOI: 10.1016/S1472-6483(10)61651-3

[46] Jenkins TG, Aston KI, Carrell DT. Sperm epigenetics and aging. Translational Andrology and Urology. 2018;**7**(Suppl. 3):S328-S335. DOI: 10.21037/tau.2018.06.10

[47] Hamad MF, Abu Dayyih WA, Laqqan M, AlKhaled Y, Montenarh M, Hammadeh ME. The status of global DNA methylation in the spermatozoa of smokers and non-smokers. Reproductive Biomedicine Online. 2018;**37**:581-589. DOI: 10.1016/j.rbmo.2018.016

[48] Donkin I, Barrès R. Sperm epigenetics and influence of environmental factors. Molecular Metabolism. 2018;**14**:1-11. DOI: 10.1016/j.molmet.2018.02.006

[49] Schoysman R, Vanderzwalmen P, Nijs M, Segal L, Segal-Bertin G, Geerts L, et al. Pregnancy after fertilisation with human testicular spermatozoa. Lancet. 1993;**342**:1237

[50] Silber SJ, Van Steirteghem AC, Liu J, Nagy Z, Tournaye H, Devroey P. High fertilization and pregnancy rate after intracytoplasmic sperm injection with spermatozoa obtained from testicular biopsy. Human Reproduction. 1995;**10**:148-152

[51] Tesarik J, Mendoza C, Testart J. Viable embryos from injection of round spermatids into oocytes. The New England Journal of Medicine. 1995;**333**:525. DOI: 10.1056/NEJM199508243330819

[52] Tesarik J, Mendoza C. Spermatid injection into human oocytes. I. Laboratory techniques and special features of zygote development. Human Reproduction. 1996;**11**:772-779

[53] Tesarik J, Rolet F, Brami C, Sedbon E, Thorel J, Tibi C, et al. Spermatid injection into human oocytes. II. Clinical application in the treatment of infertility due to non-obstructive azoospermia. Human Reproduction. 1996;**11**:780-783

[54] Barak Y, Kogosowski A, Goldman S, Soffer Y, Gonen Y, Tesarik J. Pregnancy and birth after transfer of embryos that developed from single-nucleated zygotes obtained by injection of round spermatids into oocytes. Fertility and Sterility. 1998;**70**:67-70

[55] Tanaka A, Nagayoshi M, Takemoto Y, Tanaka I, Kusunoki H, Watanabe S, et al. Fourteen babies born after round spermatid injection into human oocytes. Proceedings of the National Academy of Sciences of the United States of America. 2015;**112**:14629-14634. DOI: 10.1073/pnas.1517466112

[56] Kimura Y, Yanagimachi R. Development of normal mice from oocytes injected with secondary spermatocyte nuclei. Biology of Reproduction. 1995;**53**:855-862

[57] Tesarik J, Guido M, Mendoza C, Greco E. Human spermatogenesis in vitro: Respective effects of follicle-stimulating hormone and testosterone on meiosis, spermiogenesis, and Sertoli cell apoptosis. The Journal of Clinical Endocrinology and Metabolism. 1998;**83**:4467-4473. DOI: 10.1210/jcem.83.12.5304

[58] Tesarik J, Bahceci M, Ozcan C, Greco E, Mendoza C. Restoration of fertility by in-vitro spermatogenesis. Lancet. 1999;**353**:555-556. DOI: 10.1016/S0140-6736(98)04784-9

[59] Tanaka A, Suzuki K, Nagayoshi M, Tanaka A, Takemoto Y, Watanabe S,

et al. Ninety babies born after round spermatid injection into oocytes: Survey of their development from fertilization up to 2 years old. Fertility and Sterility. 2018;**110**:443-451. Comment by Tesarik J, Mendoza C, Mendoza-Tesarik R. https://www.fertstertdialog.com/users/16110-fertility-and-sterility/posts/32485-25452. DOI: 10.1016/j.fertnstert.2018.04.033

[60] Tesarik J, Mendoza C. In vitro fertilization by intracytoplasmic sperm injection. BioEssays. 1999;**21**:791-801. DOI: 10.1002/(SICI)1521-1878(199909)21:9<791::AID-BIES11>3.0.CO;2-Z

[61] Machaty Z. Signal transduction in mammalian oocytes during fertilization. Cell and Tissue Research. 2016;**363**:169-183. DOI: 10.1007/s00441-015-2291-8

[62] Miyazaki S. Inositol 1,4,5-trisphosphate-induced calcium release and guanine nucleotide-binding protein-mediated periodic calcium rises in golden hamster eggs. The Journal of Cell Biology. 1988;**106**:345-353

[63] Tesarik J, Sousa M. Mechanism of calcium oscillations in human oocytes: A two-store model. Molecular Human Reproduction. 1996;**2**:383-386

[64] Saunders CM, Larman MG, Parrington J, Cox LJ, Royse J, Blayney LM, et al. PLCζ: A sperm specific trigger of Ca^{2+} oscillations in eggs and embryo development. Development. 2002;**129**:3533-3544

[65] Tesarik J, Sousa M. Comparison of Ca^{2+} responses in human oocytes fertilized by subzonal insemination and by intracytoplasmic sperm injection. Fertility and Sterility. 1994;**62**:1197-1204. DOI: 10.1016/S0015-0282(16)57185-4

[66] Ozil JP, Huneau D. Activation of rabbit oocytes: The impact of the Ca^{2+} signal regime on development. Development. 2001;**128**:917-928

[67] Ozil JP, Markoulaki S, Toth S, Matson S, Banrezes B, Knott JG, et al. Egg activation events are regulated by the duration of a sustained $[Ca^{2+}]_{cyt}$ signal in the mouse. Developmental Biology. 2005;**282**:39-54. DOI: 10.1016/j.ydbio.2005.02.035

[68] Ozil JP, Banrezes B, Tóth S, Pan H, Schultz RM. Ca^{2+} oscillatory pattern in fertilized mouse eggs affects gene expression and development to term. Developmental Biology. 2006;**300**:534-544. DOI: 10.1016/j.ydbio.2006.08.041

[69] Tesarik J. Calcium signaling in human preimplantation development: A review. Journal of Assisted Reproduction and Genetics. 1999;**16**:216-220. DOI: 10.1023/A:1020321024973

[70] Ferrer-Buitrago M, Bonte D, Dhaenens L, Vermogen S, Lu Y, De Sutter P, et al. Assessment of the calcium releasing machinery in oocytes that failed to fertilize after conventional ICSI and assisted oocyte activation. Reproductive Biomedicine Online. 2019;**38**(4):497-507. DOI: 10.1016/j.rbmo.2018.12.035

[71] Hansen M, Kurinczuk JJ, Bower C, Webb S. The risk of major birth defects after intracytoplasmic sperm injection and in vitro fertilization. The New England Journal of Medicine. 2002;**346**:725-730. DOI: 10.1056/NEJMoa010035

[72] Reefhuis J, Honein MA, Schieve LA, Correa A, Hobbs CA, Rasmussen SA. National birth defects prevention study. Assisted reproductive technology and major structural birth defects in the United States. Human Reproduction. 2009;**24**:360-366. DOI: 10.1093/humrep/den387

[73] Davies MJ, Moore VM, Willson KJ, Van Essen P, Priest K, Scott H, et al. Reproductive technologies and the

risk of birth defects. The New England Journal of Medicine. 2012;**366**:1803-1813. DOI: 10.1056/NEJMoa1008095

[74] Tararbit K, Houyel L, Bonnet D, De Vigan C, Lelong N, Goffinet F, et al. Risk of congenital heart defects associated with assisted reproductive technologies: A population-based evaluation. European Heart Journal. 2011;**32**:500-508. DOI: 10.1093/eurheartj/ehq440

[75] Giorgione V, Parazzini F, Fesslova V, Cipriani S, Candiani M, Inversetti A, et al. Congenital heart defects in IVF/ICSI pregnancy: Systematic review and meta-analysis. Ultrasound in Obstetrics & Gynecology. 2017;**51**:33-42. DOI: 10.1002/uog.18932

[76] Lie RT, Lyngstadaas A, Ørstavik KH, Bakketeig LS, Jacobsen G, Tanbo T. Birth defects in children conceived by ICSI compared with children conceived by other IVF-methods; a meta-analysis. International Journal of Epidemiology. 2005;**34**:696-701. DOI: 10.1093/ije/dyh363

[77] Wen J, Jiang J, Ding C, Dai J, Liu Y, Xia Y, et al. Birth defects in children conceived by in vitro fertilization and intracytoplasmic sperm injection: A meta-analysis. Fertility and Sterility. 2012;**97**:1331-1337.e4. DOI: 10.1016/j.fertnstert.2012.02.053

[78] Pendina AA, Efimova OA, Chiryaeva OG, Tikhonov AV, Petrova LI, Dudkina VS, et al. A comparative cytogenetic study of miscarriages after IVF and natural conception in women aged under and over 35 years. Journal of Assisted Reproduction and Genetics. 2014;**31**:149-155. DOI: 10.1007/s10815-013-0148-1

[79] Ray PF, Toure A, Metzler-Guillemain C, Mitchell MJ, Arnoult C, Coutton C. Genetic abnormalities leading to qualitative defects of sperm morphology or function. Clinical Genetics. 2017;**91**:217-232. DOI: 10.1111/cge.12905

[80] Cassuto NG, Hazout A, Hammoud I, Balet R, Bouret D, Barak Y, et al. Correlation between DNA defect and sperm-head morphology. Reproductive Biomedicine Online. 2012;**24**:211-218. DOI: 10.1016/j.rbmo.2011.10.006

[81] Cassuto NG, Montjean D, Siffroi J-P, Bouret D, Marzouk F, Copin H, et al. Different levels of DNA methylation detected in human sperms after morphological selection usinf high magnification microscopy. BioMed Research International. 2016;**2016**:6372171. DOI: 10.1155/2016/6372171

[82] Rybouchkin A, Dozortsev D, Pelinck MJ, De Sutter P, Dhont M. Analysis of the oocyte activating capacity and chromosomal complement of round-headed human spermatozoa by their injection into mouse oocytes. Human Reproduction. 1996;**11**:2170-2175

[83] Bartoov B, Berkovitz A, Eltes F, Kogosovsky A, Yagoda A, Lederman H, et al. Pregnancy rates are higher with intracytoplasmic morphologically selected sperm injection than with conventional intracytoplasmic injection. Fertility and Sterility. 2003;**80**:1413-1419

[84] Berkovitz A, Eltes F, Yaari S, Katz N, Barr I, Fishman A, et al. The morphological normalcy of the sperm nucleus and pregnancy rate of intracytoplasmic sperm injection with morphologically selected sperm. Human Reproduction. 2005;**20**:185-190. DOI: 10.1093/humrep/deh545

[85] Hazout A, Dumont-Hassan M, Junca AM, Cohen Bacrie P, Tesarik J. High-magnification ICSI overcomes paternal effect resistant to conventional ICSI. Reproductive Biomedicine Online. 2006;**12**:19-25

[86] Cassuto NG, Hazout A, Bouret D, Balet R, Larue L, Benifla JL, et al. Low birth defects by deselecting abnormal spermatozoa before ICSI. Reproductive Biomedicine Online. 2014;**28**:47-53. DOI: 10.1016/j.rbmo.2013.08.01

[87] Hershko-Klement A, Sukenik-Halevy R, Biron Shental T, Miller N, Berkovitz A. Intracytoplasmic morphologically selected sperm injection and congenital birth defects: A retrospective cohort study. Andrology. 2016;**4**:887-893. DOI: 10.1111/andr.12221

[88] Gatimel N, Parinaud J, Leandri RD. Intracytoplasmic morphologically selected sperm injection (IMSI) does not improve outcome in patients with two successive IVF-ICSI failures. Journal of Assisted Reproduction and Genetics. 2016;**33**:349-355. DOI: 10.1007/s10815-015-0645-5

[89] Gaspard O, Vanderzwalmen P, Wirleitner B, Ravet S, Wenders F, Eichel V, et al. Impact of high magnification sperm selection on neonatal outcomes: A retrospective study. Journal of Assisted Reproduction and Genetics. 2018;**35**:1113-1121. DOI: 10.1007/s10815-018-1167-8

[90] Tesarik J, Mendoza C. Genomic imprinting abnormalities: A new potential risk of assisted reproduction. Molecular Human Reproduction. 1996;**2**:295-298

[91] Tsai CC, Huang FJ, Wang LJ, Lin YJ, Kung FT, Hsieh CH, et al. Clinical outcomes and development of children born after intracytoplasmic sperm injection (ICSI) using extracted testicular sperm or ejaculated extreme oligo-astheno-teratozoospermia sperm: A comparative study. Fertility and Sterility. 2011;**96**:567-571. DOI: 10.1016/j.fertnstert.2011.06.080

[92] Mariappen U, Keane KN, Hinchliffe PM, Dhaliwal SS, Yovich JL. Neither male age nor semen parameters influence clinical pregnancy or live birth outcomes from IVF. Reproductive Biology. 2018;**18**:324-329. DOI: 10.1016/j.repbio.2018.11.003

[93] Tang L, Liu Z, Zhang R, Su C, Yang W, Yao Y, et al. Imprinting alterations in sperm may not significantly influence ART outcomes and imprinting patterns in the cord blood of offspring. PLoS One. 2017;**12**:e0187869. DOI: 10.1371/journal.pone.0187869

[94] Denham J, O'Brien BJ, Harvey JT, Charchar FJ. Genome-wide sperm DNA methylation changes after 3 months of exercise training in humans. Epigenomics. 2015;**7**:717-731. DOI: 10.2217/epi.15.29

[95] Donkin I, Versteyhe S, Ingerslev LR, Qian K, Mechta M, Nordkap L, et al. Obesity and bariatric surgery drive epigenetic variation of spermatozoa in humans. Cell Metabolism. 2016;**23**: 369-378. DOI: 10.1016/j.cmet.2015

[96] Ingerslev LR, Donkin I, Fabre O, Versteyhe S, Mechta M, Pattamaprapanont P, et al. Endurance training remodels sperm-borne small RNA expression and methylation at neurological gene hotspots. Clinical Epigenetics. 2018;**10**:12. DOI: 10.1186/s13148-018-0446-7

[97] Öst A, Lempradl A, Casas E, Weigert M, Tiko T, Deniz M, et al. Paternal diet defines offspring chromatin state and intergenerational obesity. Cell. 2014;**159**:1352-1364. DOI: 10.1016/j.cell.2014.11.005

[98] Conine CC, Sun F, Song L, Rivera-Pérez JA, Rando OJ. Small RNAs gained during epididymal transit of sperm are essential for embryonic development in mice. Developmental Cell. 2018;**46**:1-11. DOI: 10.1016/j.devcel.2018.06.024

[99] Greco E, Scarselli F, Iacobelli M, Rienzi L, Ubaldi F, Ferrero S, et al. Efficient treatment of infertility due to sperm DNA damage by ICSI with testicular spermatozoa. Human Reproduction. 2005;**20**:226-230. DOI: 10.1093/humrep/deh590

[100] Tesarik J, Galán-Lázaro M. Clinical scenarios of unexplained sperm DNA fragmentation and their management. Translational Andrology and Urology. 2016;**5**:935-950. DOI: 10.21037/tau.2017.03.70

[101] Stepper P, Kungulovski G, Jurkowska RZ, Chandra T, Krueger F, Reinhardt R, et al. Efficient targeted DNA methylation with chimeric dCas9-Dnmt3a-Dnmt3L methyltransferase. Nucleic Acids Research. 2017;**45**(4):1703-1713

Chapter 6

Implantation: Cross Talk of the Developing Embryo and Endometrium

Lauren Grimm, Amber Cooper, Angie Beltsos and Roohi Jeelani

Abstract

The window of implantation has long posed as a challenge in understanding the exact synchronized cross talk that must take place in order for a developing embryo to be appropriately received by the endometrium. This is due mostly to the fact that it is difficult to study human models of implantation without sacrificing the potential for pregnancy. For many who present with a diagnosis of infertility with an otherwise unexplained etiology, recurrent implantation failure or a displaced window of receptivity may be an underlying, silent cause. As assisted reproductive technology (ART) continues to advance and offer new scientific breakthroughs allowing greater insight and understanding to reproductive failure and infertility, endometrial receptivity testing may offer answers to struggling patients.

Keywords: window of implantation, uterine receptivity, endometrium, blastocyst, embryo

1. Background

In order for pregnancy to occur, two events must take place:

1. Fertilization: the moment the sperm fertilizes the oocyte

2. Implantation: the moment the developing embryo meets the uterus, creating a nest from which to grow and develop

Following fertilization, the developing embryo must embed itself within the endometrium. In order for this to take place, both the embryo and uterus require the secretion and suppression of specific proteins that allow for implantation, including the expression of adhesion molecules on the cell surface, secretion of growth factors, and morphologic cell differentiation. Similarly, the embryo must also have developed to the blastocyst stage and be able to secrete appropriate protein factors for invasion and immunosuppression. These events between the embryo and endometrium must occur concomitantly in order for proper implantation to occur. If either the embryo or endometrium is asynchronous to the other, implantation will not take place, inducing the next cycle of menses. While great scientific advances have been made in the field of assisted reproduction since its inception in 1978, it is only within the last

10 years that we have really begun to understand this intricate network of synchronized events that allows the embryo and uterus to meet and become one.

2. The window of implantation

The uterus is constantly preparing itself for the possibility of implantation. As will be described in depth throughout this section, the uterus undergoes two phases throughout the normal menstrual cycle. To quickly summarize, following regular menses, estrogen released from the growing follicles in the ovaries causes the uterine lining to grow and thicken in what is known as the uterine proliferative phase. Following ovulation and the release of the oocyte into the canal of the fallopian tubes, the resulting corpus luteum acts to secrete progesterone, which plays a vital role in the ability of the endometrium to become receptive and available for implantation. This phase of the uterine cycle that correlates to the luteal phase of the menstrual cycle is known as the secretory phase, characterized by increased vascularization of the endometrium, uterine secretions, and reduced contractility of the surrounding smooth muscle [1]. While the uterine secretory phase lasts for about 2 weeks, coming to an end with the onset of menses, the window of implantation is thought to only occur over the course of a few hours, roughly 7–9 days following the LH surge or 6–8 days after ovulation (roughly days 20–24 of the menstrual cycle). During this time, the cells of the endometrial lining form small, finger-like protrusions, known as pinopods, which act to absorb fluid and macromolecules within the uterus. As the embryo begins to invade the endometrial tissue, a variety of cytokines, glycoproteins, and plasminogens are secreted by the embryo and uterus alike, allowing for changes in the cytoskeleton of decidual cells in the uterus and adhesion of the embryoblast to the succeeding layers of the endometrium [2]. Once implantation is complete, the embryo can continue to grow and develop into a maturing fetus, receiving blood and nutrients from the mother (**Figure 1**).

2.1 The proliferative phase

The proliferative phase of the endometrium corresponds with the follicular phase of the menstrual cycle. As estrogen is produced and released by the granulosa cells of

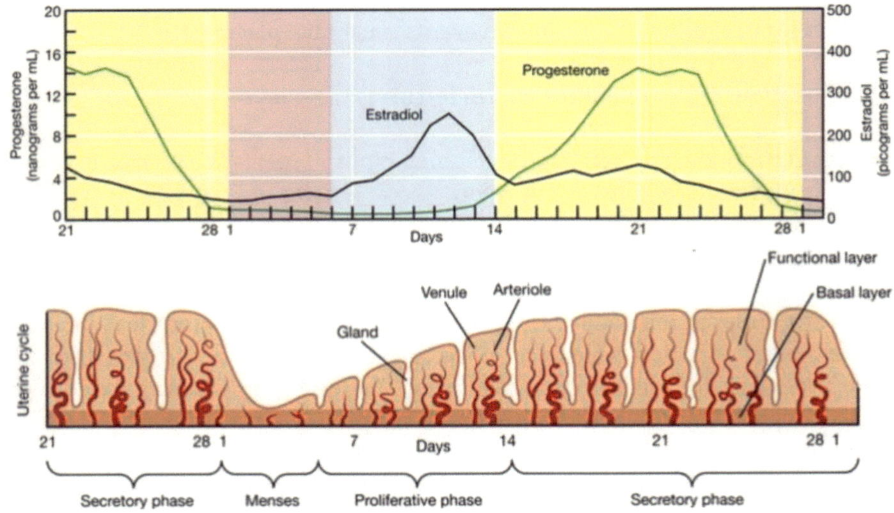

Figure 1.
The menstrual cycle: ovarian hormone production and uterine phase diagram.

the developing follicle, it is secreted into the bloodstream where it can bind a number of tissues, including the brain, breasts, uterus, and ovaries. As it pertains to the uterus, estrogen binds to estrogen receptors (ER; alpha and beta) in the cytoplasm or nucleus of endometrial glandular and epithelial stromal cells. The resulting E2-ER complex can then directly interact with the promoter regions of specific sequences of DNA related to the G1 phase of the cell cycle and induce mitotic proliferation by regulating cyclins, cyclin-dependent kinases (cdk), and cyclin-dependent kinase inhibitors [3]. One of these cyclins includes cyclin E, which increases in concentration during the endometrial proliferative phase and in response to estrogen signaling. Along with cdk2, cyclin E is believed to be the rate-limiting activator of G1 to S phase [4]. Other cyclins that are directly regulated by binding of the E2-ER complex include cyclin B1 and cyclin D1 [3]. Throughout the ovarian follicular phase, as serum estrogen levels continue to rise in response to folliculogenesis, the transcription of cell cycle-related genes in the endometrial tissue increases.

Estrogen not only has a transcriptional effect on endometrial tissue but on a variety of other important proteins is necessary for uterine preparation. This includes the induction of a variety of cytokines and growth factor proteins that help to stimulate uterine lining proliferation and endothelial growth. Many of these growth factors include transforming growth factors (TGF family), epithelial growth factor (EGF), and platelet-derived growth factor (PDGF), which all help to contribute to an overall thickened endometrium [5]. However, one of the most important growth factors that aids in the building and thickening of the endometrium is vascular endothelial growth factor (VEGF), which is believed to mediate angiogenic activity within the endometrium. The expansion of heavy vasculature throughout the endometrial lining contributes to not only an abundant supply of nutrients to the growing tissue but also a rich supply of vasculature for the growing fetus to attach to following implantation.

As the uterus continues to prepare for the moment of implantation, estrogenic binding also results in the presentation of progesterone receptors on the cell surface [3]. This effect on endometrial cells is important as the uterus begins to prepare to enter into the next uterine cycle phase.

2.2 The secretory phase

Once ovulation has occurred, estrogen levels abruptly decrease, resulting in a shift of the endometrium from the proliferative phase to the secretory phase. Once the oocyte is released from the surrounding granulosa cells, the resulting follicle turns into a corpus luteum that begins to secrete progesterone. Progesterone (p4) is one of the key steroid hormones that contributes to the ability of implantation to be successful. While estrogen ensures the endometrial lining is thick and heavily vascularized, progesterone makes the uterine lining sticky, providing the perfect environment to accept a growing embryo.

With the onset of ovulation and the dramatic decrease in estrogen levels, much of the proliferation that had previously taken place along the endometrial surface of the uterus begins to slow down. There is a slowing down of proliferation rather than a complete halt due to the small amount of estrogen the corpus luteum continues to secrete following release of the oocyte [6]. However, with the induction and secretion of progesterone now underway, the endometrial lining shifts focus in its preparation for implantation. One of the ways progesterone aids in this shift is via the activation of cyclin-dependent kinase inhibitor p27. As a reminder, following the formation of the E2-ER complex, initiation of transcription and translation of cycle E, and its partner cdk2, provides initiation of the mitotic cell cycle within the endometrial tissue. However, p27 acts as an inhibitor of this complex and thus prevents cell cycle progression [4]. Therefore, via the secretion of p4 and the induction of an active p27, endometrial proliferation is down-regulated during the uterine secretory phase (**Figure 2**).

Apart from slowing down proliferation, much of the secretory phase of the uterine cycle consists of the transcription and translation of molecules necessary for embryo implantation. Implantation can be classified into three stages: apposition, adhesion, and invasion [2]. During blastocyst apposition, the embryo makes its way across the endometrial lining and is guided towards the optimal spot for adhesion. Once the embryo subsequently anchors to the endometrial lining, the embryo-endometrial binding can no longer be dislodged from uterine flushing [2]. It is at this point the embryo can begin to invade the endometrial lining tissue. As you will see, much of this process uses many of the same biomarkers and molecules well known to the immune system and necessary for cellular migration, adhesion, and invasion during infection.

2.2.1 Apposition

Blastocyst apposition is primarily thought to take place as a result of mucins that line the basal lamina of the endometrium. Mucins are a heavy molecular weight glycoprotein that contain an intracellular cytoplasmic tail and a variable extracellular domain. Of all the mucins known to exist within the human genome, only Mucin-1 (MUC1) and Mucin-6 (MUC6) have been found in the human endometrium [7]. When highly expressed along the endometrial cell surface, MUC1 and MUC6 interfere with cellular adhesion between the embryo and uterine lining due to steric hindrance.

Normally, the apical surface of epithelial cells found throughout the body are protected by a shield of thick glycocalyx that is highly composed of mucins meant to guard the tissue surface from any surrounding pathogens. In the case of the endometrium, MUC 1 extends beyond this thick glycocalyx barrier, repelling the blastocyst from premature adhesion until it finds the optimal space and time for implantation. It has been found that the distribution and regulation of MUC1 and MUC6 varies throughout the menstrual cycle, in which both are downregulated right before implantation in the mouse model [8]. Thus, it is believed that the high progesterone levels exhibited during the window of implantation must inhibit MUC1 and MUC6 expression, thus facilitating embryo to endometrium interactions.

2.2.2 Adhesion

The primary type of molecules that contribute to cell-to-cell adhesion of the developing embryo and endometrium are cellular adhesion molecules (CAMs).

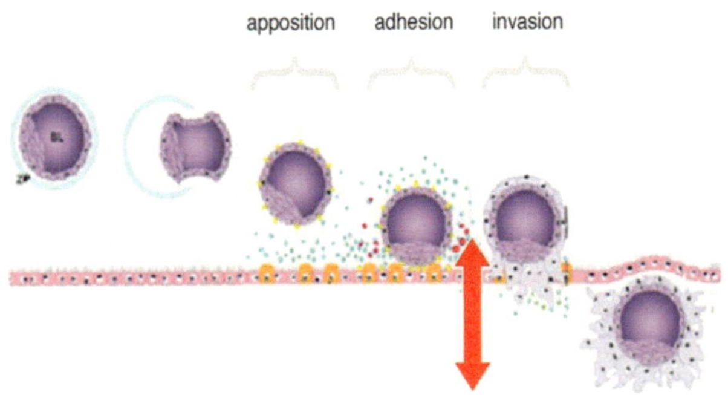

Figure 2.
Blastocyst hatching, followed by implantation via apposition, adhesion, and invasion of the endometrial tissue.

The CAM family of proteins is composed of four known members: integrins, cadherins, selectins, and immunoglobulins. How these adhesion molecules aid in embryo to endometrial linkage and embryonic invasion can be seen in **Figure 3**.

To start, a large variety of integrins have been associated with the luminal and glandular endometrial cells of the endometrium [9]. Most integrins are consistently expressed throughout the basal lamina of the uterine lining. However, some are expressed and regulated at specific times throughout the menstrual cycle. These include cycle-specific integrins a1b1, a4b1, and aVb3, which have been shown to be co-expressed during the window of implantation [10]. Similarly, integrins have been found to be expressed by the human trophoblast at the time of optimal implantation of the embryo. It is thus thought that integrins play a significant role in endometrial and embryonic adhesion, in which the integrins present on both the epithelial surface of the endometrium and the trophoblast of the developing embryo bind to specific extracellular matrix components [10, 11]. The ECM components are typically thought to include oncofetal FN secreted by the trophoblast and osteopontin, which has been positively identified by immunohistochemistry of the receptive endometrium [11].

It is true that just like the rest of the uterine cycle, ovarian steroid hormones also play a large role in the expression and inhibition of adhesion molecules like integrins. Accordingly, integrin aVb3 expression has been shown to be induced by EGF, among other growth factors, and negatively regulated by estrogenic factors [12]. Therefore, during the proliferative phase, high E2 levels effectively suppress integrin expression on the endometrial cell surface, while luteal phase progesterone acts to downregulate estrogen receptor activity, thus indirectly mediating the activation of integrin activity. Progesterone also has a direct effect on the presentation of integrin ligands, like osteopontin, by stimulating its gene expression [13].

Selectins, specifically L-selectin, of the CAM family of proteins also play a major role in blastocyst adhesion and implantation. L-selectin consists of a large, heavily glycosylated extracellular domain, and a small cytoplasmic tail, similar to that of integrins. Selectins are best known to play important roles in leukocyte

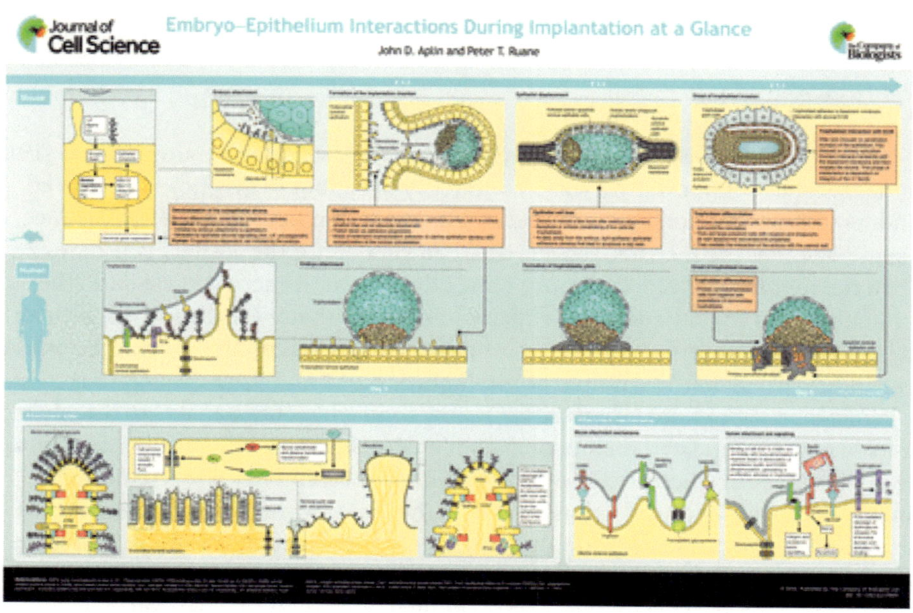

Figure 3.
Embryo epithelial interactions during implantation at a glance.

transendothelial cellular trafficking. Just like with leukocytes, selectins have been found to be heavily expressed along the trophectoderm of the blastocyst [14]. The endometrium, on the other hand, thus expresses oligosaccharide-based ligands such as HECA-452 and MECA-79 that bind selectively to L-selectin on the embryonic cell surface [14]. While MECA-79 has been shown to be immunolocalized along the luminal and glandular epithelium of the endometrium, its expression is known to intensify during the mid-secretory phase, in which implantation typically occurs [15]. Previous experimental findings suggest that the interaction between L-selectin on the trophoblast cells and its oligosaccharide ligand on the endometrium may make up the initial step in the implantation process of embryonic binding [16].

2.2.3 Invasion

Once adhesion has taken place, invasion of the embryo into the endometrial lining is necessary for continued blastocyst development. Cellular adhesion molecules play a role not only in the adhesion of the blastocyst but also in its invasion of uterine tissue. The most well-understood example of this is the downregulation of cadherins among the endometrial cells.

Biomarkers present during embryo implantation as seen in the mouse model and human endometrium.

Cadherins consist of a group of glycoproteins that are responsible for calcium (Ca^{+})-dependent cell-to-cell adhesion mechanism. Among the three subclasses, E-, P-, and N-cadherins, E-cadherin represents the most studied subclass in relation to implantation. The regulation of E-cadherin at the epithelial cell surface enables cellular control [17]. Intracellular Ca^{+} is essential in the E-cadherin regulation and assembly, in which a rise in intracellular Ca^{+} induces a signaling cascade that results in cytoskeletal reorganization and the disassembly of E-cadherins between cellular junctions. Consequently, calcitonin expression is induced by increased progesterone secretion, which results in an increase in intracellular Ca^{+} concentrations [18]. This specifically seems to take place during the mid-secretory phase, at which time the window of implantation is implicated to occur. It is thus believed that progesterone indirectly regulates E-cadherin expression via the calcitonin pathway, providing the developing blastocyst an opportunity for invasion, following initial apposition and adhesion.

2.2.4 Histologic dating

Back in 1950, Noyes et al. described histologic dating of the endometrium [19]. For decades, histologic dating was a commonly used tool to diagnose a displaced window of implantation based on the endometrial samples' physical appearance. In some women, the menstrual cycle date can lag behind the actual cycle date [2]. When the menstrual cycle lags more than 2 days from the actual cycle date, the endometrium is considered "out of phase." For those that were diagnosed with an out of phase endometrium, exogenous hormonal supplementation could be used to treat and manipulate the window of implantation.

While histologic endometrial dating is now somewhat outdated due to the advancements in new and updated methodologies of evaluating the window of implantation, one important cell structure characteristic of uterine receptivity is worth noting. Pinopodes are bulb-like projections found on the apical surface of endometrial cells that are several micrometers wide and project into the lumen of the uterus above the microvilli. Pinopod physiologic expression is specific and limited in its expression to the 2 days of the menstrual cycle corresponding to implantation [20]. Morphologic expression of pinopods has been found to be progesterone dependent. Moreover, HOXA-10, a homeobox gene whose expression is required for implantation, has been found to have an essential role in pinopod formation [21]. While the exact function of pinopods remains unknown, studies have shown developing embryos preferentially attach to and invade specific areas of the endometrium where pinopod formation was allowed to occur in vitro [22]. Further studies have also demonstrated that endometrial pinopod morphogenesis is associated with increased mid-luteal phase expression of LIF as well as progesterone and integrin aVb3 [13, 23, 24].

2.2.5 Other important biomarkers related to implantation

There are a number of other important endometrial biomarkers specifically expressed during the uterine secretory phase that have major roles in coordinating successful implantation.

One of the most important biomarkers not yet mentioned is that of cytokines. Cytokines make up a type of protein that affects a variety of cellular functions, including cellular proliferation and differentiation. Cytokines that have been found to be present during the window of implantation include LIF, IL-6, and IL-1 [2]. Studies have demonstrated the importance of all three cytokines via knockout experiments in mice, in which lack of LIF, IL-6, or IL-1 resulted in decreased implantation [2, 25]. Importantly, all three cytokines have also been shown to have temporal expression throughout the menstrual cycle, where their expression and activity peaked during the mid-secretory phase [26, 27]. Receptors for LIF and IL-6 have been found to be expressed on both the endometrium and blastocyst, suggesting a paracrine- and autocrine-like function during implantation [28]. While steroid hormone regulation of these cytokines has not been confirmed, their regulation being similar in appearance to peak progesterone secretion implies that there is most likely a linkage between them.

Another important biomarker present during the secretory phase of the uterine cycle that has been shown to affect blastocyst implantation is prostaglandins. As mentioned previously, similar to an immune reaction, implantation can be thought of as a pro-inflammatory reaction with the premise that blastocyst attachment, invasion, and further development requires connection to the maternal vasculature. Thus, prostaglandins play a vital role in endometrial vascular permeability and cellular differentiation, as well as embryo transport and invasion. While prostaglandins (PG) are constitutively expressed throughout the menstrual cycle, specific PG receptors have shown to be preferentially transcribed and translated at different times throughout the two uterine phases [2]. This means that prostaglandins can then exert specific rolls along the endometrium at different times throughout the menstrual cycle. The importance of prostaglandins during the window of receptivity has been demonstrated in the mouse model, in which knockout mice were shown to exhibit various implantation defects, including failure to implant or late implantation.

Finally, while not a specific biomarker, it is important to mention the Maximal Implantation Potential (MIP) of the endometrium. When we think about the shape of the uterus, most find it helpful to visualize as an inverted triangle, with the cervix at the apex and the fallopian tubes at either ends of the base. The MIP is a region along the endometrium at the intersecting points of the two straight lines coming out of the openings of the fallopian tubes. It is at this region of the uterus and endometrial lining that the blood supply is richest, and the biomarkers of implantation present themselves in greater concentrations. During natural implantation, the MIP is the point of the uterus that the developing embryo most often optimally and preferentially implants.

As you can see, implantation and the process of uterine preparation are extensive and delicate processes. While many of the important players in implantation have been readily identified and mentioned here, still very little is known about the exact mechanisms, effects, and processes required to achieve implantation.

2.3 Menses

If implantation does not occur, either due to asynchrony of the previously described events or the lack of fertilization of the oocyte, the onset of menses is initiated, and a new uterine cycle begins. In order for progesterone secretion during the uterine secretory phase to be maintained, the corpus luteum must receive a positive feedback, and it must be received from an implanted and developing embryo via human chorionic gonadotropin hormone (hCG). Without the presence of hCG, the corpus luteum begins to degenerate after about 10 days, resulting in a decrease in progesterone production and a breakdown of the uterine lining.

3. Recurrent implantation failure

As one of the most intricate and sensitive processes that takes place in the human body, the relative inefficiency of implantation is ironic given that continuous reproduction is critical to species survival. For those seeking fertility treatment, recurrent implantation failure remains a frustrating and difficult possible underlying cause to an otherwise unexplained diagnosis of infertility or in conjunction with another inhibitory diagnoses. While there is no universal definition for recurrent implantation failure (RIF) despite multiple publications on the topic, broadly speaking, Das et al. defined it as "the repeated transfer of morphologically good embryos to a normal uterus without achieving successful implantation or clinical pregnancy" [29].

Ordinarily, the probability that an embryo will successfully implant is about 30% [30]. This means there is a 70% chance of implantation failure. In these cases, implantation failure may be due to one of two factors: inadequate uterine receptivity and/or problems with the embryo itself. When it comes to selecting good quality embryos, few objective methods of embryo assessment exist. Most rely on embryo morphologic grading, a subjective assessment of embryonic development based on the expansion and quality of the inner cell mass and trophectoderm (see **Figure 4**). Embryo grading has long stood as the gold standard of embryonic assessment for quality and to this day continues to be a reliable indicator of embryonic competence.

Over the last decade, preimplantation genetic testing has made its way onto the market as a means of objective chromosomal evaluation of the embryo. Preimplantation genetic testing for aneuploidy (PGT-A) requires a small biopsy of a few cells from the developing embryo. Currently, this is most often done during the blastocyst stage, in which a small biopsy is taken from the cells of the trophectoderm. Yet, biopsies can also be performed at the blastomere stage, and new research suggests improved efficacy when the biopsy is taken from the inner cell mass of the blastocyst or the spent media culture where the developing embryo has grown in vitro [31, 32]. From there, chromosomal evaluation is done to attest for the number of chromosomes present, with the assumption that euploid embryos (blastocysts with a normal 46 chromosome count) are healthy and deemed optimal for embryo transfer. However, PGT-A is expensive, costing patients thousands of dollars, and imperfect, where many embryos often result as mosaic (some cells have normal chromosomal count, and some do not) or "undetermined."

Yet, for those who opt to undergo PGT-A and continue to suffer the loss of RIF, asynchrony in uterine receptivity is most often the cause. A displaced window of implantation may be caused by a variety of factors, including abnormal cytokine and hormonal signaling, among other things, in which the endometrium is not prepared to accept a blastocyst at the otherwise appropriate time. Thus, evaluation

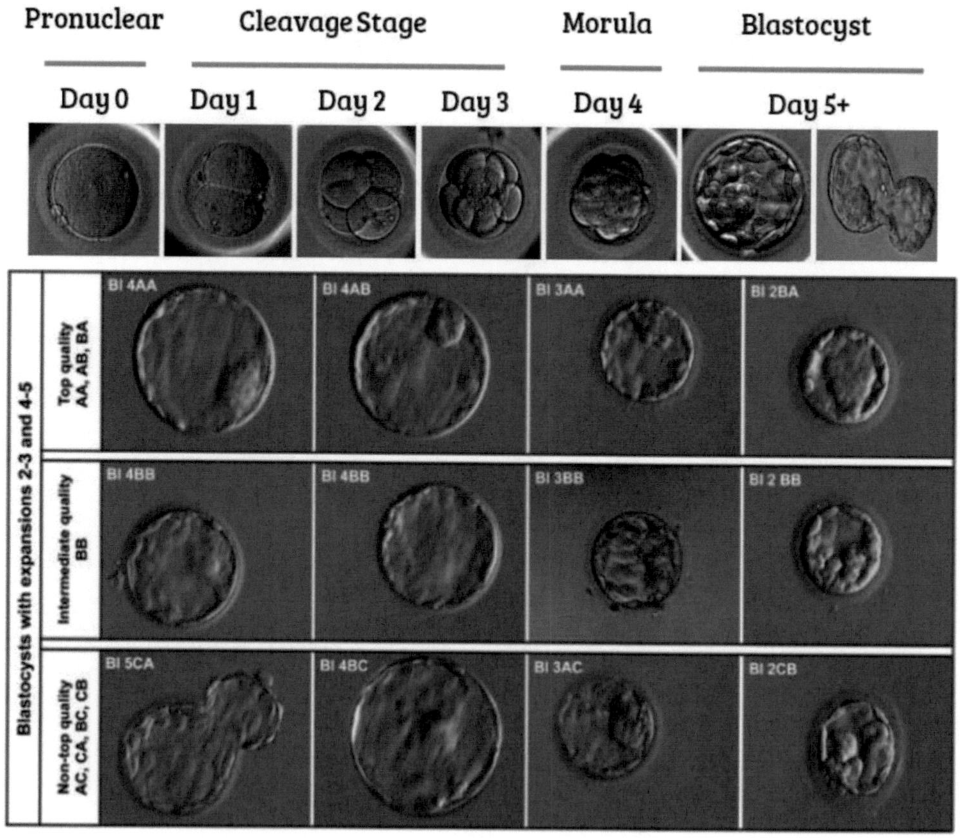

Figure 4.
Visual of embryonic development and morphologic grading according to blastocyst expansion and cellular differentiation receptivity at embryo transfer.

of implantation markers via an endometrial biopsy taken at the time of supposed implantation may be the key to predicting pregnancy outcome and adequate progesterone administration for optimal uterine.

4. Endometrial receptivity testing

Over the last decade, advancements in technology have made it possible for us to evaluate the window of implantation and diagnose displacements in one's uterine cycle activity. Of the numerous tests that exist, including the window of implantation test, which uses reverse transcriptase PCR analysis of endometrial tissue, and the endometrial function test, a histologic analysis of endometrial sampling, the most well-known example remains the endometrial receptivity array (ERA) by Igenomix. ERA utilizes next-generation sequencing (NGS) to analyze the RNA composition of the endometrial tissue to detect for expression and suppression of known endometrial biomarkers characteristic of the window of implantation. These biomarkers include LIF, MUC16, as well as various integrins and cytokines mentioned earlier in this chapter [33]. Diagnosis of a displaced window of receptivity is based on the RNA expression and transcriptomic signature found within the endometrial cell sampling. Based on this genetic analysis, technology is then able to diagnose whether or not the endometrium is receptive, pre-receptive, post-receptive, or non-receptive. **Figure 5** is a display of the transcriptomic signature of

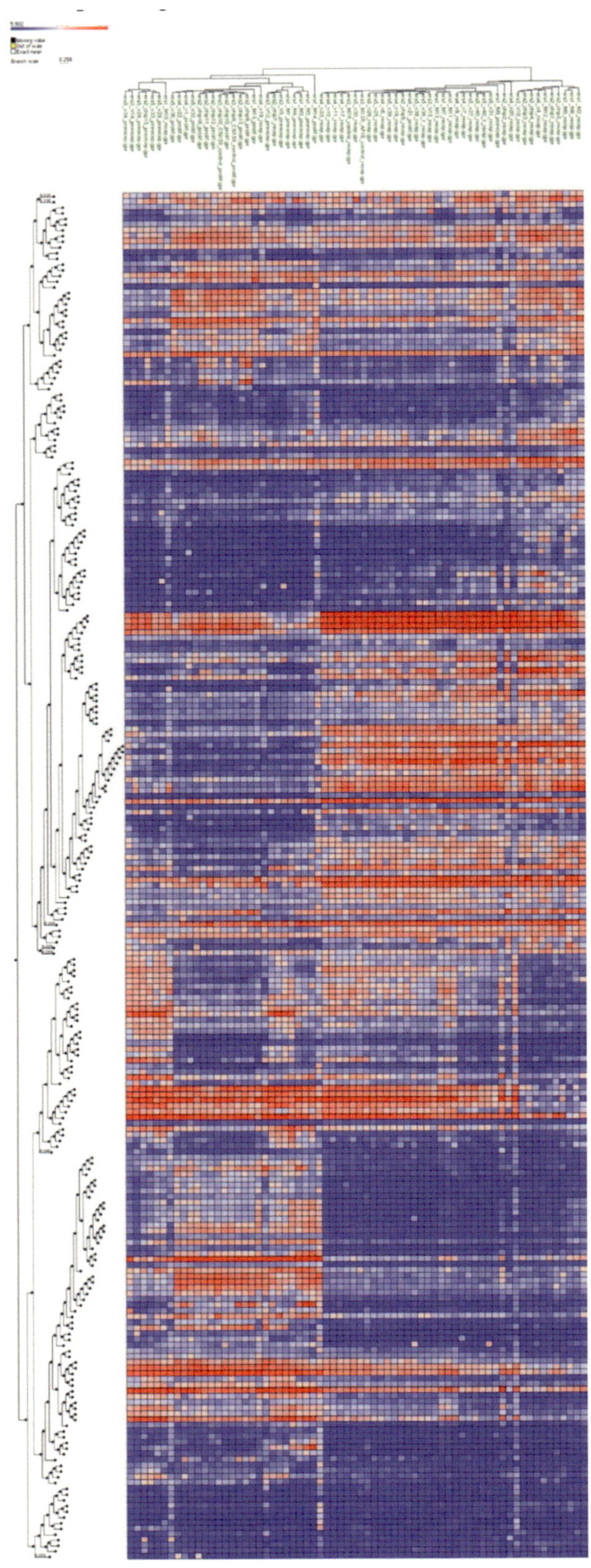

Figure 5.
Transcriptomic signature of the human endometrium based on next-generation sequencing.

the endometrium at its various phases throughout the menstrual cycle, including the proliferative phase, pre-receptive secretory phase, and receptive secretory phase.

A receptive endometrium indicates that the endometrial lining consists of all the correct biomarkers for proper implantation to take place, indicating the embryo should be transferred the same time as the biopsy took place. A non-receptive endometrial lining, on the other hand, refers to one of two cases: an endometrium that is either pre-receptive or post-receptive [34]. A pre-receptive endometrium refers to a window of implantation that takes place 12–48 h after the time of biopsy, whereas a post-receptive endometrium occurs when the window of implantation takes place at an earlier time (12–48 h) than the time of biopsy. In these cases, a corrective course of exogenous progesterone administration is typically advised wherein the embryo transfer takes place earlier or later to when the biopsy took place/the original time implantation was otherwise thought to occur, resulting in more or less overall progesterone exposure. Recently, letrozole, an aromatase inhibitor, and GnRh agonist drug therapies have also been found to correct a displaced window of receptivity, especially in women diagnosed with endometriosis, in which both letrozole and GnRh agonists have been shown to alter integrin expression in the endometrium and induce uterine receptivity [35].

Since it was first brought onto the market, endometrial receptivity testing has offered a novel approach to what had otherwise been a black hole in assisted reproductive technology treatment. For those that experience significant RIF, the ERA has been shown to increase clinical pregnancy rate to upwards of 75%, a figure previously unheard of for those facing infertility [34].

Yet, while endometrial receptivity testing has come a long way since its original inception, increasing in accuracy and offering hope to patients who otherwise had no other answers, skepticism still exists as to the clinical utility of this relatively new and evolving technology. Some have posited that the act of biopsying the endometrium has a similar effect to uterine scratching, which is a technique that involves superficial wounding of the endometrial lining and is thought to improve uterine receptivity in subsequent menstrual cycles. Others, however, point to the lack of research and evidence-based medicine to prove these tests accurately diagnose uterine receptivity and truly improve pregnancy rates, arguing more research into our understanding of the window of implantation is still needed.

5. Summary

Uterine receptivity and the window of implantation are incredibly intricate and complex processes that are meant to result in pregnancy. Following initial apposition of the embryo to the endometrium by MUC1 and MUC6, cytokines, such as LIF, recruit the blastocyst to the optimal spot for implantation along the endometrial lining. Through cellular adhesion molecules, like integrins and L-selectin, the embryo is able to bind the basal lamina of the endometrium, adhering to the uterine wall before invading the epithelial tissue and completing the process of implantation.

While this complex biological system often works accurately for the majority, giving way to a healthy pregnancy, many still experience asynchronies between the endometrium and developing embryo, resulting in infertility. As such, in an effort to optimize assisted reproductive technologies, scientists have sought out new and innovative techniques in order to understand and diagnose irregularities in the most important processes of human reproduction. The invention of endometrial receptivity testing now allows clinicians the ability to predict an individual's personalized window of implantation, offering new understanding to the field and hope for those who previously faced recurrent implantation failure (**Figure 6**).

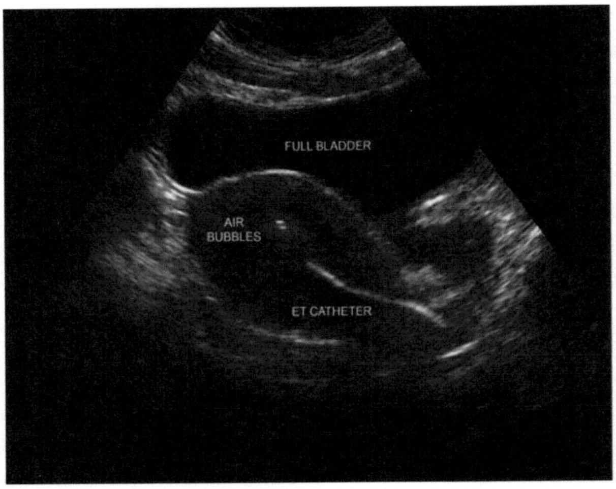

Figure 6.
Ultrasound imaging of an embryo transfer (ET).

Overall endometrial receptivity testing allows us greater insight into the understanding of reproductive infertility and the timing of the window of implantation. While research remains ongoing as to the clinical utility of these tests, including validation studies and the rate of pregnancy and live birth outcomes, endometrial receptivity testing offers another piece to the puzzle in our attempt to completely understand the underlying etiologies of infertility.

Acknowledgements

Thank you to Dr. Roohi Jeelani for the opportunity to participate in the writing of this chapter as well as to Dr. Angie Beltsos and Dr. Amber Cooper. I am forever grateful for your consistent support. Thank you as well to Jessi Anderson, Nepheli Raptis, Emma Radley, Hanna Mandell, and Christy Oso for your assistance on this project.

Notes

All adapted figures, photographs, and tables shown here have received permission for use from the original journals in which they appeared.

Author details

Lauren Grimm[1*], Amber Cooper[2], Angie Beltsos[1] and Roohi Jeelani[1]

1 Vios Fertility Institute, Chicago, IL, USA

2 Vios Fertility Institute, St. Louis, MO, USA

*Address all correspondence to: lauren.grimm@viosfertility.com

References

[1] Monard M, Marsh C, Schumacher K, Nothnick W. Secretory phase of menstruation and implantation. Frontiers in Women's Health. 2018;**3**(4). ISSN: 2398-2799. DOI: 10.15761/FWH.1000156

[2] Achache H, Revel A. Endometrial receptivity markers, the journey to successful embryo implantation. Human Reproduction Update. 2006;**12**(6):731-746

[3] da Costa e Silva RC et al. Estrogen signaling in the proliferative endometrium: Implications in endometriosis. Revista da Associação Médica Brasileira. 2016;**62**(1):72-77. DOI: 10.1590/1806-9282.62.01.72

[4] Dubowy RL et al. Improved endometrial assessment using cyclin E and p27. Fertility and Sterility. 2003;**80**(1):146-156. DOI: 10/10/16/S0015-0282(03)00573-9

[5] Zadehmodarres S, Salehpour S, Saharkhiz N, Nazari L. Treatment of thin endometrium with autologous platelet-rich plasma: A pilot study. JBRA Assisted Reproduction. 2017;**21**(1):54-56. DOI: 10.5935/1518-0557.20170013

[6] Oliver R, Pillarisetty LS. In: StatPearls, editor. Anatomy, Abdomen and Pelvis, Ovary Corpus Luteum. Treasure Island, FL: StatPearls Publishing; 2019. Available from: https://www.ncbi.nlm.nih.gov/books/NBK539704/

[7] Gipson IK, Ho SB, Spurr-Michaud SJ, Tisdale AS, Zhan Q, Torlakovic E, et al. Mucin genes expressed by human female reproductive tract epithelia. Biology of Reproduction. 1997;**56**(4):999-1011. DOI: 10.1095/biolreprod56.4.999

[8] Braga VM, Gendler SJ. Modulation of Muc-1 mucin expression in the mouse uterus during the estrus cycle, early pregnancy and placentation. Journal of Cell Science. 1993;**105**(2):397-405

[9] Lessey BA, Damjanovich L, Coutifaris C, Castelbaum A, Albelda SM, Buck CA. Integrin adhesion molecules in the human endometrium. Correlation with the normal and abnormal menstrual cycle. The Journal of Clinical Investigation. 1992;**90**(1):188-195. DOI: 10.1172/JCI115835

[10] Lessey BA, Castelbaum A, Wolfe L, Greene W, Paulson M, Meyer WR, et al. Use of Integrins to date the endometrium. Fertility and Sterility. 2000;**73**:779-787

[11] Wang J, Armant DR. Integrin-mediated adhesion and Signaling during blastocyst implantation. Cells, Tissues, Organs. 2002;**172**:190-201

[12] Somkuti SG, Yuan L, Fritz MA, Lessey BA. Epidermal growth factor and sex steroids dynamically regulate a marker of endometrial receptivity in Ishikawa cells. The Journal of Clinical Endocrinology & Metabolism. 1997;**82**(7):2192-2197. DOI: 10.1210/jcem.82.7.4102

[13] Lessey BA. Two pathways of progesterone action in the human endometrium: Implications for implantation and contraception. Steroids. 2003;**68**:809-815

[14] Genbacev OD, Prakobphol A, Foulk RA, Krtolica AR, Ilic D, Singer MS, et al. Trophoblast L-selectin-mediated adhesion at the maternal-fetal interface. Science. 2003;**2599**:405-408

[15] Lai TH, Shih IM, Vlahos N, Ho CL, Wallach E, Zhao Y. Differential expression of L-selectin ligand in the endometrium during the menstrual cycle. Fertility and Sterility. 2005;**83**(Suppl. 1):1297-1302

[16] Fazleabas AT, Kim JJ. Development. What makes an embryo stick? Science. 2003;**299**:355-356

[17] Gumbiner BM. Cell adhesion: The molecular basis of tissue architecture and morphogenesis. Cell. 1996;**84**:345-357

[18] Kumar S, Zhu L-J, Polihronis M, Cameron ST, Baird DT, Schatz F, et al. Progesterone induces calcitonin gene expression in human endometrium within the putative window of implantation. Journal of Clinical Endocrinology & Metabolism. 1998;**83**(12):4443-4450. DOI: 10.1210/jcem.83.12.5328

[19] Noyes RW, Hertig A, Rock J. Dating the endometrial biopsy. Fertility and Sterility. 1950;**1**:3-25

[20] Nikas G. Pinopodes as markers of endometrial receptivity in clinical practice. Human Reproduction. 1999;**14**(2):99-106. DOI: 10.1093/humrep/14.suppl_2.99

[21] Bagot CN, Kliman HJ, Taylor HS. Maternal Hoxa10 is required for pinopod formation in the development of mouse uterine receptivity to embryo implantation. Developmental Dynamics. 2001;**222**:538-544. DOI: 10.1002/dvdy.1209

[22] Bentin-Ley U, Sjögren A, Nilsson L, Hamberger L, Larsen JF, Horn T. Presence of uterine pinopodes at the embryo–endometrial interface during human implantation in vitro. Human Reproduction. 1999;**14**(2):515-520. DOI: 10.1093/humrep/14.2.515

[23] Aghajanova L, Stavreus-Evers A, Nikas Y, Hovatta O, Landgren BM. Coexpression of pinopods and leukemia inhibitory factor, as well as its receptor in human endometrium. Fertility and Sterility. 2003;**79**(Suppl. 1):808-8014

[24] Stavreus-Evers A, Nikas G, Sahlin L, Eriksson H, Landgren BM. Formation of pinopodes in human endometrium is associated with the concentrations of progesterone and progesterone receptors. Fertility and Sterility. 2001;**76**:782-791

[25] Simon C, Moreno C, Remohi J, Pellicer A. Cytokines and embryo implantation. Journal of Reproductive Immunology;**39**:117-131

[26] Charnock-Jones DS, Sharkey AM, Fenwick P, Smith SK. Leukaemia inhibitory factor mRNA concentration peaks in human endometrium at the time of implantation and the blastocyst contains mRNA for the receptor at this time. Journal of Reproduction and Fertility. 1994;**101**(2):421-426

[27] Simón C, Gimeno MÍJ, Mercader A, O'Connor JE, RemohÍ J, Polan ML, et al. Embryonic regulation of integrins β_3,α_4, and α_1 in human endometrial epithelial cells in vitro. The Journal of Clinical Endocrinology & Metabolism. 1997;**82**(8):2607-2616. DOI: 10.1210/jcem.82.8.4153

[28] Sharkey AM, Dellow K, Blayney M, Macnamee M, Charnock-Jones S, Smith SK. Stage-specific expression of cytokine and receptor messenger ribonucleic acids in human preimplantation embryos. Biology of Reproduction. 1995;**53**(4):974-981. DOI: 10.1095/biolreprod53.4.974

[29] Das M, Holzer HE. Recurrent implantation failure: Gamete and embryo factors. Fertility and Sterility. 2012;**97**(5):1021-1027

[30] Coughlan C, Ledger W, Wang Q, Fenghua L, Demirol A, Gurgan T, et al. Recurrent implantation failure: Definition and management. Reproductive Biomedicine Online. 2014;**28**(1):14-38

[31] Lawrenz B, El Khatib I, Liñán A, Bayram A, Arnanz A, Chopra R, et al. The clinicians' dilemma with mosaicism—An insight from inner cell mall biopsies. Human Reproduction.

2019;**34**(6):998-1010. DOI: 10.1093/humrep/dez055

[32] Huang L, Bogale B, Tang Y, Sunney Xie X, Racowsky C. Noninvasive preimplantation genetic testing for aneuploidy in spent medium may be more reliable than trophectoderm biopsy. PNAS. 2019;**116**(28):14105-14112

[33] Díaz-Gimeno P et al. A genomic diagnostic tool for human endometrial receptivity based on the transcriptomic signature. Fertility and Sterility. 2011;**95**(1):50-60.e15

[34] Mahajan N. Endometrial receptivity array: Clinical application. Journal of Human Reproductive Sciences. 2015;**8**(3):121-129. DOI: 10.4103/0974-1208.165153

[35] Sharma N. GnRH agonist and letrozole in women with recurrent implantation failure. Annals of Translational Medicine. 2019;**7**(Suppl 6):S209. DOI: 10.21037/atm.2019.08.100

Section 2

Assisted Reproductive Technologies

Chapter 7

The Low-Molecular-Weight Ligands of the Gonadotropin Receptors as the New Generation of the Regulators of the Reproductive Functions and Steroidogenesis

Alexander O. Shpakov, Kira V. Derkach, Andrey A. Bakhtyukov and Dmitry V. Dar'in

Abstract

In clinic, the luteinizing (LH) and follicle-stimulating (FSH) hormones and human chorionic gonadotropin (hCG) are used to treat reproductive dysfunctions and in assisted reproductive technology. They are the αβ-heterodimeric complexes and specifically bind to ectodomain of G protein-coupled LH and FSH receptors. This leads to activation of many signaling cascades; some of which are responsible for steroidogenesis, folliculogenesis, and spermatogenesis, while the others, such as β-arrestin pathways, trigger the downregulation of gonadotropin receptors. A low selectivity of the intracellular signaling of gonadotropins and a large number of their isoforms are the main causes of undesirable effects of gonadotropins, limiting their clinical applications. Unlike gonadotropins, the low-molecular-weight (LMW) ligands interact with an allosteric site located in the transmembrane domain of the LH and FSH receptors and selectively activate the certain signaling pathway, preventing a number of side effects of gonadotropins. The LMW ligands are characterized by activity of the full and inverse agonists and neutral antagonists, as well as the positive and negative modulators, and they have the in vivo activity, including when administered orally. This review focuses on the advances in the development of LMW allosteric ligands of the LH and FSH receptors and the prospects for their use in reproductive medicine.

Keywords: sex steroid hormone, steroidogenesis, low-molecular-weight agonist, luteinizing hormone, follicle-stimulating hormone, receptor of luteinizing hormone

1. Introduction

The most important areas of clinical applications of the gonadotropins, such as the luteinizing (LH) and follicle-stimulating (FSH) hormones and human chorionic gonadotropin (hCG), are (i) the stimulation of the steroidogenesis, folliculogenesis, and spermatogenesis in patients with the dysfunctions in the hypothalamo-pituitary-gonadal axis, (ii) the induction of ovulation in the assisted reproductive technologies, and (iii) the treatment of sex hormone-dependent tumors [1–4]. The gonadotropins with LH activity are isolated from the urine of pregnant women (the urinary forms of hCG) or produced in the specialized cellular cultures (the recombinant forms of LH and hCG), while FSH is isolated from the urine of postmenopausal women (the urinary forms of FSH) or produced by genetic engineering approaches (the recombinant forms of FSH) [1, 5, 6]. Despite the fact that these forms of gonadotropins are widely used in the clinic, they have the significant side effects. In the case of urinary forms of hCG and FSH, the main disadvantages are the presence of biologically active impurities in the gonadotropin preparations and a low degree of its standardization [2, 7]. The placental hCG differs significantly in both the structure and functions from the LH and sulfated hCG which are secreted by the pituitary gonadotrophs and circulate in the blood of adult men and women [2, 8]. Furthermore, the placental hCG is produced only during pregnancy and regulates the growth and development of the embryo [9]. The urinary FSH contains mainly highly glycosylated forms of this gonadotropin with the reduced activity, which associated with the impaired reproductive functions and infertility at the postmenopausal period [10]. At the same time, the recombinant forms of gonadotropins differ from their natural forms in the posttranslational modifications, primarily in the number, structure, and charge of N-glycans, which significantly changes their specific biological activity and pharmacological profile. All this not only significantly limits the use of natural and recombinant forms of gonadotropins in the treatment of androgen deficiency, hypogonadotropic hypogonadism, and amenorrhea but also reduces their effectiveness in the controlled induction of ovulation and in other assisted reproductive technologies.

Thus, one of the urgent tasks of reproductive medicine is to minimize the side effects of gonadotropins and to increase their effectiveness and specificity. An alternative approach is the development of a new generation of the selective regulators of the LH and FSH receptors, the most suitable among which are the low-molecular-weight (LMW) allosteric ligands of these receptors.

2. The LH and FSH receptors and their binding with the gonadotropins and the low-molecular-weight allosteric ligands

The LH and FSH receptors belong to the δ group of the rhodopsin family of the G protein-coupled receptors (GPCR) and contain seven membrane-penetrating hydrophobic regions that form the heptahelical transmembrane channel [11–16]. Unlike most GPCRs with a short extracellular N-terminal region, the gonadotropin receptors have a large-size extracellular domain (an ectodomain) containing the leucine-rich repeats (LRRs). The LRRs are involved in the formation of an orthosteric site responsible for a high-affinity binding of the receptors with gonadotropins. The gonadotropins are the αβ-heterodimeric complexes, in which the α-subunit encoded by a single gene is identical in all gonadotropins, while the β-subunits are encoded by separate genes and differ in the primary structure and modifications. The αβ-heterodimeric complexes of gonadotropins are stabilized by the cystine knots that ensure a close contact between the central regions of the α- and β-subunits [12, 16]. The β-subunit is responsible for the specificity of gonadotropins binding with the LH and FSH receptors, while the α-subunit provides the physical contacts between the ligand-bound ectodomain and the transmembrane domain. The binding of gonadotropin with an ectodomain induces conformational changes in both the transmembrane channel and the intracellular regions of the LH and FSH receptors, which are responsible for their functional coupling with the heterotrimeric G proteins (G_s, $G_{q/11}$, and $G_{i/o}$) and β-arrestins, resulting in the activation of a large number of the intracellular signaling cascades and the transcriptional factors [15–18] (**Figure 1**).

By activating the G_s proteins, the gonadotropins stimulate the enzyme adenylyl cyclase (AC), which leads to an increase in the intracellular cAMP levels and the activation of protein kinase A (PKA) and exchange protein directly activated by cyclic AMP (Epac). The stimulation of PKA leads to activation of the transcriptional factor cAMP-response element binding protein (CREB), which controls the expression of a large number of PKA-dependent genes, while the activation of Epac induces the stimulation of phosphatidylinositol-3-kinase, mitogen-activated protein kinases (MAPKs), and the other effector enzymes. The gonadotropin-induced activation of the cAMP-dependent pathways is the key mechanism for triggering the steroidogenesis, spermatogenesis, and folliculogenesis (**Figure 1**). By activating $G_{q/11}$ proteins, the gonadotropins stimulate the phosphoinositide-specific phospholipase Cβ (PLCβ), which catalyzes the formation of inositol-3,4,5-triphosphate and diacylglycerol, the important second messengers. This induces the activation of calcium-dependent signaling and different isoforms of protein kinase C [15–19]. A specific interaction between the β-arrestins and the GPCR kinases-phosphorylated sites located within the intracellular loops of the LH and FSH receptors induces G

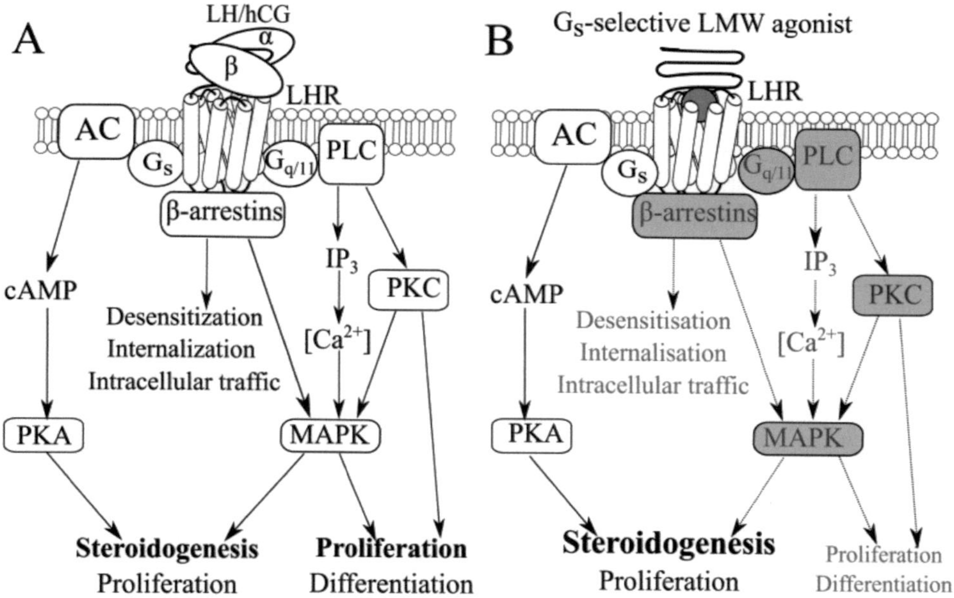

Figure 1.
The signaling pathways of the gonadotropins with LH-like activity and the G_s protein-selective LMW agonists. (A) The gonadotropins, LH and hCG, specifically bind to an ectodomain of LH receptor, which triggers the conformational changes in its serpentine domain and provokes the interaction of the intracellular regions of the receptor with the G proteins (G_s and $G_{q/11}$) and β-arrestins. The result of this is activation of the cAMP-dependent and phosphoinositide signaling pathways and the cascade of mitogen-activated protein kinases, which control the steroidogenesis, growth, differentiation, and apoptosis in the cells of reproductive tissues. A specific interaction of gonadotropin-activated LH receptor with β-arrestins induces the endocytosis of LH receptor, its degradation, or recycling. (B) The G_s-selective LMW agonists bind to the allosteric site located within the transmembrane channel of LH receptor and activate the G_s protein, triggering cAMP-signaling pathways. At the same time, these agonists do not have a significant effect on other signaling pathways. Abbreviations: AC, adenylyl cyclase; hCG, human chorionic gonadotropin; LH, luteinizing hormone; MAPK, mitogen-activated protein kinase; PKA, protein kinase A; PLC, phosphoinositide-specific phospholipase Cβ.

protein-independent stimulation of the MAPK cascade and is involved in the internalization, endocytosis, and recyclization of the gonadotropin receptor complexes [18–22]. The Ca^{2+}- and β-arrestin-dependent pathways, as well as the AC signaling system, are involved in the regulation of the synthesis and secretion of sex steroid hormones and also control the growth, differentiation, and survival of the testicular and ovarian cells (**Figure 1**). About two-thirds of gonadotropin-dependent genes are regulated through cAMP-dependent mechanisms, while the expression of another third of the genes is regulated through cAMP-independent mechanisms [23].

The choice of the intracellular signaling pathway depends on the stability and the ratio of active conformations of the LH and FSH receptors, which, in turn, is determined by (i) the type of gonadotropin and the structural features of its α- and β-subunits (the N-glycosylation, site-specific proteolysis, etc.), (ii) the structural features of the LH and FSH receptors (the posttranslational modifications, mutations, polymorphisms, etc.), and their ability to form the dimeric and oligomeric complexes, as well as (iii) the functional activity of the downstream regulatory and accessory proteins (the G proteins, β-arrestins, etc.) [6, 19, 24, 25]. A specific binding of gonadotropin to ectodomain generates a large set of the active conformations of receptor, which triggers some intracellular pathways at once and, as a result, induces multiple cell responses. For example, the placental hCG with a high efficiency stimulates the cAMP-dependent signaling pathways, being a powerful activator of the steroidogenesis, but its stimulating effect on the $G_{q/11}$-mediated signaling is realized to a much lesser extent. Moreover, the recombinant LH with a high efficiency stimulates the PLCβ- and β-arrestin-dependent signaling pathways, but weakly, in comparison with hCG, stimulates the cAMP-signaling and steroidogenesis [18].

Unlike gonadotropins, the ligands of the allosteric site that is located within the transmembrane channel of the LH and FSH receptors more selectively regulate the intracellular signaling cascades. This is due to the fact that, by binding to the allosteric site, they stabilize, as a rule, only one conformation of the gonadotropin receptor, either active or inactive. In the first case, they function as the full allosteric agonists or as the positive allosteric modulators (PAMs), enhancing the stimulating effects of gonadotropins, or as the ago-PAM, combining the effects of allosteric agonists and "pure" PAMs. In the second case, they function as the allosteric antagonists or as the negative allosteric modulators (NAMs) that prevent the activation of the LH and FSH receptors by gonadotropins [26]. Since the binding sites for the gonadotropins and the LMW allosteric ligands do not overlap, there is no competition between them. Due to this, in the case of co-administration of the gonadotropin and LMW agonist, their stimulating effects can be additive and even synergistic. Below we consider the most effective LMW allosteric ligands of the LH and FSH receptors, which were developed by us and the other authors.

3. Thienopyrimidine-based low-molecular-weight agonists of the luteinizing hormone receptor

Screening of a large number of organic compounds allowed to identify the 1,3,5-substituted pyrazole and terphenyl derivatives, which have the activity of the full and inverse allosteric agonists of LH receptor [27–30]. It was shown that a derivative of terphenyl, the compound LUF5771, inhibited the gonadotropin- and LMW agonist-induced stimulation of LH receptor, indicating that the LUF5771 belongs to the inverse agonists. This compound can be used as a prototype to develop the contraceptives and the anticancer drugs for treatment of hormone-dependent tumors [29]. The 1,3,5-substituted pyrazole derivative, 8-(1-(4-(*tert*-butyl)phenyl)-3-(pyridin-3-yl)-1*H*-pyrazol-5-yl)-2-(4-hydroxybenzyl)-4-oxooctanamide (1) (**Figure 2**), had activity of the full agonist of LH receptor [27]. It stimulated the AC activity (EC_{50}, 20 nM) and increased the synthesis and secretion of testosterone by the Leydig cells (ED_{50}, 1.31 μM), and when

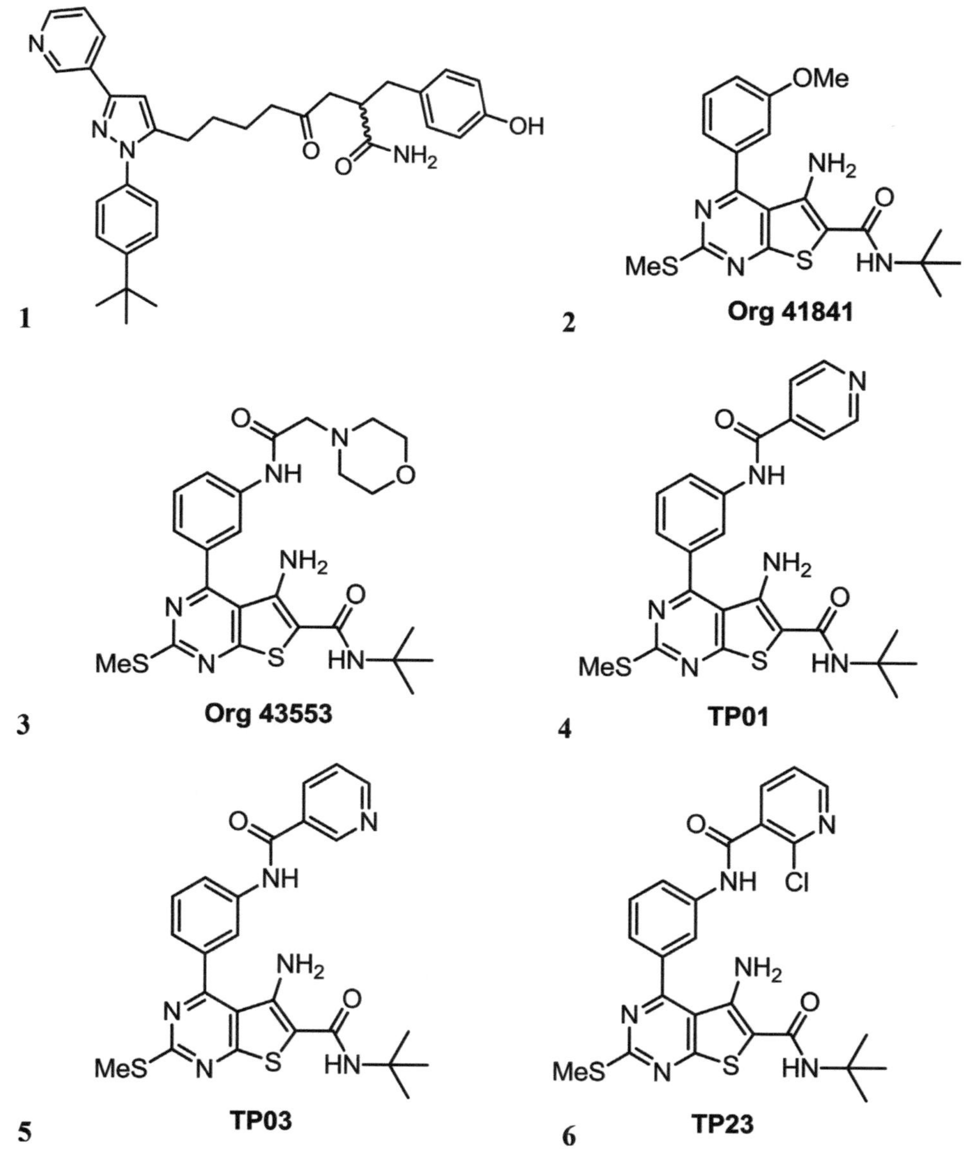

Figure 2.
The pyrazole- and thienopyrimidine-based low-molecular-weight agonists of LH receptor. (1) 8-(1-(4-(tert-butyl)phenyl)-3-(pyridin-3-yl)-1H-pyrazol-5-yl)-2-(4-hydroxybenzyl)-4-oxooctanamide [27]; (2) Compound Org 41,841, N-tert-butyl-5-amino-4-(3-methoxyphenyl)-2-(methylthio)thieno[2,3-d]pyrimidine-6-carboxamide [31]; (3) Compound Org 43,553, 5-amino-N-(tert-butyl)-2-(methylthio)-4-(3-(2-morpholinoacetamido)phenyl)thieno[2,3-d]pyrimidine-6-carboxamide [31]; (4) Compound TP01, 5-amino-N-(tert-butyl)-4-(3-(isonicotinamido)phenyl)-2-(methylthio)thieno[2,3-d]pyrimidine-6-carboxamide [32]; (5) Compound TP03, 5-amino-N-tert-butyl-2-(methylsulfanyl)-4-(3-(nicotinamido)phenyl)thieno[2,3-d]pyrimidine-6-carboxamide [33]; (6) Compound TP23, 5-amino-N- (tert-butyl)-4-(3-(2-chloronicotinamido)phenyl)-2-(methylthio)thieno[2,3-d]pyrimidine-6-carboxamide [34].

administered intraperitoneally to male rats, this compound stimulated the testosterone production in them [27]. However, the greatest success was achieved in the development of the thienopyrimidine-based agonists of LH receptor.

In 2002, as a result of screening of a large number of the organic compounds, the Dutch scientists from the Organon Company discovered the first compounds with activity of LH receptor agonists belonging to the thienopyrimidines [31]. The most effective among them were the compound Org 41,841 and its analogue Org 43,553 (**Figure 2**). Later, the pharmacological characteristics of Org 43,553 and the mechanisms of its action were studied, and this compound was considered as the "gold" standard for the allosteric agonists of LH receptor [35–39]. Based on Org 43,553 structure, we have developed and studied the series of the thienopyrimidine derivatives that with a high efficiency stimulated the AC activity and steroidogenesis in the Leydig cells in both the in vitro and in vivo conditions [33–35, 40–42]. The most active among these derivatives were the compounds TP01, TP03, and TP23 (**Figure 2**). The study of thienopyrimidine-based LMW agonists of LH receptor allowed identifying the mechanisms of their action and the pharmacological profile, which can be an advantage when using these compounds in the clinic.

Using the Org 41,841 and Org 43,553, the allosteric sites in the transmembrane channels of gonadotropins receptors and related to them thyroid-stimulating hormone (TSH) receptor were carried out. This allowed to detect the structural features of the active and inactive conformations of the serpentine domain of gonadotropins receptors, to identify the amino acid residues involved in the formation of their allosteric sites, and to decipher the mechanisms of signal transduction through these receptors [43, 44]. Based on the site-directed mutagenesis, the amino acid residues in the second extracellular loop (ECL2) and within the fifth and sixth transmembrane regions (TM5 and TM6) of TSH receptor, which form its allosteric site, were replaced with the corresponding amino acids of LH receptor, which made the allosteric site of TSH receptor similar to that in LH receptor. It was found that a single substitution, $Leu^{570}Phe$, in the ECL2 of TSH receptor resulted in the Org 41,841 binding with a mutant receptor with the EC_{50} of 800 nM, while the double substitutions, the $Leu^{570}Phe/Phe^{585}Thr$ and $Leu^{570}Phe/Tyr^{643}Phe$, led to the Org 41,841 binding with the EC_{50} of 1000 nM. These data indicate an important role of the residues $Lyr^{570}Phe$, $Phe^{585}Thr$, and $Tyr^{643}Phe$ in the formation of the allosteric site in LH receptor [43]. The simultaneous replacement of nine amino acids ($Ile^{560}Val$ and $Leu^{570}Phe$ in the ECL2; $Prp^{577}Thr$, $Ala^{579}Ser$, $Leu^{580}Gln$, $Ala^{581}Val$, and $Phe^{585}Thr$ in the TM5; and $Tyr^{643}Phe$ and $Ile^{648}Ala$ in the TM6) that form the allosteric site of TSH receptor with the corresponding amino acids of LH receptor induced a high-affinity binding of Org 41,841 with mutant TSH receptor, similar to that of LH receptor. In the cells with expressed mutant TSH receptor, the AC stimulating effects induced by the Org 41,841 and TSH were similar [43]. It was also shown that the negatively charged Glu^{506} located in the TM3 of the LH and TSH receptors has a key role in specific interaction with Org 41,841, since the substitution of $Glu^{506}Ala$ inhibits both the Org 41,841 binding to mutant LH receptor and the AC stimulating effect of Org 41,841 [43, 44].

The allosteric LMW agonists stabilize any one active conformation and, thereby, selectively stimulate preferably one intracellular cascade. It was shown that the Org 43,553 (1–10 μM) stimulated the activity of PLCβ by 33–37%, which is less than 5% of the corresponding effect of LH [36]. Moreover, the Org 43,553 effectively stimulated the activity of AC and cAMP-dependent transcription factors at lower concentrations. Based on these data, a conclusion was made on the selectivity of stimulating influence of Org 43,553 on the AC signaling system, which is realized through the G_s proteins and on the inefficiency of this compound in regard to the $G_{q/11}$ proteins and PLCβ-dependent signaling [36].

Using the bacterial toxin-induced ADP ribosylation and the peptide strategy, we showed the selectivity of the thienopyrimidine derivative TP03, as a stimulator of the AC signaling system in the rat testicular and ovarian membranes [45]. In the membranes treated with cholera toxin that hyperactivates the G_s proteins and prevents the signal transduction through them, the stimulating effects of TP03 on the AC activity and the GTP binding were suppressed. At the same time, the treatment of the plasma membranes with pertussis toxin, which inhibits the G_i proteins, and their incubation with the peptide 349–359 of $G\alpha_{q/11}$-subunit, which leads to uncoupling of the LH receptor and $G_{q/11}$ proteins, did not affect the regulatory effects of TP03. Only at high concentrations (10–100 μM), the TP03 effect on the GTP binding of $G_{q/11}$ proteins was detected but to a small extent. Under the same conditions, the regulatory effects of hCG were not specific for different types of G proteins [45]. It should be noted that the thienopyrimidine derivatives and the other allosteric ligands of LH receptor, which did not affect the AC activity and the steroidogenesis, are usually excluded from further research. However, they can activate G_s-independent signaling cascades, including the $G_{q/11}$ proteins and β-arrestins. As a consequence, these compounds may be of interest for studying the molecular mechanisms of the allosteric regulation of LH receptors and can be used in medicine.

The selectivity of signal transduction may have an important role in maintaining the tissue sensitivity to both the gonadotropins and LMW agonists, which was demonstrated by us in the case of TP03 [42]. Despite the fact that hCG and TP03 increased the testosterone levels during the 7-day treatment of male rats, a dynamics of this effect differed significantly. In long-term hCG treatment, an increase in the plasma testosterone concentration was the maximum on the first day, and then it decreased. At the same time, the steroidogenic effect of TP03, on the contrary, gradually increased, reaching a maximum on the seventh day of treatment. On the first day of treatment, TP03-induced increase in the testosterone concentration was 4 times lower than that in the case of hCG, while at the end of the experiment, the steroidogenic effects of hCG and TP03 were comparable [42]. One of the causes for this may be the specific changes in the LH receptor sensitivity to gonadotropins and thienopyrimidines, as well as the different mechanisms of their action on steroidogenesis.

A long-term administration of hCG to male rats leads to a significant decrease in the testicular expression of the *Lhr* gene encoding LH receptor, while a long-term administration of TP03 induces an increase in the *Lhr* gene expression, which is one of the factors maintaining the sensitivity of the Leydig cells to gonadotropins [42]. It should be noted that the gonadotropin resistance of the reproductive tissues is one of the urgent problems of the LH and hCG applications to treat the reproductive dysfunctions and in the assisted reproductive technologies [17, 46]. In our experiments, both the hCG and TP03 increased the expression of the *Star* gene, which encodes the steroidogenic acute regulatory protein (StAR) responsible for cholesterol transport into mitochondria, the rate-limiting stage of steroidogenesis, and gonadotropin in this regard was more active [42]. It was shown that the more the *Lhr* gene expression and the steroidogenic effect of the drug on testosterone production were decreased, the more the *Star* gene expression was increased. This may indicate a compensatory mechanism for increasing the *Star* gene expression in the conditions of the impaired gonadotropin signaling and the reduced PKA-induced stimulation of the StAR protein in the Leydig cells.

In the case of a long-term treatment of male rats with hCG, the intratesticular expression of the *Cyp11a1* gene encoding the C27 cholesterol side-chain cleavage cytochrome P450 (cytochrome $P450_{scc}$) that converts cholesterol to pregnenolone was significantly increased, and on the seventh day, the expression of the *Hsd3b* gene encoding the 3β-hydroxysteroid dehydrogenase/Δ5–4 isomerase (3β-HSD) that converts pregnenolone to progesterone was also increased. When the TP03 was used, there were no significant changes in the expression of the *Cyp11a1* and *Hsd3b* genes, which indicates a stable functioning of the steroidogenesis system in the conditions of a long-term treatment of animals with LMW agonist [42].

Along with the selectivity of the intracellular signaling induced by the thienopyrimidine derivatives, which identifies them as the selective bias agonists of LH receptor, their pharmacokinetic characteristics also contribute to the stability of the steroidogenic effect of these LMW agonists. When administered to rats, the Org 43,553 shows a half-life time of 3.4 hours, while the half-life time for hCG is 6.6 hours, indicating the more rapid degradation and excretion of LMW agonist than gonadotropin [37]. Reducing the half-life time for thienopyrimidines is of great practical importance, since it contributes to maintaining the tissue sensitivity to endogenous gonadotropins and, in addition, reduces the risk of ovarian hyperstimulation syndrome, a severe complication of gonadotropin-induced ovarian stimulation in the assisted reproductive technologies. Unlike gonadotropins, both the single and long-term treatments of female rats with Org 43,553 did not cause an increase in the ovarian diameter and the vascular permeability in the ovary and did not provoke the development of ovarian hyperstimulation syndrome [38]. Also, there were no signs of the ovarian hyperstimulation syndrome in women who received Org 43,553 orally at the doses from 25 to 900 mg. In 83% of women, the administration of Org 43,553 at a single dose of 300 mg caused the ovulation and the production of high-quality oocytes [47].

Since the orthostatic and allosteric sites in LH receptor do not overlap, the LMW allosteric agonists do not inhibit the specific LH and hCG binding [27, 35, 36]. Moreover, the AC stimulating effects of the LMW agonists and gonadotropins are additive, at least in a range of their concentrations lower than the EC_{50} values [33, 35, 36, 41]. As shown by us, the steroidogenic effect of hCG in male rats pretreated with the TP03 was enhanced significantly, and this potentiating effect of TP03 was most pronounced at the low doses of hCG (Shpakov, Bakhtyukov and Derkach, unpublished data). This effect of thienopyrimidines can be due to their chaperone-like properties (**Figure 3**). It was shown that the Org 42,599, the trifluoroacetate salt of Org 43,553, restored the activity of the mutant LH receptors with the Ala^{593}Pro and Ser^{616}Tyr replacements [48]. The incubation of the cells expressing these receptors with Org 42,599 led to an increase in the expression of the mutant receptors, the number of the receptors with the appropriate folding, and membrane topology and the receptor density on the cell surface. The chaperone-like properties of Org 42,599 are due to its ability to penetrate the plasma membrane and specifically bind to an allosteric site of intracellularly located LH receptors, which promotes their efficient translocation into the plasma membrane of the Leydig cells [48]. It should be emphasized that the LH receptors with the Ala^{593}Pro and Ser^{616}Tyr mutations in the transmembrane regions are not capable of translocation into the cell surface and cannot be activated by gonadotropins. These mutations were found in patients with hypoplasia of the Leydig cells [49–52].

The allosteric sites of closely related GPCRs are known to be characterized by the variability of the primary structure and the three-dimensional organization, which in most cases makes the allosteric regulators more specific than the orthosteric regulators [26, 53]. In the case of the receptors of pituitary glycoprotein

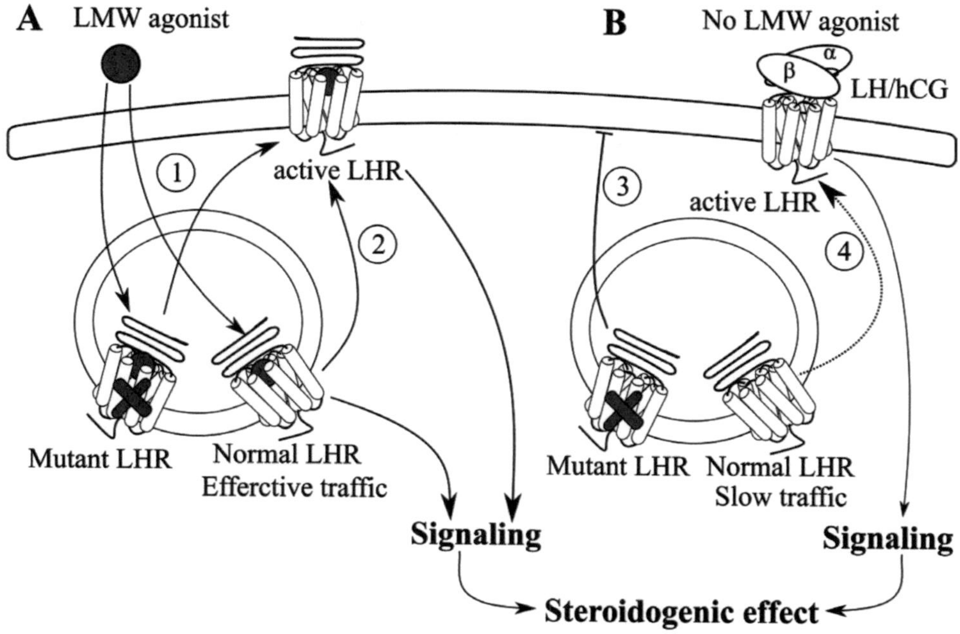

Figure 3.
The chaperone-like properties of the LMW allosteric agonists. (A) The LMW agonist, being a hydrophobic substance, penetrates the plasma membrane, interacts with normal LH receptors located in the intracellular vesicles, and ensures their effective translocation into the plasma membrane of Leydig cells (1). This effect can be realized in the case of the mutant LH receptors that are not capable of normal posttranslational processing and translocation into the membrane (2). As a result, the treatment with the LMW agonists leads to the preservation and even to an increase in the sensitivity of LH-competent cells to LH and hCG. B. In the absence of agonists, the mutant LH receptors are not able to translocate into the membrane (3), while the normal forms of the receptor are retained within the cell for a longer time (4). All this leads to a weakened response to gonadotropins with LH activity.

hormones, the specificity of LMW agonists to their allosteric site is not so high that it can be assumed to be due to the inverted position of the orthosteric and allosteric sites in these receptors as compared to other GPCRs belonging to class A [26]. At the same time, we and other authors showed that the Org 43,553, TP01, TP03, and TP23 have a very weak effect on the activity of the FSH and TSH receptors [36, 54]. When administered to male rats, the TP01, TP03, and TP23 did not affect the basal and thyroliberin-stimulated levels of thyroid hormones [54].

4. The low-molecular-weight ligands of the follicle-stimulating hormone receptor

The first LMW allosteric agonist of FSH receptor, a piperidine carboxamide, was developed in 2001. It stimulated the AC activity in the CHO cells expressing the FSH receptor (EC_{50}, 3.9 nM) but was not active in the in vivo conditions [55]. A search for new LMW ligands of FSH receptor revealed a large number of the compounds with different pharmacological activity [39, 56–58]. They belong to different classes of the organic compounds, such as the thiazolidines [59–62], substituted γ-lactams [63], diketopiperazines [64, 65], *N*-alkylated sulfonyl piperazines [66], tetrahydroquinolines [67], hexahydroquinolines [68, 69], thienopyrimidines [70], and benzamides [69]. Among the developed LMW ligands, the thiazolidines, hexa- and tetrahydroquinolines, and benzamides with activity of the full and inverse agonists and the neutral antagonists of FSH receptor are of the greatest interest.

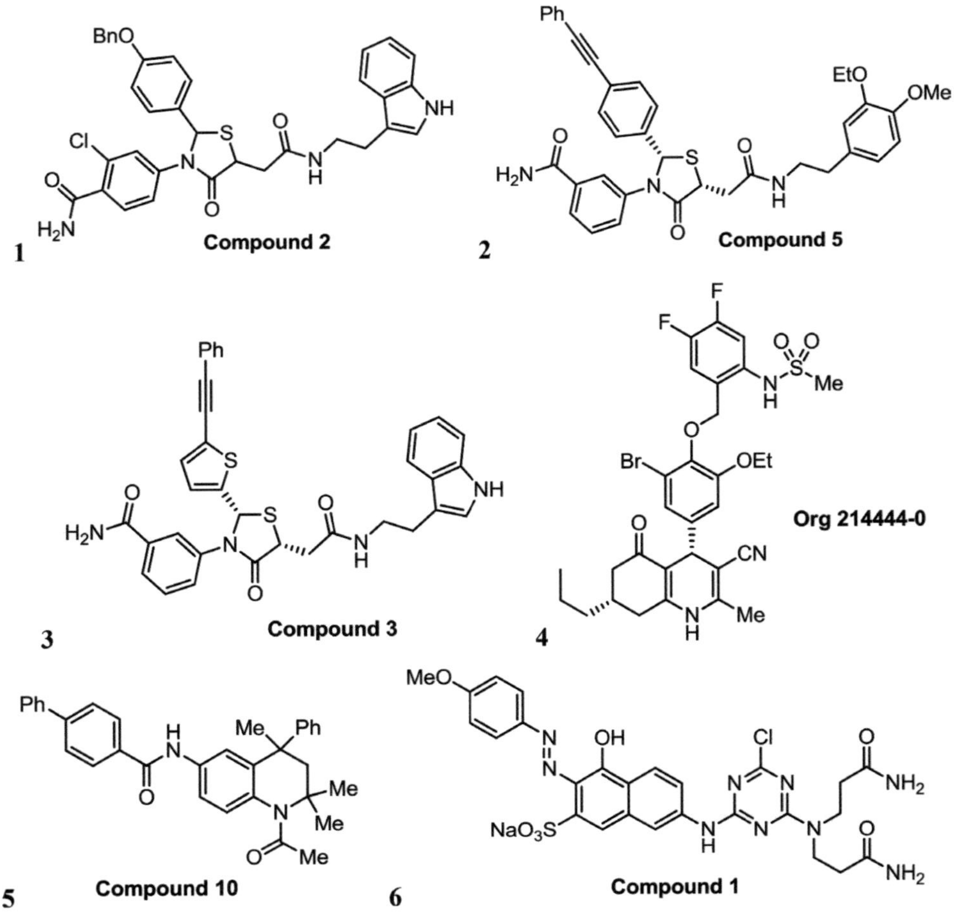

Figure 4.
The low-molecular-weight allosteric agonists and antagonists of the FSH receptor. (1) Compound 2, 4-(5-(2-((2-(1H-indol-3-yl)ethyl)amino)-2-oxoethyl)-2-(4-(benzyloxy)phenyl)-4-oxothiazolidin-3-yl)-2-chlorobenzamide [59]; (2) Compound 5, 3-(2S,5R)-5-(2-((3-ethoxy-4-methoxyphenethyl)amino)-2-oxoethyl)-4-oxo-2-(4-(phenylethynyl)phenyl)thiazolidin-3-yl)benzamide [61]; (3) Compound 3, 3-(2S,5R)-5-(2-((2-(1H-indol-3-yl)ethyl)amino)-2-oxoethyl)-4-oxo-2-(5-(phenylethynyl)thiophen-2-yl)thiazolidin-3-yl)benzamide [62]; (4) Compound Org214444–0, N-(2-((2-bromo-4-((4R,7S)-3-cyano-2-methyl-5-oxo-7-propyl-1,4,5,6,7,8-hexahydroquinolin-4-yl)-6-ethoxyphenoxy)methyl)-4,5-difluorophenyl)methanesulfonamide [68]; (5) Compound 10, N-(1-acetyl-2,2,4-trimethyl-4-phenyl-1,2,3,4-tetrahydroquinolin-6-yl)-[1,1'-biphenyl]-4-carboxamide [67]; (6) Compound 1, 7-{4-[bis-(2-carbamoyl-ethyl)-amino]-6-chloro-(1,3,5)-triazin-2-ylamino)-4-hydroxy-3-(4-methoxy-phenylazo)-naphthalene}-2-sulfonic acid sodium salt [71].

In 2004, compound 2 belonging to the thiazolidines was developed (**Figure 4**). It suppressed FSH-induced stimulating effects and, by its pharmacological profile, was classified as an inverse agonist [59]. Based on its structure, the thiazolidine derivatives with the activity of the full agonists were developed [60, 61, 63], including highly active compound 5 (**Figure 4**). This compound stimulated the cAMP-dependent cascades and the steroidogenesis in the cell cultures and in the in vivo conditions induced the development of preovulatory follicles and stimulated the ovulation in immature female rats [61, 72]. Compound 5 was able to enhance the stimulating effects of low-dose FSH, acting as the PAM for FSH receptor. Another thiazolidine derivative, compound 3 (**Figure 4**), at the low concentrations activated the G_s proteins and stimulated the cAMP-dependent cascades in the cells expressing the FSH receptor, functioning as a full agonist. At the same, at the high concentrations, compound 3 inhibited FSH-induced activation of G_s proteins and stimulated the G_i proteins, reducing the activity of AC and cAMP-dependent transcription factors, functioning as the NAM [62, 73].

In 2006, the compound Org214444–0, a derivative of 4-phenyl-5-oxo-1,4,5,6,7,8-hexahydroquinolines (**Figure 4**), was developed, which in the absence of FSH caused the AC activation in CHO cells expressing the FSH receptor (EC_{50} about 1 nM) and stimulated the steroidogenesis in the human and rat granulosa cells [68, 69]. Moreover, Org214444-0 increased the FSH affinity to receptor and the efficiency of FSH-induced AC stimulation, which makes it possible to identify this compound as ago-PAM. Oral administration of Org214444-0 led to the stimulation of the folliculogenesis and induced the ovulation in mature female rats, indicating the stability and effective absorption of Org214444-0 in the gastrointestinal tract [69].

Compound 10, a tetrahydroquinoline derivative (**Figure 4**), with a high efficiency inhibited FSH-induced follicular growth and ovulation in mice [67]. There is reason to believe that compound 10 prevents the functional interaction between the extracellular and serpentine domains of FSH receptor and, thereby, disrupts the signal transduction from the ligand-binding site located within an ectodomain to the intracellular regions of receptor that are involved in the interaction with the G_s proteins. This characterizes this compound as NAM for FSH receptor [67]. Additionally, it has been shown that the 7-{4-[bis-(2-carbamoyl-ethyl)-amino]-6-chloro-(1,3,5)-triazin-2-ylamino)-4-hydroxy-3-(4-methoxy-phenylazo)-naphthalene}-2-sulfonic acid (compound 1) (**Figure 4**), also belonging to NAM for FSH receptor, in a dose-dependent manner reduced the specific FSH binding to the receptor, suppressed the stimulating effects of FSH on the AC activity and steroidogenesis, and in the in vivo conditions prevented FSH-induced ovulation in female rats [71, 74].

Among the benzamide derivatives, the most active were the compounds ADX61623, ADX68692, and ADX68693, which demonstrated the activity of allosteric antagonists of FSH receptor [75, 76]. These compounds had an unusual pharmacological profile, which, as may be supposed, was due to the complexity of their effect on the FSH-stimulated signaling in the target cells. In the in vitro conditions, the *N*-(4-(2-cyanopropane-2-yl)phenyl)-3,4-dimethoxybenzamide (ADX61623) at the low concentrations inhibited FSH-induced production of cAMP and progesterone in follicular cells, while at the high concentrations, it increased the production of estradiol [75]. Of the three benzamide derivatives, only the ADX68692 was active when administered orally and subcutaneously to mature female rats, dysregulating the sexual cycle and reducing the number of matured oocytes [76]. However, it should be noted that the ADX68692 was able to modulate the activity of LH receptor, enhancing the production of progesterone and reducing the synthesis of testosterone in the rat Leydig cells [77].

In conclusion, it should be noted that despite the large number of the investigated allosteric ligands of FSH receptor, they are not yet used in the clinic due to the many unresolved problems with their bioavailability, the mechanisms of action, and possible undesirable effects [57, 58]. However, the limitations with the use of commercial FSH drugs in the clinic and the need to develop the selective FSH receptor inhibitors are a good stimulus to further development of the LMW ligands of FSH receptor and their implementation into clinical practice.

5. Conclusion and future perspectives

Summing up the current results in the development and study of the LMW allosteric ligands of the LH and FSH receptors, it is necessary to focus on the following advantages, which are important for their application for reproduction and molecular and clinical endocrinology, including the assisted reproductive technologies.

i. The LMW allosteric agonists of the gonadotropins receptors do not compete with the gonadotropins for the binding sites and, thus, do not suppress the effects of LH, hCG, and FSH, and in some cases they enhance them, acting as PAM or ago-PAM. The inhibition of the stimulating effect of gonadotropins by the LMW allosteric inverse agonists and NAMs is due to their allosteric effects, but not the result of the competition for receptor binding sites.

ii. The LMW ligands of the LH and FSH receptors are characterized by the selectivity for intracellular signaling cascades, functioning as the bias ligands, which allows predicting and determining the functional response of cells to their action and prevents a number of undesirable side effects that are detected when gonadotropins are used.

iii. Since the LMW agonists are selective, they, unlike gonadotropins, have a little effect on the β-arrestin signaling pathways responsible for downregulation of the receptors. As a result, under conditions of treatment with the LMW allosteric agonists, the sensitivity of the tissues to endogenous gonadotropins is preserved, which makes it possible to use the long-term courses of LMW agonists as well as to use them with the gonadotropins.

iv. The LMW allosteric ligands of the LH and FSH receptors can be active not only with their parenteral routes of administration but also with their oral delivery, since they are stable in the gastrointestinal tract and are well absorbed by intestinal cells.

v. The LMW agonists have chaperone-like properties in relation to the LH and FSH receptors, preventing their intracellular degradation and increasing their translocation to the plasma membrane. In this regard, the LMW agonists can be used to enhance the response of the reproductive system to the gonadotropins in the case of the mutant LH and FSH receptors that are not capable of translocation as well as in the conditions of the metabolic, inflammatory, and autoimmune disorders inducing the impaired posttranslational processing of these receptors. It should be noted that the mutations and polymorphisms in the gonadotropin receptors lead to a decrease in the sensitivity of the testes and ovaries to gonadotropins [78, 79]. In the assisted reproductive technologies, they reduce the response of the ovaries to the gonadotropin stimulation, which leads to the impaired folliculogenesis, the reduced output of high-quality oocytes, and the deterioration of the development and implantation of the embryo [78, 80]. Since both gonadotropins, LH and FSH, play an important role in the development and maturation of the follicles and oocytes, the polymorphisms in the LH and FSH receptors can be the main causes of an impairment of folliculogenesis and oogenesis, including their late stages [79, 81, 82].

Despite the advantages listed above, the LMW allosteric ligands of the LH and FSH receptors have not yet found use in the clinic. The main reason is insufficient knowledge of the pharmacokinetics and the distribution of these compounds in the body, as well as the problems with the development of their dosage forms, especially since most of these compounds are highly hydrophobic and dissolve in DMSO. The attempts to reduce the hydrophobicity of LMW ligands by modifying their structure lead to the partial or complete loss of their specific activity, due to their reduced ability of penetration into the transmembrane channel of the gonadotropins receptors. The most promising approach to solve this problem is to use the solubilizing agents that can increase the water solubility of these compounds.

Thus, the development of the LMW allosteric ligands of the gonadotropin receptors, which have a high specificity in regulating certain signaling pathways and effector systems in the testicular and ovarian cells, opens up a promising way to create a new generation of highly selective drugs that can be used to treat and prevent the reproductive disorders and in assisted reproductive technologies, both separately and in combination with gonadotropins and other regulators of the hypothalamic-pituitary-gonadal axis.

Acknowledgements

This work was supported by the Russian Science Foundation (project No 19-75-20122).

Disclosure

Conflicts of interest are absent.

Abbreviations

AC	adenylyl cyclase
ECL_2	second extracellular loop
FSH	follicle-stimulating hormone
GPCR	G protein-coupled receptor
hCG	human chorionic gonadotropin
LH	luteinizing hormone
LMW ligand	low-molecular-weight ligand
MAPK	mitogen-activated protein kinases
NAM	negative allosteric modulator
PAM	positive allosteric modulator
PLCβ	phosphoinositide-specific phospholipase Cβ
TSH	thyroid-stimulating hormone

Author details

Alexander O. Shpakov[1*], Kira V. Derkach[1], Andrey A. Bakhtyukov[1] and Dmitry V. Dar'in[2]

1 Sechenov Institute of Evolutionary Physiology and Biochemistry, Russian Academy of Sciences, St. Petersburg, Russia

2 Institute of Chemistry, St. Petersburg State University, Russia

*Address all correspondence to: alex_shpakov@list.ru

References

[1] De Leo V, Musacchio MC, Di Sabatino A, Tosti C, Morgante G, Petraglia F. Present and future of recombinant gonadotropins in reproductive medicine. Current Pharmaceutical Biotechnology. 2012;**13**(3):379-391. DOI: 10.2174/138920112799361918

[2] Ezcurra D, Humaidan P. A review of luteinising hormone and human chorionic gonadotropin when used in assisted reproductive technology. Reproductive Biology and Endocrinology. 2014;**12**:95. DOI: 10.1186/1477-7827-12-95

[3] Plant TM. 60 years of neuroendocrinology: The hypothalamo-pituitary-gonadal axis. The Journal of Endocrinology. 2015;**226**:T41-T54. DOI: 10.1530/JOE-15-0113

[4] Ulloa-Aguirre A, Lira-Albarrán S. Clinical applications of gonadotropins in the male. Progress in Molecular Biology and Translational Science. 2016;**143**:121-174. DOI: 10.1016/bs.pmbts.2016.08.003

[5] Levi Setti PE, Alviggi C, Colombo GL, Pisanelli C, Ripellino C, Longobardi S, et al. Human recombinant follicle stimulating hormone (rFSH) compared to urinary human menopausal gonadotropin (HMG) for ovarian stimulation in assisted reproduction: A literature review and cost evaluation. Journal of Endocrinological Investigation. 2015;**38**(5):497-503. DOI: 10.1007/s40618-014-0204-4

[6] Fournier T. Human chorionic gonadotropin: Different glycoforms and biological activity depending on its source of production. Annales de Endocrinologie. 2016;**77**(2):75-81. DOI: 10.1016/j.ando.2016.04.012

[7] Van Dorsselaer A, Carapito C, Delalande F, Schaeffer-Reiss C, Thierse D, Diemer H, et al. Detection of prion protein in urine-derived injectable fertility products by a targeted proteomic approach. PLoS One. 2011;**6**:e17815. DOI: 10.1371/journal.pone.0017815

[8] Cole LA. hCG, the wonder of today's science. Reproductive Biology and Endocrinology. 2012;**10**:24. DOI: 10.1186/1477-7827-10-24

[9] Theofanakis C, Drakakis P, Besharat A, Loutradis D. Human chorionic gonadotropin: The pregnancy hormone and more. International Journal of Molecular Sciences. 2017;**18**(5):pii: E1059. DOI: 10.3390/ijms18051059

[10] Bousfield GR, Dias JA. Synthesis and secretion of gonadotropins including structure-function correlates. Reviews in Endocrine and Metabolic Disorders. 2011;**12**(4):289-302. DOI: 10.1007/s11154-011-9191-3

[11] Ji I, Lee C, Jeoung M, Koo Y, Sievert GA, Ji TH. Trans-activation of mutant follicle-stimulating hormone receptors selectively generates only one of two hormone signals. Molecular Endocrinology. 2004;**18**:968-978. DOI: 10.1210/me.2003-0443

[12] Puett D, Li Y, DeMars G, Angelova K, Fanelli F. A functional transmembrane complex: The luteinizing hormone receptor with bound ligand and G protein. Molecular and Cellular Endocrinology. 2007;**260-262**:126-136. DOI: 10.1016/j.mce.2006.05.009

[13] Puett D, Angelova K, da Costa MR, Warrenfeltz SW, Fanelli F. The luteinizing hormone receptor: Insights into structure-function relationships and hormone-receptor-mediated changes in gene expression in ovarian cancer cells. Molecular and Cellular

Endocrinology. 2010;**329**(1-2):47-55. DOI: 10.1016/j.mce.2010.04.025

[14] Angelova K, Felline A, Lee M, Patel M, Puett D, Fanelli F. Conserved amino acids participate in the structure networks deputed to intramolecular communication in the lutropin receptor. Cellular and Molecular Life Sciences. 2011;**68**(7):1227-1239. DOI: 10.1007/s00018-010-0519-z

[15] Ulloa-Aguirre A, Dias JA, Bousfield G, Huhtaniemi I, Reiter E. Trafficking of the follitropin receptor. Methods in Enzymology. 2013;**521**:17-45. DOI: 10.1016/B978-0-12-391862-8.00002-8

[16] De Pascali F, Tréfier A, Landomiel F, Bozon V, Bruneau G, Yvinec R, et al. Follicle-stimulating hormone receptor: Advances and remaining challenges. International Review of Cell and Molecular Biology. 2018;**338**:1-58. DOI: 10.1016/bs.ircmb.2018.02.001

[17] Riccetti L, De Pascali F, Gilioli L, Potì F, Giva LB, Marino M, et al. Human LH and hCG stimulate differently the early signalling pathways but result in equal testosterone synthesis in mouse Leydig cells *in vitro*. Reproductive Biology and Endocrinology. 2017;**15**(1):2. DOI: 10.1186/s12958-016-0224-3

[18] Riccetti L, Yvinec R, Klett D, Gallay N, Combarnous Y, Reiter E, et al. Human luteinizing hormone and chorionic gonadotropin display biased agonism at the LH and LH/CG receptors. Scientific Reports. 2017;**7**(1):940. DOI: 10.1038/s41598-017-01078-8

[19] Landomiel F, De Pascali F, Raynaud P, Jean-Alphonse F, Yvinec R, Pellissier LP, et al. Biased signaling and allosteric modulation at the FSHR. Frontiers in Endocrinology. 2019;**10**:148. DOI: 10.3389/fendo.2019.00148

[20] Kara E, Crépieux P, Gauthier C, Martinat N, Piketty V, Guillou F, et al. A phosphorylation cluster of five serine and threonine residues in the C-terminus of the follicle-stimulating hormone receptor is important for desensitization but not for beta-arrestin-mediated ERK activation. Molecular Endocrinology. 2006;**20**(11):3014-3026. DOI: 10.1210/me.2006-0098

[21] Reiter E, Ahn S, Shukla AK, Lefkowitz RJ. Molecular mechanism of beta-arrestin-biased agonism at seven-transmembrane receptors. Annual Review of Pharmacology and Toxicology. 2012;**52**:179-197. DOI: 10.1146/annurev.pharmtox.010909.105800

[22] Casarini L, Reiter E, Simoni M. β-Arrestins regulate gonadotropin receptor-mediated cell proliferation and apoptosis by controlling different FSHR or LHCGR intracellular signaling in the hGL5 cell line. Molecular and Cellular Endocrinology. 2016;**437**:11-21. DOI: 10.1016/j.mce.2016.08.005

[23] Ulloa-Aguirre A, Crepieux P, Poupon A, Maurel MC, Reiter E. Novel pathways in gonadotropin receptor signaling and biased agonism. Reviews in Endocrine and Metabolic Disorders. 2011;**12**(4):259-274. DOI: 10.1007/s11154-011-9176-2

[24] Fournier T, Guibourdenche J, Evain-Brion D. Review: hCGs—Different sources of production, different glycoforms and functions. Placenta. 2015;**36**(Suppl 1):S60-S65. DOI: 10.1016/j.placenta.2015.02.002

[25] Nwabuobi C, Arlier S, Schatz F, Guzeloglu-Kayisli O, Lockwood CJ, Kayisli UA. hCG: Biological functions and clinical applications. International Journal of Molecular Sciences. 2017;**18**(10):pii: E2037. DOI: 10.3390/ijms18102037

[26] van der Westhuizen ET, Valant C, Sexton PM, Christopoulos A.

Endogenous allosteric modulators of G protein-coupled receptors. The Journal of Pharmacology and Experimental Therapeutics. 2015;**353**:246-260. DOI: 10.1124/jpet.114.221606

[27] Jorand-Lebrun C, Brondyk B, Lin J, Magar S, Murray R, Reddy A, et al. Identification, synthesis, and biological evaluation of novel pyrazoles as low molecular weight luteinizing hormone receptor agonists. Bioorganic and Medicinal Chemistry Letters. 2007;**17**(7):2080-2085. DOI: 10.1016/j.bmcl.2006.12.062

[28] Heitman LH, Ijzerman AP. G protein-coupled receptors of the hypothalamic-pituitary-gonadal axis: A case for Gnrh, LH, FSH, and GPR54 receptor ligands. Medicinal Research Reviews. 2008;**28**:975-1011. DOI: 10.1002/med.20129

[29] Heitman LH, Narlawar R, de Vries H, Willemsen MN, Wolfram D, Brussee J, et al. Substituted terphenyl compounds as the first class of low molecular weight allosteric inhibitors of the luteinizing hormone receptor. Journal of Medicinal Chemistry. 2009;**52**:2036-2042. DOI: 10.1021/jm801561h

[30] Heitman LH, Kleinau G, Brussee J, Krause G, Ijzerman AP. Determination of different putative allosteric binding pockets at the lutropin receptor by using diverse drug-like low molecular weight ligands. Molecular and Cellular Endocrinology. 2012;**351**(2):326-336. DOI: 10.1016/j.mce.2012.01.010

[31] van Straten NC, Schoonus-Gerritsma GG, van Someren RG, Draaijer J, Adang AE, Timmers CM, et al. The first orally active low molecular weight agonists for the LH receptor: Thienopyr(im)idines with therapeutic potential for ovulation induction. Chembiochem: A European Journal of Chemical Biology. 2002;**3**(10):1023-1026. DOI: 10.1002/1439-7633(20021004)3:10<1023::AID-CBIC1023>3.0.CO;2-9

[32] Shpakov AO, Dar'in DV, Derkach KV, Lobanov PS. The stimulating influence of thieno pyrimidine compounds on the adenylyl cyclase systems in the rat testes. Doklady Biochemistry and Biophysics. 2014;**456**:104-107. DOI: 10.1134/S1607672914030065

[33] Derkach KV, Dar'in DV, Bakhtyukov AA, Lobanov PS, Shpakov AO. In vitro and in vivo studies of functional activity of new low molecular weight agonists of the luteinizing hormone receptor. Biochemistry (Moscow). Supplement Series A: Membrane and Cell Biology. 2016;**10**(4):294-300. DOI: 10.1134/S1990747816030132

[34] Derkach KV, Legkodukh AS, Dar'in DV, Shpakov AO. The stimulating effect of thienopyrimidines structurally similar to Org 43553 on adenylate cyclase activity in the testes and on testosterone production in male rats. Cell and Tissue Biology. 2017;**11**(1):73-80. DOI: 10.1134/S1990519X17010035

[35] Heitman LH, Oosterom J, Bonger KM, Timmers CM, Wiegerinck PHG, Ijzerman AP. [^{3}H]org 43553, the first low-molecular-weight agonistic and allosteric radioligand for the human luteinizing hormone receptor. Molecular Pharmacology. 2008;**73**(2):518-524. DOI: 10.1124/mol.107.039875

[36] van Koppen CJ, Zaman GJ, Timmers CM, Kelder J, Mosselman S, van de Lagemaat R, et al. A signaling-selective, nanomolar potent allosteric low molecular weight agonist for the human luteinizing hormone receptor. Naunyn-Schmiedeberg's Archives of Pharmacology. 2008;**378**(5):503-514. DOI: 10.1007/s00210-008-0318-3

[37] van de Lagemaat R, Timmers CM, Kelder J, van Koppen C, Mosselman S, Hanssen RG. Induction of ovulation by a potent, orally active, low molecular weight agonist (Org 43553) of the luteinizing hormone receptor. Human Reproduction. 2009;**24**(3):640-648. DOI: 10.1093/humrep/den412

[38] van de Lagemaat R, Raafs BC, van Koppen C, Timmers CM, Mulders SM, Hanssen RG. Prevention of the onset of ovarian hyperstimulation syndrome (OHSS) in the rat after ovulation induction with a low molecular weight agonist of the LH receptor compared with hCG and rec-LH. Endocrinology. 2011;**152**(11):4350-4357. DOI: 10.1210/en.2011-1077

[39] van Straten NC, Timmers CM. Non-peptide ligands for the gonadotropin receptors. Annual Reports in Medicinal Chemistry. 2009;**44**:171-188. DOI: 10.1016/S0065-7743(09)04408-X

[40] Derkach KV, Dar'in DV, Lobanov PS, Shpakov AO. Intratesticular, intraperitoneal, and oral administration of thienopyrimidine derivatives increases the testosterone level in male rats. Doklady Biological Sciences. 2014;**459**(1):326-329. DOI: 10.1134/S0012496614060040

[41] Shpakov AO, Derkach KV, Dar'in DV, Lobanov PS. Activation of adenylyl cyclase by thienopyrimidine derivatives in rat testes and ovaries. Cell and Tissue Biology. 2014;**8**(5):400-406. DOI: 10.1134/S1990519X14050071

[42] Bakhtyukov AA, Derkach KV, Dar'in DV, Shpakov AO. Conservation of steroidogenic effect of the low-molecular-weight agonist of luteinizing hormone receptor in the course of its long-term administration to male rats. Doklady Biochemistry and Biophysics. 2019;**484**:78-81. DOI: 10.1134/S1607672919 010216

[43] Jäschke H, Neumann S, Moore S, Thomas CJ, Colson AO, Costanzi S, et al. A low molecular weight agonist signals by binding to the transmembrane domain of thyroid-stimulating hormone receptor (TSHR) and luteinizing hormone/chorionic gonadotropin receptor (LHCGR). The Journal of Biological Chemistry. 2006;**281**(15):9841-9844. DOI: 10.1074/jbc.C600014200

[44] Moore S, Jaeschke H, Kleinau G, Neumann S, Costanzi S, Jiang JK, et al. Evaluation of small-molecule modulators of the luteinizing hormone/choriogonadotropin and thyroid stimulating hormone receptors: Structure-activity relationships and selective binding patterns. Journal of Medicinal Chemistry. 2006;**49**(13):3888-3896. DOI: 10.1021/jm060247s

[45] Derkach KV, Bakhtyukov AA, Shpakov AA, Dar'in DV, Shpakov AO. Specificity of heterotrimeric G protein regulation by human chorionic gonadotropin and low-molecular agonist of luteinizing hormone receptor. Cell and Tissue Biology. 2017;**11**(6):475-482. DOI: 10.1134/S1990519X17060037

[46] Banker M, Garcia-Velasco JA. Revisiting ovarian hyper stimulation syndrome: Towards OHSS free clinic. Journal of Human Reproductive Sciences. 2015;**8**:13-17. DOI: 10.4103/0974-1208.153120

[47] Gerrits M, Mannaerts B, Kramer H, Addo S, Hanssen R. First evidence of ovulation induced by oral LH agonists in healthy female volunteers of reproductive age. The Journal of Clinical Endocrinology and Metabolism. 2013;**98**:1558-1566. DOI: 10.1210/jc.2012-3404

[48] Newton CL, Whay AM, McArdle CA, Zhang M, van Koppen CJ, van de Lagemaat R, et al. Rescue of expression and signaling of human luteinizing hormone G protein-coupled

receptor mutants with an allosterically binding small-molecule agonist. Proceedings of the National Academy of Sciences of the United States of America. 2011;**108**(17):7172-7176. DOI: 10.1073/pnas.1015723108

[49] Kremer H, Kraaij R, Toledo SP, Post M, Fridman JB, Hayashida CY, et al. Male pseudohermaphroditism due to a homozygous missense mutation of the luteinizing hormone receptor gene. Nature Genetics. 1995;**9**(2):160-164. DOI: 10.1038/ng0295-160

[50] Latronico AC, Anasti J, Arnhold IJ, Rapaport R, Mendonca BB, Bloise W, et al. Brief report: Testicular and ovarian resistance to luteinizing hormone caused by inactivating mutations of the luteinizing hormone-receptor gene. The New England journal of medicine. 1996;**334**(8):507-512. DOI: 10.1056/NEJM199602223340805

[51] Mizrachi D, Segaloff DL. Intracellularly located misfolded glycoprotein hormone receptors associate with different chaperone proteins than their cognate wild-type receptors. Molecular Endocrinology. 2004;**18**(7):1768-1777. DOI: 10.1210/me.2003-0406

[52] Ulloa-Aguirre A, Zariñán T, Dias JA, Conn PM. Mutations in G protein-coupled receptors that impact receptor trafficking and reproductive function. Molecular and Cellular Endocrinology. 2014;**382**(1):411-423. DOI: 10.1016/j.mce.2013.06.024

[53] Lindsley CW, Emmitte KA, Hopkins CR, Bridges TM, Gregory KJ, Niswender CM, et al. Practical strategies and concepts in GPCR allosteric modulator discovery: Recent advances with metabotropic glutamate receptors. Chemical Reviews. 2016;**116**(11):6707-6741. DOI: 10.1021/acs.chemrev.5b00656

[54] Bakhtyukov AA, Derkach KV, Dar'in DV, Shpakov AO. Thienopyrimidine derivatives specifically activate testicular steroidogenesis but do not affect thyroid functions. Journal of Evolutionary Biochemistry and Physiology. 2019;**55**(1):30-39. DOI: 10.1134/S0022093019010046

[55] El Tayer N, Reddy A, Buckler D. Applied Research Systems ARS Holding NA, Assignee FSH Mimetics for the Treatment of Infertility. Unites States Patent US 6,235,755; 2001

[56] Nataraja SG, Yu HN, Palmer SS. Discovery and development of small molecule allosteric modulators of glycoprotein hormone receptors. Frontiers in Endocrinology. 2015;**6**:142. DOI: 10.3389/fendo.2015.00142

[57] Anderson RC, Newton CL, Anderson RA, Millar RP. Gonadotropins and their analogs: Current and potential clinical applications. Endocrine Reviews. 2018;**39**(6):911-937. DOI: 10.1210/er.2018-00052

[58] Anderson RC, Newton CL, Millar RP. Small molecule follicle-stimulating hormone receptor agonists and antagonists. Frontiers in Endocrinology. 2019;**9**:757. DOI: 10.3389/fendo.2018.00757

[59] Maclean D, Holden F, Davis AM, Scheuerman RA, Yanofsky S, Holmes CP, et al. Agonists of the follicle stimulating hormone receptor from an encoded thiazolidinone library. Journal of Combinatorial Chemistry. 2004;**6**(2):196-206. DOI: 10.1021/cc0300154

[60] Wrobel J, Jetter J, Kao W, Rogers J, Di L, Chi J, et al. 5-alkylated thiazolidinones as follicle-stimulating hormone (FSH) receptor agonists. Bioorganic and Medicinal Chemistry. 2006;**14**(16):5729-5741. DOI: 10.1016/j.bmc.2006.04.012

[61] Yanofsky SD, Shen ES, Holden F, Whitehorn E, Aguilar B, Tate E, et al.

Allosteric activation of the follicle-stimulating hormone (FSH) receptor by selective, nonpeptide agonists. The Journal of Biological Chemistry. 2006;**281**(19):13226-13233. DOI: 10.1074/jbc.M600601200

[62] Arey BJ. Allosteric modulators of glycoprotein hormone receptors: Discovery and therapeutic potential. Endocrine. 2008;**34**:1-10. DOI: 10.1007/s12020-008-9098-2

[63] Pelletier JC, Rogers J, Wrobel J, Perez MC, Shen ES. Preparation of highly substituted gamma-lactam follicle stimulating hormone receptor agonists. Bioorganic and Medicinal Chemistry. 2005;**13**:5986-5995. DOI: 10.1016/j.bmc.2005.07.025

[64] Guo T, Adang AE, Dolle RE, Dong G, Fitzpatrick D, Geng P, et al. Small molecule biaryl FSH receptor agonists. Part 1: Lead discovery via encoded combinatorial synthesis. Bioorganic and Medicinal Chemistry Letters. 2004;**14**(7):1713-1716. DOI: 10.1016/j.bmcl.2004.01.043

[65] Guo T, Adang AE, Dong G, Fitzpatrick D, Geng P, Ho KK, et al. Small molecule biaryl FSH receptor agonists. Part 2: Lead optimization via parallel synthesis. Bioorganic and Medicinal Chemistry Letters. 2004;**14**(7):1717-1720. DOI: 10.1016/j.bmcl.2004.01.043

[66] Magar S, Goutopoulos A, Liao Y, Schwarz M, Russell TJ. Piperazine Derivatives and Methods of Use. Patent WO2004031182A1; 2002

[67] Van Straten NC, van Berkel TH, Demont DR, Karstens WJ, Merkx R, Oosterom J, et al. Identification of substituted 6-amino-4-phenyltetrahydroquinoline derivatives: Potent antagonists for the follicle-stimulating hormone receptor. Journal of Medicinal Chemistry. 2005;**48**(6):1697-1700. DOI: 10.1021/jm049676l

[68] Grima Poveda PM, Karstens Willem FJ, Timmers CM. Inventors, NV Organon, Assignee 4-Phenyl-5-Oxo-1,4,5,6,7,8-Hexahydroquinoline Derivatives for the Treatment of Infertility. United States patent US 8,022,218; 2006

[69] van Koppen CJ, Verbost PM, van de Lagemaat R, Karstens WJ, Loozen HJ, van Achterberg TA, et al. Signaling of an allosteric, nanomolar potent, low molecular weight agonist for the follicle-stimulating hormone receptor. Biochemical Pharmacology. 2013;**85**(8):1162-1170. DOI: 10.1016/j.bcp.2013.02.001

[70] Hanssen RGJM, Timmers CM. Thieno[2,3-d]pyrimidines with combined LH and FSH agonistic activity. World Patent WO2003020726. 2003

[71] Arey BJ, Deecher DC, Shen ES, Stevis PE, Meade EH, Wrobel J, et al. Identification and characterization of a selective, nonpeptide follicle-stimulating hormone receptor antagonist. Endocrinology. 2002;**143**:3822-3829

[72] Sriraman V, Denis D, de Matos D, Yu H, Palmer S, Nataraja S. Investigation of a thiazolidinone derivative as an allosteric modulator of follicle stimulating hormone receptor: Evidence for its ability to support follicular development and ovulation. Biochemical Pharmacology. 2014;**89**(2):266-275. DOI: 10.1016/j.bcp.2014.02.023

[73] Zoenen M, Urizar E, Swillens S, Vassart G, Costagliola S. Evidence for activity-regulated hormone-binding cooperativity across glycoprotein hormone receptor homomers. Nature Communications. 2012;**3**:1007. DOI: 10.1038/ncomms1991

[74] Wrobel J, Green D, Jetter J, Kao W, Rogers J, Pérez MC, et al. Synthesis of (bis)sulfonic acid, (bis)benzamides as follicle-stimulating hormone (FSH) antagonists. Bioorganic and Medicinal Chemistry. 2002;**10**(3):639-656. DOI: 10.1016/S0968-0896(01)00324-8

[75] Dias JA, Bonnet B, Weaver BA, Watts J, Kluetzman K, Thomas RM, et al. A negative allosteric modulator demonstrates biased antagonism of the follicle stimulating hormone receptor. Molecular and Cellular Endocrinology. 2011;**333**:143-150. DOI: 10.1016/j.mce.2010.12.023

[76] Dias JA, Campo B, Weaver BA, Watts J, Kluetzman K, Thomas RM, et al. Inhibition of follicle-stimulating hormone-induced preovulatory follicles in rats treated with a nonsteroidal negative allosteric modulator of follicle-stimulating hormone receptor. Biology of Reproduction. 2014;**90**:19. DOI: 10.1095/biolreprod.113.109397

[77] Ayoub MA, Yvinec R, Jégot G, Dias JA, Poli SM, Poupon A, et al. Profiling of FSHR negative allosteric modulators on LH/CGR reveals biased antagonism with implications in steroidogenesis. Molecular and Cellular Endocrinology. 2016;**436**:10-22. DOI: 10.1016/j.mce.2016.07.013

[78] Riccetti L, De Pascali F, Gilioli L, Santi D, Brigante G, Simoni M, et al. Genetics of gonadotropins and their receptors as markers of ovarian reserve and response in controlled ovarian stimulation. Best practice & research. Clinical Obstetrics and Gynaecology. 2017;**44**:15-25. DOI: 10.1016/j.bpobgyn.2017.04.002

[79] Chen C, Xu X, Kong L, Li P, Zhou F, Zhao S, et al. Novel homozygous nonsense mutations in LHCGR lead to empty follicle syndrome and 46, XY disorder of sex development. Human Reproduction. 2018;**33**(7):1364-1369. DOI: 10.1093/humrep/dey215

[80] Binder H, Strick R, Zaherdoust O, Dittrich R, Hamori M, Beckmann MW, et al. Assessment of FSHR variants and antimüllerian hormone in infertility patients with a reduced ovarian response to gonadotropin stimulation. Fertility and Sterility. 2012;**97**(5):1169-75.e1. DOI: 10.1016/j.fertnstert.2012.02.012

[81] Lisi F, Caserta D, Montanino M, Berlinghieri V, Bielli W, Carfagna P, et al. Recombinant luteinizing hormone priming in multiple follicular stimulation for in-vitro fertilization in downregulated patients. Gynecological Endocrinology. 2012;**28**(9):674-677. DOI: 10.3109/09513590.2011.652716

[82] Rahman A, Francomano D, Sagnella F, Lisi F, Manna C. The effect on clinical results of adding recombinant LH in late phase of ovarian stimulation of patients with repeated implantation failure: A pilot study. European Review for Medical and Pharmacological Sciences. 2017;**21**(23):5485-5490. DOI: 10.26355/eurrev_201712_13939

Chapter 8

Proteomics as a Future Tool for Improving IVF Outcome

Goran Mitulović and Tanja Panić-Janković

Abstract

New technical and methodical and more efficient approaches beyond preimplantation genetic screening (PGS) are needed to elevate success rates in in vitro fertilization (IVF). One new approach could be the characterization of the embryos' proteome during the IVF process. This means that specific proteins secreted by the embryo in the surrounding cultivating medium can be analyzed and compared between embryos in order to identify potential markers for a successful embryo transfer and resulting pregnancy. Furthermore, this procedure could result with understanding the processes during the whole time of incubation, from the moment of oocyte fertilization until embryo transfer and subsequently implantation by analyzing the culturing medium used in multiple culture medium exchange during the cultivation period. This procedure of embryo transfer to a new culture medium is essential for the embryo's development and is performed daily or at least when the embryos reached the stage of embryoblast at day 4. The remaining medium after embryo removal is routinely discarded. However, this medium still can be useful for a detailed analysis of proteins and lipids that were secreted by the embryo during the previous incubation process and could help gaining information on the embryos' current developmental status.

Keywords: in vitro fertilization, proteomics, pregnancy, oocyte, pregnancy outcome

1. Introduction

The European Society of Human Reproduction and Embryology (ESHRE) report from February 2018 shows that Europe continues to lead the world with approximately 50% of all reported in vitro fertilization (IVF) cycles. The latest figures are available for 2014, and these show that 39 European countries reported almost 800.000 cycles, which compare to 150.000 cycles in the USA or 65.000 cycles in Australia and New Zealand (https://www.eshre.eu/~/media/sitecore-files/Guidelines/ART-fact-sheet_vFebr18_VG.pdf?la=en). Although there are no official reports from China, it is estimated that this country performs more than 800.000 IVF cycles with a tendency to grow. In summary, the ESHRE estimates that around 2.5 million IVF cycles is performed every year and that about 500.000 babies are born following the IVF.

The pregnancy rate depends on the embryo quality, and in Europe in 2014, the mean pregnancy rate per embryo transfer was 35% after IVF, 33% after ICSI, 30% after frozen embryo transfer, and 59% after egg donation. It is observed that pregnancy rates are higher in younger patients (<35 years).

IntechOpen

There are large differences between countries concerning the number of embryos transferred and the resulting multiple births that can occur following the multiple embryo transfer. Multiple pregnancies are classified as high-risk pregnancies and pose a significant health risk to both the mother and baby. However, regardless of that, the practice of multiple embryo transfer is still present, and it is being widely used in order to increase the chances of pregnancy. Currently, efforts are made to reduce the number of multiple embryo transfer, and a mean of 1.81 embryos per transfer is being reported. In Europe, according to the report of the European Society of Human Reproduction and Embryology, the number of multiple delivery rates for embryo transfers dropped from 26.9% in year 2000 to 17.5% in 2014 (latest data available), and it is expected to decline further. Some countries, e.g., Sweden, has reached a very low multiple delivery rate, and the single embryo transfer was performed in more than two-thirds of all transfers.

The importance of IVF in society is also highlighted by the 2010 Nobel Prize which has been awarded to Robert Edwards who is, together with Robert Steptoe, the "father" of the fist "IVF-Baby."

The IVF process is an utmost stressful, both physically and psychologically, for both parents but primarily for the mother-in-being. A number of physical examinations and medical procedures are being performed in order to ensure that the process will lead to a successful pregnancy.

During the IVF process, especially when decisions are made which embryo shall be transferred in order to ensure the greatest chance for success, the best possible decision, based on the fast and accurate information on the status of the embryo, is needed. Due to the increasing age of mothers-to-be, during the past years, a steady increase in pregnancies following artificial reproductive techniques (ART), namely, IVF and intra-cytoplasmatic sperm injection (ICSI), was observed. The reasons for this development must be seen in economic, educational, and social factors, which lead to steadily rising rates of elderly patients. With increasing age, fecundability and fertility decrease. However, the advances made in reproductive medicine itself might be one of the reasons, why an increasing number of women delay childbearing, hoping for late babies and consciously making decisions to use the help of reproductive medicine.

The elevation of pregnancy rates for IVF procedures is certainly needed in order to reduce the burden on patients and lower costs affiliated with the procedures, which very often must be repeated until a pregnancy is reached and the embryo develops to successful birth. New technologies and methods more efficient than the current approach using PGS are needed. One new approach could be the analysis of the embryos' proteome during the IVF process. This means to analyze the specific proteins that are secreted by the embryo in the IVF surrounding of the culture medium. Routinely, the medium left after embryo transfer is being discarded. The multiple embryo transfer occurring during the IVF procedure is necessary after the fertilization step, and the spent media are a rich source of biological material that can be used for diagnostic purpose. This procedure of embryo transfer to a new culture medium is essential for the embryo's development and occurs daily or at least when the embryos have achieved the stage of embryoblast at day 4.

The spent medium can be useful for a detailed examination of proteins and lipids that were secreted by the embryo during each stage of development and can be used for the estimation of the "embryo quality" and selection of corresponding embryos for primary transfer.

An overview of technologies and approaches being used and a simplified experimental approach are presented in this chapter. The method used in our laboratory is used just as an example of the technologies used, and a number of different approaches will be discussed.

2. Materials and methods

2.1 Analyzed embryo cultivation medium: source of the material

Embryo cultivation medium is usually being discarded during the IVF procedure although it can be used for multiple diagnostic and prognostic procedures. Certainly, ethical and moral guidelines and procedures must be observed, and the ethical board or other corresponding bodies must approve of the use of this material. The following experiments have been performed by using cultivation media from IVF media upon approval from the ethical boards of the Medical University in Vienna and the University of Linz in Austria. Samples were collected during different stages of embryo development and analyzed using methods established for analysis of low samples amounts.

2.2 Proteomics sample preparation

Trypsin for protein digestion was purchased from Promega Inc. (Vienna, Austria). Solvents for HPLC—methanol (MeOH), acetonitrile (AcN), 2,2,2-trifluoroethanol (TFE), formic acid (FA), heptafluorobutyric acid (HFBA), iodoacetamide (IAA), triethylammonium bicarbonate (TEAB), and dithiothreitol—were purchased from Sigma-Aldrich (Vienna, Austria).

One of the most important steps when analyzing embryo cultivation media is the depletion of serum albumin present in these samples. Tarasova et al. [1] described the innovative method of using immobilized antihuman albumin antibodies for depletion of small sample volumes. Briefly, for depletion of culture media samples from selected embryos, the sample was diluted using the phosphate buffered saline buffer (pH 7.4) consisting of 0.01 M phosphate buffer, 0.0027 M KCl, and 0.14 M NaCl. This buffer was further also used as a washing buffer A upon the sample loading. In order to ensure full sample recovery from the depletion column, a ready-to-use elution buffer from Agilent (pH 2.25) (Agilent Technologies, CA, USA) was used as buffer B. We have developed a new column for the depletion of human albumin by immobilizing the antihuman albumin antibodies to the monolithic support disk, the CIMac-HSA column, especially for analysis of small sample amounts, which also occur in IVF samples. This column was used in an ICS-5000 inert HPLC system (Dionex-Thermo Scientific, Germering, Germany) for albumin depletion with a column flow rate of 0.3 mL/min. Upon sample injection, the loading and washing buffer A was pumped through the column for 5 min, and the flow-through fraction was collected (V = 350 μL). This fractions' volume corresponds to the full absorbance peak and contains all proteins that were not trapped on the column. The albumin was trapped by the interaction with the antibodies on the column's surface, and it was eluted by increasing the amount of the eluting mobile phase from 5 to 10 min. The column was, finally, flushed with the loading buffer A for additional 4 min, and this step was followed by an additional washing step with buffer B and, finally, equilibrating step using, again, the loading buffer A for 13 min. The total time for completing this depletion protocol is 30 min when applying the column flow rate of 0.3 mL/min. During this time, the very important column wash step and the complete re-equilibration of the column preceding the next depletion run is being perfromed. The flow rate used was selected for maximizing the protein's interaction time and was a compromise between the speed and efficacy of operation. If desired, higher column flow rates can be used without losing much of the column's performance [2], but this shall be carefully examined and optimized.

Proteins in both collected fractions and non-depleted samples were depleted using a standard protocol with trypsin. Due to a high concentration of phosphate buffer in collected fractions, 1 M triethylammonium bicarbonate (TEAB) was added to the fractions in order to reach a final concentration of 50 mM TEAB and to dilute the phosphate buffer. For protein denaturation, 10 μL of 0.1% (w/v) Rapigest in 50 m MTEAB were added to all fractions, and reduction of disulfide bonds was performed using dithiothreitol (final concentration of 5 mM DTT) and incubating the reaction mixture for 30 min at 60°C.

For a successful trypsinization, alkylation was performed using iodoacetamide at a final concentration of 15 mM IAA. Upon addition of IAA, the sample was incubated at room temperature, in the dark, for 30 min. An excess of iodoacetamide is inhibiting the trypsin action and needs to be neutralized, which was achieved by adding 2 μL of 50 mM DTT in 50 mM TEAB, vigorous mixing for 2 min at room temperature. Finally, 10 μL of 0.2 μg/μL trypsin solution were added, and samples were incubated for 16 h at 37°C in an incubation oven. Tryptic activity was stopped by acidifying the solution with 1% TFA solution.

For LC–MS/MS analysis, 20 μL of the digested and diluted sample (aqueous 0.1% TFA at a ratio of 2:3 (v/v)) were injected for LC–MS/MS analysis.

2.3 Chromatographic separation and mass spectrometry detection

A Dionex UltiMate 3000 RSLC nanoLC system (Dionex-Thermo Scientific) was used for the nanoHPLC separation of tryptic peptides. Mobile phases used for chromatographic separation of tryptic peptides were as follows: (A) 5% of acetonitrile in aqueous 0.1% formic acid and (B) methanol, trifluoroethanol, water and acetonitrile (30:10:10:50 (v/v/v/v) and 0.1% of formic acid). The sample was loaded onto the trap column for washing the residula salts and focusing of the analytes as a small sample front by using loading mobile phase consisting of 0.1% aqueous TFA chilled to 3°C.

The nonlinear gradient of 75 min total running time was used for HPLC separations of tryptic peptides. The gradient was composed using sequential linear steps:

1. 1.0% B min^{-1} for 7 min.

2. 0.5% B min^{-1} gradient for 38 min.

3. 1.5% B min − 1 for 20 min.

4. 3.0% B min^{-1} for 10 min.

The HPLC flow was introduced into the maXis Impact UHR TOF mass spectrometer (Bruker Daltonics, Bremen, Germany), and the LC–MS/MS analysis was performed in triplicate for each sample. For peptide fragmentation (MS/MS), collision-induced dissociation was used, and all MS/MS data were acquired in a 300–2000 m/z range using a three-second cycle without further optimization of the instrument's parameters. In order to prevent unnecessary fragmentation of ions with low intensity, the lower threshold for precursor ions was set to 1000 counts. Due to tailing of some peptides and frequently observed co-elution of peaks, a dynamic exclusion was employed, and the duration was set to 120 s. In case where the precursor ion showed higher intensity after the exclusion period of 120 s, it was reconsidered for an additional MS/MS event.

Database search for protein identification was performed using the all-taxonomy Swiss-Prot database (http://www.uniprot.org). For this search, X! Tandem [3] with following parameters was used:

1. Precursor mass tolerance of ±10 ppm.

2. Fragment mass tolerance of ±0.3 Da.

3. Maximum of two missed cleavages were allowed.

Some posttranslational modifications of peptides due to the sample preparation and due to biological processes can be expected. For the experiment described, cysteine carbamidomethylation was selected as the fixed modification and methionine oxidation; phosphorylation of serine, threonine, and tyrosine residues, as well as the acetylation of lysine and N-terminal residues, were selected as variable modifications.

2.4 Data analysis

All data analysis for the experiments described in this manuscript was analyzed using the method described by Tarasova et al. [1]. The use of pyteomics.pepxmltk converter (https://pypi.python.org/pypi/pyteomics.pepxmltk) and search was described elsewhere [4]. Briefly, this platform was used to convert X! Tandem files to the standard pep.xml format and perform data analysis. All identifications, upon database search, were filtered to meet the requirement of the 1.0% FDR at peptide level. Search results were submitted for a post-search validation using the MPscore software, described earlier [5]. Quantitative information on identified proteins is a substantial requirement for determining the differences between biological samples, and all proteins fulfilling the identification and validation requirements were quantified using the label-free quantitation approach called normalized spectral index (SIn) (Griffin et al.) [6].

3. Results and discussion

3.1 Albumin depletion in IVF cultivation medium

The presence of albumin in cultivating medium is necessary for the normal development of embryos. However, its presence is a significant burden for proteomics analysis, and it must be removed prior to further analysis steps. The removal of albumin has been extensively discussed and described in a number of publications [1, 2, 7–9]. Different groups have used a number of methods such as immunodepleting chromatography, molecular weight cutoff filters, peptide libraries, size exclusion chromatography, etc. All these methods have some advantages but also show disadvantages. In case of depleting the albumin from IVF cultivating medium, the very low sample volume (max. of 40 μl) must be taken into consideration. Furthermore, depletion method must be performed fast and must be reproducible over a large number of samples, if intended to be used for fast analysis of clinical samples that shall help making the decision on which fertilized oocyte shall be transferred first and which ones shall be frozen for later procedures. The use of a novel immunoaffinity-based convective interaction media analytical columns (CIMac) for depletion of HSA (CIMac-HSA) was performed in this study, and it proved that it can be used for fast and reproducible albumin depletion from minute sample amounts. The column's architecture and the convective flow-through columns' channels enable a flow rate-independent binding capacity and excellent chromatographic resolution. These characteristics give CIMac-αHSA column some important analytical benefits like shorten time of analysis in comparison to common chromatographic depletion of albumin using silica-based columns, which is an extraordinary important parameter for clinical use. The albumin content in different batches of cultivating medium differs strongly, and it also differs strongly between different suppliers. Therefore, the depletion method must be selected in a way that can be applied for a variety of samples. However, independently of the selected methods, the removal of albumin from the cultivating medium results with a number of identified proteins of which some can be of importance for embryo development and for later pregnancy development.

Figure 1 shows two SDS-gel lanes for the separation of two media upon embryo transfer. Since albumin originates from different donors and is being mixed at the manufacturing site, it will certainly contain a number of other proteins that may interfere with proteins secreted from the developing embryo. Also, secreted proteins might bind on albumin and, therefore, be "invisible" for proteomics analysis.

In addition to that, the human proteome, as any proteome, is dynamic, and it is constantly changing through internal and external stimuli. Proteins being translated from RNA are directly responsible for cellular function, but different gene expression studies have, unfortunately, shown that a reliable prediction of proteins' function or abundance cannot be made. As for the human proteome, significant advances have been made for the analysis of the whole proteome and of the proteome of different disease states [3, 5, 10–20]. Bearing all of it in mind, the analysis of proteins obtained from the cultivating media is challenging, and the results are not always conclusive.

Figure 2 shows the results obtained upon analyzing four different cultivating media used in routine IVF procedures and upon embryo transfer.

Dyrlund et al. [21] have performed the analysis of unconditioned commercial embryo culture media and have identified a number of proteins upon depletion and digestion of a total of 5 mL of media. The amount of 5 mL, however, will never be available if samples are retrieved during the actual IVF process. However, this analysis showed that this amount contains an astounding amount of 25 mg of albumin. Here, a total of 111 proteins with different concentrations in different batches of the media were identified in addition to albumin. The sample of unconditioned media also contained eight proteins previously suggested as possible markers of

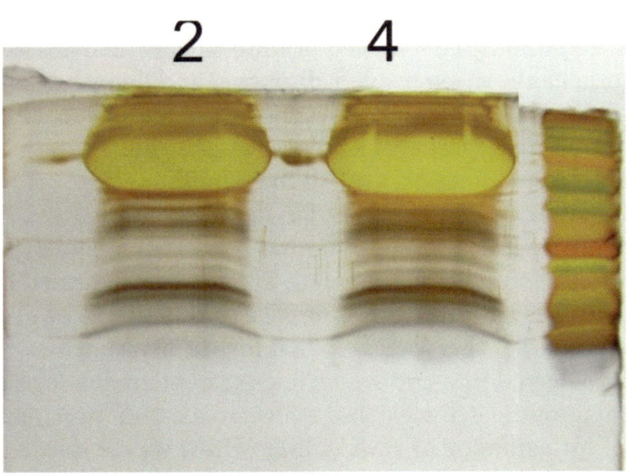

Figure 1.
Lanes 2 and 4 show an example of the separation of proteins secreted in culturing media on silver-stained SDS gel. As expected, large spots for human serum albumin (HSA) are observed for both samples with significantly lower amounts of other proteins. Since the culturing media have been declared to contain only HSA, the proteins below are secreted from the fertilized oocyte (lane 2) and unfertilized oocyte (lane 4).

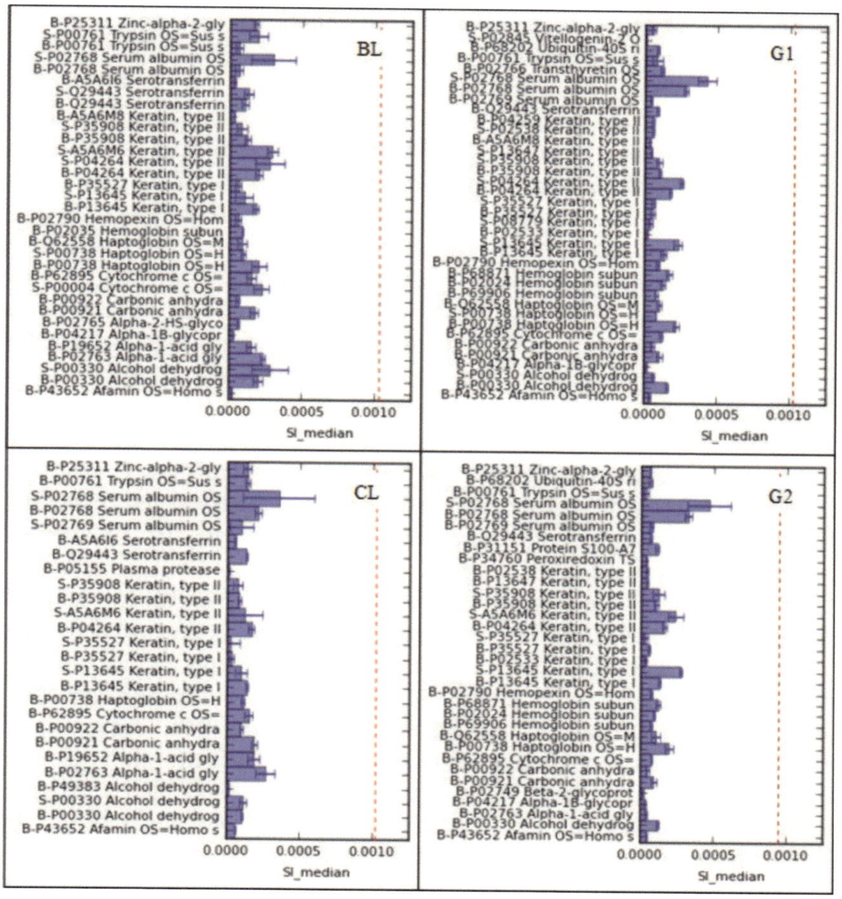

Figure 2.
Identified proteins and their relative quantities in albumin-free fractions after performing albumin depletion of culturing media samples on two different depletion columns. Proteins identified either in the CIMac-αHSA FT or the Seppro FT1 fractions are labeled with B and S, followed by Swiss-Prot protein ID. Median values of normalized spectral indexes (SI) and standard deviations are shown. Median SIHSA in non-depleted samples is marked with red dashes. More than two peptide-spectrum matches were assumed for each of the listed proteins according to Tarasova et al. [1].

embryonic viability, e.g., proteoglycan-4, serotransferrin, vitamin-D-binding protein, ubiquitin, etc.

Another study performed on IVF medium examined the batch-to-batch variations and showed that variation in both protein amounts and protein identifications can be expected [22]. When studying these media, it is important to pay attention to the fact that both media, the control and the media where embryos grow, must be from the same batch in order to make valid comparison.

Spent IVF medium is a valuable source for proteins that can be used as putative biomarkers in IVF. The major focus of researchers has been on secreted proteins, but the proteins already present in the medium can be equally valuable and must be considered in the pursuit for biomarkers of embryos' "quality." It is very possible that proteins already present in the medium may be necessary for embryo development, and the uptake or degradation of specific proteins might correlate to ascertain embryo development or lack thereof. Therefore, these media must be evaluated for their potential to differentiate embryos' success rates and track the proteins, which can be potential biomarkers. Additionally, the safety of these proteins in culture media for the offspring should also be evaluated.

3.2 Identification of proteins in IVF cultivation medium and their possible role for embryo development

Proteins identified by Dyrlund et al. were also reported by Katze-Jaff upon analysis of the secretome of the individually cultured human embryos, and a hint was made that these proteins could be related to embryo's morphology and thus its viability [23–25]. They have reported that ubiquitin was upregulated in developing blastocytes as compared to degenerating blastocytes. However, there was no correlation between the ubiquitin upregulation and the observed pregnancy rates.

Cortezzi et al. [26] reported the identification of proteins in both positive and negative groups of embryos, i.e., embryos termed viable for transfer and does who were not selected. For positive-implantation group, protein, called Jumonji (JARID2), was reported. This protein composes a histone methyltransferase complex called polycomb repressive complex 2 (PRC2), which modifies chromatin methylation to silence many embryonic patterning genes, acting as a negative regulator of cell proliferation signaling. This results with a restricted gene expression to an appropriate cell population that is essential for development, differentiation, and maintenance of cell fates.

In the same study, the testis-specific gene 10 protein (TSGA10) was identified only in negative samples. TSGA10 is a perinuclear protein, and it was described to participate in actively dividing and fetal differentiating tissues in mice embryos.

Katz-Jaffe et al. reported the identification of heparin-binding epidermal growth factor EGF-like growth factor precursor (HB-EGF) [24]. This growth factor precursor belongs to the EGF family growth factors, and it is found in the membrane-anchored form (proHB-EGF) and the soluble form (sHB-EGF). The soluble form is produced from the proteolytic cleavage of proHB-EGF at the extracellular domain. Furthermore, soluble HB-EGF has been observed to be a growth stimulator, and it does significantly improve the blastocyst development and hatching when added to serum-free medium. However, other studies from an in vitro model system indicate that proHB-EGF might function in cell-to-cell signaling by a juxtacrine mechanism inhibiting growth activity [27]. Since this protein was identified in degenerating blastocytes, its upregulation might contribute to the lack of further development.

A cystatin-like precursor is needed for successful mammalian implantation for a controlled trophoblastic invasion of the maternal uterine epithelium. It must be available and functional [28] since this invasion involves the extracellular degradation of the uterine matrix by a variety of proteinases, and one of the crucial ones are cysteine proteinases. Cystatins are known to inhibit cysteine proteinases, and their upregulation will most probably contribute to failure of implantation of degenerating blastocysts. Therefore, it is not only of importance to identify these proteins, the possible biomarkers, but also to validate these findings in the human.

4. Conclusion

Proteomics is a promising technology for the identification and validation of possible biomarkers for embryo selection in ART. As listed by Dyrlund et al., a growing list of secreted proteins has been identified that could further contribute to this field [21]. However, the challenge ahead of the research still includes the reliable and reproducible identification of a proteomics secretome signature. This signature shall be directly associated with embryo viability and the success of the procedure, i.e., successful pregnancy, and child's birth. This is a very challenging task not only due to the complexity, heterogeneity, and diversity of human embryos but also because of irreproducibility of used culturing media and contaminant proteins therein.

Another challenge for the clinical use of proteomics methods is the speed of the proteomics analysis. Sample preparation, measurement, and data analysis of a sample is currently not feasible within the time window needed for IVF. Current sample analysis methods require at least half a day for the fastest proteomics method available, which is too long. Nevertheless, proteomics methods can contribute to identification and validation of putative biomarkers, which once clinically confirmed, can be analyzed using other, faster, methods upon building corresponding antibodies.

Author details

Goran Mitulović[1,2*] and Tanja Panić-Janković[1]

1 Clinical Department of Laboratory Medicine, Medical University of Vienna, Vienna, Austria

2 Proteomics Core Facility, Medical University of Vienna, Vienna, Austria

*Address all correspondence to: goran.mitulovic@meduniwien.ac.at

References

[1] Tarasova IA, Lobas AA, Cernigoj U, Solovyeva EM, Mahlberg B, Ivanov MV, et al. Depletion of human serum albumin in embryo culture media for in vitro fertilization using monolithic columns with immobilized antibodies. Electrophoresis. 2016;**37**(17-18):2322-2327

[2] Tanja Panić -Janković UČ, Nemec B, Vidič U, Vidč J, Sekirnik R, Krajnc NL, et al. Goran Mitulović CIMac- aHSA monoliths increase throughput and sensitivity of proteomic studies of IVF media by rapid albumin depletion. Chromatography Today. 2015;**8**(13):36-40

[3] Shevchenko V, Arnotskaya N, Korneyko M, Zaytsev S, Khotimchenko Y, Sharma H, et al. Proteins of the Wnt signaling pathway as targets for the regulation of CD133+ cancer stem cells in glioblastoma. Oncology Reports. 2019;**41**(5):3080-3088

[4] Goloborodko AA, Levitsky LI, Ivanov MV, Gorshkov MV. Pyteomics—a python framework for exploratory data analysis and rapid software prototyping in proteomics. Journal of the American Society for Mass Spectrometry. 2013;**24**(2):301-304

[5] Archer TC, Ehrenberger T, Mundt F, Gold MP, Krug K, Mah CK, et al. Proteomics, post-translational modifications, and integrative analyses reveal molecular heterogeneity within Medulloblastoma subgroups. Cancer Cell. 2018;**34**(3):396-410.e8

[6] Griffin NM, Yu J, Long F, Oh P, Shore S, Li Y, et al. Label-free, normalized quantification of complex mass spectrometry data for proteomic analysis. Nature Biotechnology. 2010;**28**(1):83-89

[7] Vaezzadeh AR, Briscoe AC, Steen H, Lee RS. One-step sample concentration, purification, and albumin depletion method for urinary proteomics. Journal of Proteome Research. 2010;**9**(11):6082-6089

[8] Afkarian M, Bhasin M, Dillon ST, Guerrero MC, Nelson RG, Knowler WC, et al. Optimizing a proteomics platform for urine biomarker discovery. Molecular & Cellular Proteomics. 2010;**9**(10):2195-2204

[9] Baussant T, Bougueleret L, Johnson A, Rogers J, Menin L, Hall M, et al. Effective depletion of albumin using a new peptide-based affinity medium. Proteomics. 2005;**5**(4):973

[10] Thul PJ, Lindskog C. The human protein atlas: A spatial map of the human proteome. Protein Science. 2018;**27**(1):233-244

[11] Ma Z, Cui X, Lu L, Chen G, Yang Y, Hu Y, et al. Exosomes from glioma cells induce a tumor-like phenotype in mesenchymal stem cells by activating glycolysis. Stem Cell Research & Therapy. 2019;**10**(1):60

[12] Tsangaris GT, Papathanasiou C, Adamopoulos PG, Scorilas A, Vorgias CE, Prodromou N, et al. Pediatric ependymoma: A proteomics perspective. Cancer Genomics & Proteomics. 2017;**14**(2):127-136

[13] Marie SK, Oba-Shinjo SM, da Silva R, Gimenez M, Nunes Reis G, Tassan JP, et al. Stathmin involvement in the maternal embryonic leucine zipper kinase pathway in glioblastoma. Proteome Science. 2016;**14**:6

[14] Gato M, Blanco-Luquin I, Zudaire M, de Morentin XM, Perez-Valderrama E, Zabaleta A, et al. Drafting the proteome landscape of myeloid-derived suppressor cells. Proteomics. 2016;**16**(2):367-378

[15] Sun Y, Cheng L, Gu Y, Xin A, Wu B, Zhou S, et al. A human Lectin

microarray for sperm surface glycosylation analysis. Molecular & Cellular Proteomics. 2016;**15**(9):2839-2851

[16] Benkhalifa M, Madkour A, Louanjli N, Bouamoud N, Saadani B, Kaarouch I, et al. From global proteome profiling to single targeted molecules of follicular fluid and oocyte: Contribution to embryo development and IVF outcome. Expert Review of Proteomics. 2015;**12**(4):407-423

[17] Kim M-S, Pinto SM, Getnet D, Nirujogi RS, Manda SS, Chaerkady R, et al. A draft map of the human proteome. Nature. 2014;**509**(7502):575-581

[18] Wilhelm M, Schlegl J, Hahne H, Gholami AM, Lieberenz M, Savitski MM, et al. Mass-spectrometry-based draft of the human proteome. Nature. 2014;**509**(7502):582-587

[19] Legare C, Droit A, Fournier F, Bourassa S, Force A, Cloutier F, et al. Investigation of male infertility using quantitative comparative proteomics. Journal of Proteome Research. 2014;**13**(12):5403-5414

[20] Frapsauce C, Pionneau C, Bouley J, Delarouziere V, Berthaut I, Ravel C, et al. Proteomic identification of target proteins in normal but nonfertilizing sperm. Fertility and Sterility. 2014;**102**(2):372-380

[21] Dyrlund TF, Kirkegaard K, Poulsen ET, Sanggaard KW, Hindkjaer JJ, Kjems J, et al. Unconditioned commercial embryo culture media contain a large variety of non-declared proteins: A comprehensive proteomics analysis. Human Reproduction. 2014;**29**(11):2421-2430

[22] Xiao Y, Isaacs SN. Enzyme-linked immunosorbent assay (ELISA) and blocking with bovine serum albumin (BSA)—not all BSAs are alike. Journal of Immunological Methods. 2012;**384**(1-2):148-151

[23] Katz-Jaffe MG, Schoolcraft WB, Gardner DK. Analysis of protein expression (secretome) by human and mouse preimplantation embryos. Fertility and Sterility. 2006;**86**(3):678-685

[24] Katz-Jaffe MG, Gardner DK, Schoolcraft WB. Proteomic analysis of individual human embryos to identify novel biomarkers of development and viability. Fertility and Sterility. 2006;**85**(1):101-107

[25] Katz-Jaffe MG, Linck DW, Schoolcraft WB, Gardner DK. A proteomic analysis of mammalian preimplantation embryonic development. Reproduction. 2005;**130**(6):899-905

[26] Cortezzi SS, Garcia JS, Ferreira CR, Braga DP, Figueira RC, Iaconelli A Jr, et al. Secretome of the preimplantation human embryo by bottom-up label-free proteomics. Analytical and Bioanalytical Chemistry. 2011;**401**(4):1331-1339

[27] Iwamoto R, Mekada E. Heparin-binding EGF-like growth factor: A juxtacrine growth factor. Cytokine & Growth Factor Reviews. 2000;**11**(4):335-344

[28] Afonso S, Romagnano L, Babiarz B. The expression and function of cystatin C and cathepsin B and cathepsin L during mouse embryo implantation and placentation. Development. 1997;**124**(17):3415-3425

Chapter 9

Autologous Platelet-Rich Plasma Infusion to Improve Pregnancy Outcome in Suboptimal Endometrium: A Review

Casey Zeffiro, Silvina Bocca, Helena Russell and Mitchel C. Schiewe

Abstract

Over the past decade, platelet-rich plasma (PRP) has been used in several fields of medicine to promote cell growth and expedite wound healing for the treatment of arthritis, nerve injury, tendinitis, bone regeneration, cardiac muscle repair, and oral & plastic surgery. Recently, researchers have been applying autologous PRP to bolster the growth of endometrial lining in patients with a history of endometrium-related failed embryo transfers. Evidence reveals that PRP is a rich source of active cytokines and various growth factors, which come from an autologous source that can be easily attained from peripheral blood without risk of disease transmission to the patient. In this review, several studies were analyzed that involved patients 18–42 years of age undergoing hormone replacement therapy (HRT) in preparation for embryo transfer and serial transvaginal ultrasound in conjunction with PRP infusions into the endometrium via an intrauterine insemination (IUI) catheter. Exclusion criteria included patients with endometritis, polyps, or adhesions. Embryo transfers (ET) were performed when the endometrial lining achieved a thickness of >7 mm. The database indicates that PRP infusion therapy is a promising low-cost treatment for HRT patients that significantly increases endometrial thickness and improves pregnancy success in a previous suboptimal ET patient population.

Keywords: cytokines, embryo transfer, endometrial lining, endometrium, growth factors, hormone replacement therapy, infusion, platelet-rich plasma, suboptimal lining

Key Points

Evidence shows that PRP infusion directly into the endometrium enhances lining development in patients suffering from chronically refractive or underdeveloped endometrium. Chemical pregnancy in patients that underwent PRP infusion with frozen embryo transfer was 50% (108/216) in comparison to 17.1% (16/93) in patients that did not receive PRP treatment.

1. Introduction

The overall objective of this review was to determine if platelet-rich plasma (PRP) infusions are viable alternatives to current treatments for thin endometrial lining, and to distinguish if PRP infusions increase endometrial thickness and implantation in patients that underwent treatment in eight different case studies.

Platelet-rich plasma is prepared from autologous whole blood collected from a patient's peripheral vein, mixed with an acid citrate dextrose solution A (ACD-A) anticoagulant, and processed to separate platelets from remaining blood components [1]. Platelet-rich plasma is recognized as plasma from autologous blood with 4–5 times the concentration of normal platelet levels; these high concentrations of PRP contain cytokines and growth factors including: vascular endothelial growth factor (VEGF), transforming growth factor (TGF), platelet-derived growth factor (PDGF) and epidermal growth factor (EGF) [2, 3]. Because of the expression of several regenerative growth factors, PRP is being used in several fields of medicine to promote wound regeneration including: arthritis, nerve injury, tendinitis, bone regeneration, cardiac muscle repair, alopecia, and plastic and oral surgery recovery [4, 5]. When the body is injured, a natural healing process occurs that floods the wound site with activated platelets that instantly promote cell regeneration and proliferation. It is theorized that PRP may be used to promote the same growth and proliferation in endometrium that have previous suboptimal growth patterns. Similar research, such as endometrial scratching, has been studied to promote the generation of growth factors to increase implantation; however, the concentration of platelet levels within direct PRP infusion into the endometrium is vastly superior to the natural, localized endometrial healing process that occurs with the scratching method.

Other treatment strategies for thin endometrial lining have varied throughout recent years, but have been inclusive of extended use of exogenous estradiol, low-dose aspirin, vitamin E supplementation, and use of granulocyte colony stimulation factor (G-CSF), but not all have been proven effective [6–9]. The minimal endometrial thickness suggested for successful implantation at embryo transfer is 7 mm [10], however, there are those that argue endometrial lining is a poor indicator for pregnancy outcomes and therefore should not be heavily considered [11]. During typical HRT cycles, estradiol administration is regulated from day 2 or day 3 of an average 28 day cycle and continues until the endometrial lining reaches optimal thickness for transfer (typically >7 mm) at which time progesterone administration then occurs [12]. This model is utilized in IVF clinics globally; however, patients who fail to reach the recommended endometrial thickness often undergo canceled cycles in which they have wasted valuable time, medications, and expenses without receiving an embryo transfer.

Thin endometrial lining or suboptimal endometrial growth is a problem that affects up to 5% of the patients undergoing IVF treatment [13]. These patients often experience the emotionally and physically traumatizing effects of canceled cycles or repeated implantation failure (RIF). It is proven that growth factors expressed in the endometrium of women with RIF are less than those expressed in normal fertile women [14]. These growth factors can be stimulated by infusion of autologous PRP into the endometrium in conjunction with HRT prior to embryo transfer. However, many factors are involved in successful embryonic implantation, not limited to embryo quality, but also a synchrony between the embryo and the endometrium in addition to any immunological factors [15]. Without optimal endometrial growth, this synchrony becomes far less likely as the endometrium does not express the adequate genes nor growth factors involved in embryonic implantation [16, 17].

2. PRP collection and infusion

Through multiple studies, PRP processing was performed similarly. On the 10th day of HRT, Chang and coworkers drew 15 ml of autologous blood into a tube with 5 ml of Acid Citrate A Anticoagulant (ACD-A) and centrifuged; separating red blood cells, a gel buffy coat, and cellular plasma. The plasma and buffy coat were then transferred to a second tube and centrifuged again, yielding 0.5–1 ml of PRP [18]. Both Zadehmodarres and Nazari and their colleagues drew 17.5 ml of blood on day 9 or 10 of HRT into 2.5 ml of ACD-A and similarly centrifuged twice to obtain 0.5 ml of PRP [19, 20]. Tandulwadkar et al. used 10 ml of autologous blood into an unspecified amount of ACD-A; which was centrifuged sequentially utilizing first a soft spin for 15 minutes, followed by a hard spin for 6 minutes, again yielding between 0.5 and 0.8 ml of PRP [21]. Eftekhar and others used an alternative approach, collecting PRP on the 13th day of HRT by drawing 8.5 ml of peripheral venous blood into a syringe containing 1.5 ml of ACD-A that was then centrifuged for 10 minutes; following first centrifugation, the buffy coat and plasma layer were then removed and centrifuged again, yielding 1.5 ml of PRP [22]. Meanwhile, Hounyoung et al. collected 18 ml of venous blood in a 30 ml syringe prepared with 2 CC of ACD-A and then centrifuged twice to obtain 0.7–1.0 ml of PRP [23]. Nazari and coworkers performed a follow-up study utilizing a double-blinded trial in which 30 patients underwent PRP infusion, prepared in the same manner as the initial pilot study [19], and 30 patients underwent placebo PRP infusions [24]. Chang et al. performed a secondary study as well, involving a larger cohort of patients compared against a control group, and performed PRP collection as previously reported [18, 25]. All studies transfused the PRP into the endometrium using an IUI catheter, and then repeated intravaginal ultrasound 48 hours later to measure endometrial growth; patients who did not reach the desired lining thickness (>7 mm deemed adequate in all studies) were then treated with a second round of PRP infusion [18–25].

2.1 Hormone replacement therapy

In the past, IVF clinics allowed for natural cycle frozen embryo transfer in which they permitted endometrial lining to develop on its own, but it resulted in many timing issues with need for frequent monitoring and cancelation due to anovulation and poor development of the endometrium. Today, most clinics have moved fully to HRT protocols that allow for artificial stimulation of the endometrium that can be easily tracked utilizing blood serum and ultrasound assessment to time an embryo transfer concordant with a receptive endometrium. In humans, estrogen stimulates endometrial growth and induces progesterone receptors as it moves naturally through the menstrual cycle. After ovulation, the endometrium is exposed to progesterone which induces morphological and biochemical changes that alter the endometrium from the proliferative phase to the secretory phase [17]. In HRT cycles, estradiol administration (typically Estradiol Valerate) occurs until the lining has reached a thickness of greater than 7 mm, at which time progesterone is then administered for the number of days proportional to the embryo being transferred (i.e., a day 6 blastocyst will receive progesterone for 6 days) and then the embryo is transferred to a supposedly receptive endometrium [26, 27]. In these HRT cycles, patients receive estradiol during the follicular phase that inhibits gonadotropin secretion and prevents follicular development and ovulation. The start of the luteal phase can be exactly pinpointed, as it starts when progesterone is added to estradiol dosages.

2.2 Methodology

HRT allows for artificial stimulation of endometrial growth via hormone administration orally, transdermally, intramuscularly, vaginally, subcutaneously, or a combination of both. Most clinics administer estradiol for several days until the endometrial lining has reach a point of optimal growth, at which time they will then administer progesterone to induce the secretory phase of cycle that promotes embryo implantation [21]. Each of the studies examined in this review conducted HRT protocols concordant with physician recommendation as follows:

Chang et al.: In the pilot study, Estradiol Valerate (E_2V) started at 3 mg/d on day 3 of menses and increased every 4 days up to a max of 12 mg/d; and in the cohort study, E_2V started at 6 mg/d and subsequently increased to 12 mg/d [18, 25]. The pilot study included five patients suffering from chronically non-responsive thin endometrium (5.9–6.6 mm) who underwent PRP infusion on the 10th day of HRT and lining was measured via transvaginal ultrasound. In the cohort study, platelet-rich plasma infusion was also performed on the 10th day of HRT, and endometrial thickness was measured in both the control group and study group.

Zadehmodarres et al.: Estradiol Valerate started at 6 mg/d on day 3 of menses, and increased to 8–9 mg/d. Suppository progesterone was started when endometrial thickness reached >7 mm and continued for 2 weeks after ET [19]. PRP infusion was administered on the 11th or 12th day of cycle and assessed 48 hours later.

Nazari et al.: Estradiol Valerate started on day 2 or 3 of menses at 6 mg/d and was increased to 8 mg/d if lining did not reach >7 mm. When thickness reached 7 mm, progesterone suppositories, 4000 mg, were started twice daily [20, 24]. In the pilot study, 0.5 ml of PRP was infused into the endometrium of patients 48 hours prior to frozen embryo transfer in conjunction with an HRT cycle. In the follow-up RCT, PRP infusion or mock infusion was performed on day 11 or 12 of HRT cycle, modified from the initial pilot study, and lining was measured using transvaginal ultrasonography.

Tandulwadkar et al.: Estradiol Valerate started at 6–8 mg/d concordant with baseline endometrial vascularity as measured by Power Doppler on day 1 of menses and increased to 12 mg/d if growth was not seen. Transvaginal ultrasounds were performed starting on day 7/8 [21]. Day of PRP infusion was not given in the initial study.

Eftekhar et al.: In this study, the case group was treated with PRP and increased HRT, and the control group was just treated with increased HRT. For all women, E_2V was started at 6 mg/d, then increased to 10 mg/d [22]. PRP infusion occurred on the 13th day of cycle and endometrial lining was measured transvaginally.

Hounyoung et al.: Patients treated within this study began E_2V administration on the second day of menses, starting at 4-6 mg/d and followed by PRP infusion on cycle day 10 [23]. PRP infusion was administered via IUI catheter and repeated 2–3 times in 3 day intervals until optimal endometrial thickness was achieved (>7 mm).

3. Sample size and selection of samples

Eight clinical trials were selected, all of which were inclusive of a total of 346 patients that underwent HRT in conjunction with PRP infusion. Of 346 patients, 313 underwent embryo transfer at either cleavage or blastocyst stage. The remaining 33 patients dropped out of the studies prior to embryo transfer due to persistently poor endometrial development [18–25].

3.1 Inclusion criteria

Inclusion criteria remained relatively constant through all eight studies. All patients had a history of thin endometrial lining, repeat implantation failure, or two or more canceled cycles due to poor endometrial growth. All patients were between the ages of 18–42 years old and all had a normal BMI of <30%; donor egg cycles were not included due to the potential to skew the results. All patients that underwent embryo transfer post-PRP infusion reached an endometrial thickness of >7 mm, as deemed acceptable by the performing physicians.

3.2 Exclusion criteria

All patients with hematological and immunological disorders, hormonal disorders, chromosomal and genetic abnormalities and uterine abnormalities were excluded from the studies. All patients who did not reach optimal endometrial thickness post-PRP infusion were excluded from embryo transfer. Any patient of advanced maternal age (>42 years old) or increased BMI (>30%) was excluded from the studies.

4. Results and data analysis

Five patients were included in the initial pilot study by Chang et al. [18]. 48–72 hours post PRP, all five patients reached a minimum lining of 7 mm (7.0–8.0). All patients underwent frozen embryo transfer, and all five patients were pregnant (5/5) with an ongoing pregnancy rate of 80% (4/5).

Zadehmodarres and colleagues [19] performed their study on 10 patients with previous canceled cycles due to thin endometrial development, four of which were diagnosed with Asherman's Syndrome. All 10 patients reached adequate lining thickness for embryo transfer (7.0–7.5). All patients underwent frozen embryo transfer resulting in chemical pregnancy in 50% of patients (5/10) with an ongoing pregnancy rate of 40% (4/10).

The pilot study by Nazari and coworkers [20] was based upon a study group of 20 patients suffering from RIF due to thin endometrial lining. All patients received a blastocyst stage transfer of one to two embryos that were graded morphologically normal. Chemical pregnancy was reported in 90% of patients (18/20) with an ongoing pregnancy rate of 80% (16/20).

Tandulwadkar et al. [21] assessed not only endometrial thickness, but endometrial vascularity as well post PRP infusion as measured by serial transvaginal ultrasound. Of the 68 patients included in the study, 64 went on to achieve optimal lining thickness for frozen embryo transfer. Average mean lining thickness before PRP infusion was 5 mm, and 7.22 mm after PRP infusion. Of the 64 patients that received a frozen embryo transfer, endometrial vascularity increased in all patients. 60.1% (39/64) reported chemical pregnancy with an ongoing pregnancy rate of 45.3% (26/64).

A randomized control trial was performed by Eftekhar and others [22] in which 83 women participated; 40 were allocated to the study group and received PRP infusion, while 43 were placed in the control group and did not receive PRP. Prior to PRP infusion on the 13th day of cycle, there were no significant differences in endometrial lining as measured between the two groups; however, after PRP infusion, significant differences were noted (8.80 vs. 8.04 mm). Of the 40 women in the study group, 7 did not receive an embryo transfer due to persistently thin endometrium, whereas 10 women in the control group were excluded from frozen embryo transfer for the same reason. Thirty-three women in the study group and 33 women in the control group underwent cleavage stage frozen embryo transfer. In the study group, chemical pregnancy was reported in 42.2% (14/33) in comparison to the control group, which recorded chemical pregnancy in only 24.2% (8/33) of patients. Ongoing pregnancy rates were 33.3% (11/33) versus 18.2% (6/33), respectively.

Hounyoung and colleagues [23] performed a pilot study on 24 patients with a history of refractory endometrium. Of the 24 patients initially included in the study, two patients were canceled, and two were lost to follow-up. Data was collected for the remaining 20 patients, all of whom received a frozen embryo transfer of 2–3 day 3 cleavage stage embryos. Among the study group, a chemical pregnancy rate of 30% (6/20) was reported with an ongoing pregnancy rate of 20% (4/20).

After an initial pilot study, Nazari et al. [24] performed a follow-up double blinded randomized control trial to validate their previous findings. Sixty patients were selected for inclusion in the study; 30 were randomly assigned to the study group to receive PRP infusion, and 30 were aliquoted to the control group in which a sham-catheter was utilized for mock PRP infusion. In the PRP group, lining increased to 7.21 ± 0.18 mm respectively, and in the mock infusion group, lining reached 5.76 ± 0.97 mm. Of the 30 patients in the study group, all patients received a frozen embryo transfer in comparison to just 6 that reached optimal lining (>7 mm) for frozen embryo transfer in the control group. Chemical pregnancy was recorded in 40% (12/30) of cases in the study group, and in 6.7% (2/30) in the control group. Ongoing pregnancy rate was 33.3% (10/30) in the PRP group, and 3.3% (1/30) in the control group.

Chang and others [25] performed a follow-up randomized control trial to their initial pilot study as well, assigning 34 patients to the PRP infusion group and 30 patients to the control group, which received only HRT without PRP. In the study group, endometrial thickness reached an average of 7.65 ± 0.22 mm versus 6.52 ± 0.31 mm in the control group. The cycle cancelation rate was 19.0% in the study group, and 41.2% in the control group, which was statistically significant. All patients that reached optimal endometrial thickness received a frozen blastocyst transfer of one or two morphologically good blastocyst stage embryos. In the PRP group, clinical pregnancy was reported as 44.1% (15/34), and 20% (6/30) in the control group.

All patients within study groups that underwent embryo transfer reached optimal lining thickness (>7 mm) after one or multiple rounds of PRP infusion. Patients that underwent PRP infusion in the study groups reached an average endometrial thickness of 7.36 mm with an average increase of 1.68 mm post PRP infusion. In the control groups presented by studies performing RCT, the control patients reached an average endometrial thickness of 6.77 mm with an average increase of 0.91 mm after HRT. Among patients within study groups, the overall chemical pregnancy rate was 50% (108/216) in contrast to 17.1% (16/93) following conventional HRT without PRP infusion.

5. Discussion

Platelet-rich plasma infusion is a novel approach to endometrium enhancement. This autologous therapy strives to increase endometrial thickness among patients with histories of canceled cycles and repeat implantation failure due to chronically refractive endometrium. While there is no universally agreed upon treatment for this patient population, the search to find an effective solution for non-reactive

STUDY	Type of Study	Participants	Age	Day of PRP	Average EMT Before PRP (Study Group)	Average EMT Before PRP (Control Group)	Average EMT After PRP (Study Group)	Average EMT After HRT (Control Group)	Clinical Pregnancy Rate
Chang et al. 2015	Pilot	5	35.0 ± 4.0	10	6.22mm	N/A	7.52mm	N/A	5/5
Zadehmodarres et al. 2017	Pilot	10	35.0 ± 5.0	11 - 12	5.82mm	N/A	7.25mm	N/A	5/10
Nazari et al. 2016	Pilot	20	36.0 ± 3.0	16 - 18	N/A	N/A	N/A	N/A	18/20
Tandulwadkar et al. 2017	Pilot	64	31.0 ± 9.0	15 - 16	5.0mm	N/A	7.22mm	N/A	39/64
Eftekhar et al. 2018	RCT	66	32.5 ± 2.0	13	6.09mm ± .47mm	6.15mm ± 0.37mm	8.67mm + 0.64mm	8.04mm + 0.27mm	14/33 (s) vs. 8/33 (c)
Hounyoung et al. 2019	Pilot	20	37.5 ± 7.5	12, 15, 18	5.4mm ± 0.8mm	N/A	6.0mm + 1.1mm	N/A	6/20
Nazari et al. 2019	RCT	60	33.11 ± 3.77	11 - 12	4.92mm	5.06 mm	7.21mm	5.76mm	12/30 (s) vs. 2/30 (c)
Chang et al. 2019	RCT	64	33.5 ± 1.5	10	6.32mm + 0.54mm	6.39mm + 0.72mm	7.65mm + 0.22mm	6.52mm + 0.31mm	15/34 (s) vs. 6/30 (c)

* (s) denotes study group

** (c) denotes control group

Table 1.
Eight studies were compared for the measurement of endometrial thickness before and after PRP infusion in study groups vs. control groups. Clinical pregnancy outcomes are included following PRP treatment.

endometrial lining should be at the forefront of clinical researchers within the ART industry. Platelet-rich plasma is easily attained, cost-effective, minimally invasive, rich in cytokines and growth factors, and carries very little risk of disease or infection transmission as the patient uses their own blood to attain PRP. Infusion into the endometrium takes place in conjunction with traditional HRT and therefore can be administered during the average cycle while patients are already present for serial ultrasounds and serum hormone level measurements.

In the eight studies discussed above, PRP infusion into the endometrium proved effective when administered on various days of an HRT cycle as well as in variable quantities. While the majority of studies reviewed were clinical applications, which presents a weakness in the data as there was no comparative control group, the randomized controlled trials that were performed offered arguably conclusive, supportive evidence of PRP effectiveness. All the patients that underwent PRP infusion experienced a significantly marked increase in endometrial thickness, allowing for frozen embryo transfer. In the studies that did utilize a study population versus a control population, results among the study participants were significantly improved with greater cycle completion. Although most studies utilized frozen blastocyst transfers, there were some that elected to use frozen cleavage stage embryo transfers, which can also be considered a limiting factor among the data. The studies here agreed upon 7 mm as the minimal lining thickness for embryo implantation success, but some physicians argue that endometrial thickness is a poor marker for transfer outcome. While this argument can be made and supported, as it was by Griesinger and colleagues [11], there is a wide consensus that endometrial thickness does play a vital role in receptivity (**Table 1**).

The patient populations presented in these studies, including those among the study group and those in the control group, were all patients that had suffered two or more failed previous cycles due to poor lining development. The inclusion criteria for these studies were consistent through all eight trials and provided an unbiased patient group in order to obtain reliable results. The data conclusively shows that endometrial thickness among patients with chronically poor endometrial development is greatly increased with PRP infusion therapy in comparison to traditional HRT alone. The primary outcome of each study was satisfied by the significant increase in endometrial lining development with the secondary satisfaction of improved clinical pregnancy outcomes in the PRP group versus the control group.

Another diagnostic tool to be considered in patients with a history of suboptimal endometrial development and repeat implantation failure is the use of the Endometrial Receptivity Array (ERA). The ERA is a customized array that allows to test for 248 different genes expressed during the endometrial cycle and works concordantly with a computational algorithm that identifies the receptivity status of an endometrial biopsy to diagnose a personalized window of implantation [28]. ERA is performed with a mock embryo transfer cycle. Utilizing the ERA, Ruiz-Alonso and colleagues were able to validate conclusively that 25% of RIF patients had a displaced window of implantation and went on to coin the phrase "personalized embryo transfer" (pET) to increase the chance of a successful pregnancy in women suffering from mistimed endometrial receptivity [29]. Potentially, ERA can be utilized in conjunction with PRP infusion to determine receptivity of the endometrium in PRP patients. In the study by Tandulwadkar et al. [21], not only was lining thickness assessed, but endometrial vascularity was observed as well utilizing 3D Doppler ultrasound. Blood flow to the endometrium as well as the uterine biophysical profile can be measured via a combination between abdominal and transvaginal ultrasound. Greater blood flow to the uterus has been associated with higher implantation rates and can be seen in color utilizing Doppler ultrasound methods [27]. PRP infusion has the potential to increase lining development as well as endometrial vascularity as proven by Tandulwadkar, and future studies should observe an increase in vascularity concordant with lining and uterine biophysical profile. Utilizing the ERA and 3D Doppler system in conjunction with PRP in future studies can be therefore linked to the immune, genetic, and biophysical pathways of the endometrium.

While the use of PRP infusion into the endometrium to increase lining growth and vascularity is a relatively new area of research, the initial trials show encouraging results. The patients that were included within these studies are patients who had suffered from multiple failed or canceled cycles and would not have received embryo transfers otherwise. In a patient population that has had multiple failures, PRP infusion into the endometrium provides a suitable solution that effectively allows for embryo transfer, giving these patients a chance at pregnancy that they otherwise would not have had utilizing traditional HRT alone. Although the data is still new and there is need for additional research and much larger randomized controlled trials, the initial use of PRP as a universal means of treating poor responders to HRT shows a promising treatment method for the future.

6. Conclusion

The review of the initial data presented in these eight early studies of PRP infusion into the endometrium in conjunction with traditional HRT reveals statistically significant outcomes. Patients with previous failures that did not reach the minimal lining thickness needed to perform embryo transfer (>7 mm) underwent PRP infusion into the endometrium and reached an average endometrial thickness of 7.36 mm in comparison to the control group, which reached an average of only 6.77 mm. Clinical pregnancy rates within the study group were also significantly higher than the control group, 50% (108/216) versus 17.1% (16/93), respectively. For patients that have had multiple failures and canceled cycles, offering an absolute solution that at minimum guarantees them an embryo transfer can potentially increase the success of frozen embryo transfers in clinics globally, while decreasing patient stress and costs, and reducing the potential for embryo wastage.

Acknowledgements

The author would like to acknowledge and recognize the support of her co-authors and their institutions, the Eastern Virginia Medical School and Ovation Fertility-Newport Beach.

Conflict of interests

The author declares no conflict of interest.

Author details

Casey Zeffiro[1,2*], Silvina Bocca[1], Helena Russell[1*] and Mitchel C. Schiewe[2]

1 Eastern Virginia Medical School, Norfolk, United States

2 Ovation Fertility, Newport Beach, United States

*Address all correspondence to: czeffiro@ovationfertility.com
and russelhi@evms.edu

References

[1] Amable PR, Carias RB, Teixeira MV, da Cruz Pacheco I, Correa do Amaral RJ, Granjeiro JM, et al. Platelet-rich plasma preparation for regenerative medicine: Optimization and quantification of cytokines and growth factors. Stem Cell Research & Therapy. 2013;**4**:67

[2] Lee JW, Kwon OH, Kim TK, Cho YK, Choi KY, Chung HY, et al. Platelet rich plasma: Quantitative assessment of growth factor levels and comparative analysis of activated and inactivated groups. Archives of Plastic Surgery. 2013;**40**:530-535

[3] Christgau M, Moder D, Hiller KA, Dada A, Schmitz G, Schmalz G. Growth factors and cytokines in autologous platelet concentrate and their correlation to periodontal regeneration outcomes. Journal of Clinical Periodontology. 2006;**33**:837-845

[4] Barrione P, Gianfrancesco AD, Pereira MT, Pigozzi F. Platelet-rich plasma in muscle healing. American Journal of Physical Medicine & Rehabilitation. 2010;**89**:854-861

[5] Patel AN, Slezman CH, Kumpati GS, McKellar SH, Bull DA. Evaluation of autologous platelet rich plasma for cardiac surgery: Outcome analysis of 2000 patients. Journal of Cardiothoracic Surgery. 2016;**11**:62

[6] Chen MJ, Yang JH, Peng FH, Chen SU, Ho HN, Yang YS. Extended estrogen administration for women with thin endometrium in frozen-thawed in-vitro fertilization programs. Journal of Assisted Reproduction and Genetics. 2006;**23**:337-342

[7] Khiaru M, Banerjee K, El-Touhky T, Coomarasamy A, Khalaf Y. Aspirin in women undergoing in vitro fertilization treatment; a systemic review and meta-analysis. Fertility and Sterility. 2007;**88**:822-831

[8] Takasaki A, Tamura H, Miwa I, Taketani T, Shimamura K, Sugino N. Endometrial growth and uterine blood flow: A pilot study for improving endometrial thickness in the patients with a thin endometrium. Fertility and Sterility. 2010;**93**:1851-1858

[9] Gleicher N, Vidali A, Barad DH. Successful treatment of unresponsive thin endometrium. Fertility and Sterility. 2011;**95**(6):2123.e13-2123.e17

[10] Khalifa E, Brzyski RG, Oehninger S, Acosta AA, Muasher SJ. Sonographic appearance of the endometrium: The predictive value for the outcome of in-vitro fertilization in stimulated cycles. Human Reproduction. 1992;**7**:677-680

[11] Griesinger G, Trevisan S, Cometti B. Endometrial thickness on the day of embryo transfer is a poor predictor of IVF treatment outcome. Human Reproduction Open. 2018;**1**:1-8

[12] Zawar MP, Deshpande NM, Gadgil PA, Mahanta AA. Histopathological study of endometrium in infertility. Indian Journal of Pathology & Microbiology. 2003;**46**:630-633

[13] Mahajan N, Sharma S. The endometrium in assisted reproductive technology: How thin is thin? Journal of Human Reproductive Sciences. 2016;**9**(1):3-8

[14] Sak ME, Gul T, Evsen MS, Soydinc HE, Sak S, Ozler A, et al. Fibroblast growth factor-1 expression in the endometrium of patients with repeated implantation failure after in vitro fertilization. European Review for Medical and Pharmacological Sciences. 2013;**17**:398-402

[15] Green CJ, Fraser ST, Day ML. Insulin-like growth factor 1 increases apical fibronectin in blastocysts to

increase blastocyst attachment to endometrial epithelial cells in vitro. Human Reproduction. 2015;**30**:284-298

[16] Casper RF, Yanushpolsky EH. Optimal endometrial preparation for frozen embryo transfer cycles: Window of implantation and progesterone support. Fertility and Sterility. 2016;**105**:867-872

[17] Lessey BA, Killam AP, Metzger DA, Haney AF, Greene GL, McCarty KS Jr. Immunohistochemical analysis of human uterine estrogen and progesterone receptors throughout the menstrual cycle. The Journal of Clinical Endocrinology and Metabolism. 1988;**67**:334-340

[18] Chang Y, Li J, Chen Y, Wei L, Pang J, Liang X. Autologous platelet-rich plasma promotes endometrial growth and improves pregnancy outcome during in-vitro fertilization. International Journal of Clinical and Experimental Medicine. 2015;**8**(1):1286-1290

[19] Zadehmodarres S, Salehpour S, Saharkhiz N, Nazari L. Treatment of thin endometrium with autologous platelet-rich plasma: A pilot study. JBRA Assisted Reproduction. 2017;**21**:54-56

[20] Nazari L, Salehpour S, Hoseini S, Zadehmodarres S, Ajori L. Effects of autologous platelet-rich plasma on implantation and pregnancy in repeated implantation failure: A pilot study. International Journal of Reproductive BioMedicine. 2016;**14**:625-628

[21] Tandulwadkar SR, Naralkar MV, Surana AD, Slevakarthick M, Kharat AH. Autologous intrauterine platelet-rich plasma instillation for suboptimal endometrium in frozen embryo transfer cycles: A pilot study. Journal of Human Reproductive Sciences. 2017;**10**:208-212

[22] Eftekhar M, Neghab N, Naghshineg E, Khani P. Can autologous platelet rich plasma expand endometrial thickness and improve pregnancy rate during frozen-thawed embryo transfer cycle? A randomized clinical trial. Taiwanese Journal of Obstetrics & Gynecology. 2018;**57**:810-813

[23] Hounyoung K, Eun Shin J, Seon Koo H, Kwon H, Choi DH, Kim JH. Effect of autologous platelet-rich plasma treatment on refractory thin endometrium during the frozen embryo transfer cycle: A pilot study. Frontiers in Endocrinology. 2019;**10**:61

[24] Nazari L, Salehpour S, Hoseini S, Zadehmodarres S, Azargashb E. Effects of autologous platelet-rich plasma on endometrial expansion in patients undergoing frozen-thawed embryo transfer: A double-blind RCT. International Journal of Reproductive BioMedicine. 2019;**17**(6):443-448

[25] Chang Y, Li J, Wei L, Pang J, Chen J, Liang X. Autologous platelet-rich plasma infusion improves clinical pregnancy rate in frozen embryo transfer cycles for women with thin endometrium. Medicine (Baltimore). 2019;**98**(3):140-162

[26] Paulson RJ. Hormonal induction of endometrial receptivity. Fertility and Sterility. 2011;**96**:530-535

[27] Malhorta N, Malhorta J, Malhorta N, Rao JP, Mishra N. Endometrial receptivity and scoring for prediction of implantation and newer markers. Donald School Journal of Ultrasound in Obstetrics and Gynecology. 2010;**4**(4):439-446

[28] Diaz-Gimeno P, Horcajadas JA, Marinez-Conejero JA, Esteban FJ, Alma P, Pelicer A. A genomic diagnostic tool for human endometrial receptivity based on the transcriptomic signature. Fertility and Sterility. 2011;**95**:50-60

[29] Ruiz-Alonso M, Belsa D, Diaz-Gimeno P, Gomez E. The endometrial receptivity array for diagnosis and personalized embryo transfer as a treatment for patients with repeated implantation failure. Fertility and Sterility. 2013;**100**:818-824

Chapter 10

Recurrent Pregnancy Loss: Investigations and Interventions

Vinicius M. Lopes, Murilo C. Souza-Oliveira, Amanda Evelyn C. Goulart, Eduardo S. Pimentel, Natalia I. Zavattiero Tierno, Tatianna Q. F. Ribeiro, Cristina T. Medina, Valéria L. Mathias Castro, Leilane G. Noleto Lima, Anna Luiza M. Souza and Jean Pierre B. Brasileiro

Abstract

Recurrent pregnancy loss (RPL) affects 0.8–1.4% of couples, and this prevalence increases with aging. However, etiology is commonly unknown, and most therapies are not supported by strong evidence. There are many examinations that investigate causes of RPL: hormonal status, spermatozoa morphology and DNA fragmentation, immunologic status, uterine assessment, thrombophilia, and others. Recently different types of treatment have emerged, most lacking good evidence. As for example, we may mention the use of anticoagulants, aspirin, corticosteroids, progesterone, and antioxidants and psychological support. It is argued that some procedures such as preimplantation genetic testing for aneuploidy and intracytoplasmic morphologically selected sperm injection would impact on the outcomes and help RPL management. This chapter will discuss the current evidence concerning examinations and treatments that would improve the outcomes in patients with RPL, with recommended practice.

Keywords: recurrent pregnancy loss, recurrent miscarriage, in vitro fertilization, infertility, preimplantation *genetic* testing for aneuploidy, thrombophilia, sperm DNA fragmentation, natural killer cells, reproductive techniques, maternal KIR, paternal HLA-C

Keypoints

The practice of physical activity, healthy eating, quitting smoking, and reduction of alcohol consumption are factors that interfere in the reproductive outcomes. Medical understanding and ability to listen to patients about their obstetric past are fundamentally important for the treatment.

The genetic investigation is controversial and consists of chromosomal evaluation of the conception products and the couple's karyotype. The goal is to identify the etiology of the loss and may be useful for future guidance of the couple. There is no consensus on performing IVF-PGT, and this option should be discussed case by case. In extreme cases IVF using donated gametes may be the last option.,

Patients with RPL without other risk factors for thrombosis should not be screened for inherited thrombophilias, and those with positive screening have no benefit from available treatment. The only thrombophilia that should be routinely investigated for early miscarriage is APS. The recommended treatment is the use of low-dose AAS preconception and LMWH in a prophylactic dose initiated when diagnosing pregnancy.,

Screening immunological factors for patients with RPL is not recommended. There is also no recommendation to use venous immunoglobulin or corticosteroids empirically. Only antinuclear antibody can be ordered for prognostic purposes, according to ESHRE.,

Screening for congenital uterine anomalies is part of the investigation of women with a history of RPL. Nuclear magnetic resonance is the gold standard for diagnosis. The only finding that can be surgically corrected and prognosis improved is the septate uterus.,

The diagnosis of cervical incompetence is based on clinical history. The classic treatment is transvaginal cerclage between 12 and 16 weeks after first trimester morphological ultrasound.,

Patients with RPL should undergo through endometrial cavity evaluation. The gold standard is hysteroscopy. Although there is limited evidence linking submucosal fibroids, endometrial polyps, and synechiae with RPL, surgical correction in patients with RPL without other identifiable factors is suggested.,

There are no research and treatment benefits for PCOS patients and their associated endocrine disorders. Thyroid evaluation should be performed with serum TSH and anti-TPO, and clinical hypothyroidism should be treated. For prolactin, the test is not indicated in the absence of signs of hyperprolactinemia, but if this condition is diagnosed, treatment is indicated. Vitamin D test is not routinely recommended, but the preconception counseling in women with RPL may include prophylactic vitamin D supplementation due to the high prevalence of hypovitaminosis D in this population.,

The relationship of chronic endometritis with RPL is unclear. The current gold standard for the diagnosis of chronic endometritis is the pathological anatomy of immunohistochemically endometrial biopsy for the CD138 marker. A therapeutic option would be the use of doxycycline alone or in combination with other antibiotics.,

For male factor, measurement of spermatic DNA fragmentation index and Kruger morphology would be indicated. The use of antioxidants is a clinical treatment that can improve DNA fragmentation. In the presence of ICSI indication associated with increased spermatic DNA fragmentation, the use of testicular, IMSI, or PICSI sperm can be considered.

1. Introduction

Recurrent pregnancy loss (RPL) is defined by two or more losses with gestational age less than 20–24 weeks [1, 2]. Its prevalence varies between 0.8 and 1.4% considering only patients who have had a clinical pregnancy [2]. The pathogenesis is multifactorial, and in only 50% of the cases, the causal factor can be identified: immunological, endocrine, genetic, metabolic, and anatomical, among others [3]. The identification of etiology is not always possible, and recurrence of miscarriage seems to influence negatively the couple's psychological profile [2]. Thus, the understanding of diagnostic methods that can identify etiological factors and treatments that can improve the outcome is fundamental for the follow-up of couples with RPL.

2. Risk factors

Some personal factors such as lifestyle and even environmental exposure may be associated with obstetric complications and gestational loss. Advanced maternal age is one of the best-established risk factors in the literature for RPL [2]. Approximately 50–70% of early gestational losses are associated with chromosomal abnormalities, and their incidence increases with maternal age, reaching 50% in women over 40 years [3]. The European Society of Human Reproduction and Embryology (ESHRE) recommends that women should be informed of the highest risk of miscarriage after age 40 [2].

Obesity also has a major impact on women's reproductive health. High body mass index (BMI) is associated with worse outcomes in infertility treatments and a higher incidence of gestational loss [4]. One study with obese women showed a higher frequency of euploid miscarriages than nonobese women (58% vs. 37%) [5].

This is probably due to the association of obesity with several endocrine disorders, such as diabetes, hypothyroidism, and polycystic ovary syndrome and possibly endometrial changes [5]. The Royal College of Obstetricians and Gynecologists (RCOG) recommends prepregnancy weight loss due to the associated increased risk of miscarriage, stillbirth, preeclampsia, diabetes, and postpartum hemorrhages [6]. The practice of regular physical activity presents improvement in the obstetric outcome; however, there are no studies investigating the impact of exercise in patients with RPL [2].

Smoking seems to be related to defects in trophoblastic function, thus increasing the risk of gestational loss, in addition to poor obstetric prognosis [2]. Assisted reproduction societies recommend quitting smoking because of the negative impact on the chances of a live birth [2, 3]. Several studies have shown that drinking alcohol during pregnancy also increases the risk of gestational loss [2]. Although further studies are needed to establish if there is any safe dose for drinking in pregnancy, there are recommendations for couples with RPL not to drink alcohol.

Caffeine abuse can also affect fertility as well as be a risk factor for gestational losses. Ingestion of high caffeine levels (500 mg per day or > 5 cups per day) is associated with decreased fertility [7]. During pregnancy, drinking between 200 and 300 mg/day (2–3 cups) may increase the risk of miscarriage [3]. Thus, it seems sensible to guide this population to reduce caffeine consumption.

Few studies assess environmental exposure as a risk factor for RPL, one of which suggests that exposure to heavy metals and lack of micronutrients may cause gestational loss [8]. Another study suggests that ingestion of high concentrations of organochlorine pesticides may be associated with RPL [9].

It has been suggested in the past that stress could be associated with worsening the reproductive outcomes. There is a higher prevalence of depression in patients with RPL [10], but it is not known if this picture is not the cause or effect of RPL [2]. The American Society for Reproductive Medicine (ASRM) advises psychological support for these women who are more prone to feelings of grief, sadness, depression, anxiety, and guilt [3].

3. Genetic factors

The human conception is a vulnerable event—a large proportion of all conceptions are cytogenetically abnormal, and most of such pregnancies evolve to abortion. In couples with RPL, research can be divided into two main categories: genetic analysis of products of conception and parental genetic analysis.

3.1 Genetic analysis of products of conception

Studies in which products of conception were analyzed showed that genetic alterations, mainly aneuploidies, contribute to a significant portion of the causes of gestational losses, accounting for 50% of recurrent losses [11]. Despite the importance of genetic alterations as causes of miscarriage, there is still no consensus as to whether routine evaluation of pregnancy tissue should be performed. ASRM does not recommend genetic evaluation of conception products [3]. ESHRE, in turn, suggests that this analysis should not be done routinely but that it may be promoted for the purpose of clarifying the etiological factor and to assist in deciding whether further investigation or treatment is needed [2]. Other studies and guidelines, however, have proposed new algorithms in which the assessment of gestational repetition losses should be initiated with chromosome testing in conception products [12].

New chromosomal tests such as the chromosomal microarray analysis (CMA) have the potential to reduce costs since, in the presence of altered examination, costly and unnecessary evaluations will not be employed [13]. In addition, when a cause is identified, the tendency is to reduce the use of empirical treatments that have no scientific evidence [13]. Research has shown that in couples with previous embryonic aneuploidy, the likelihood of a child's birth during subsequent pregnancies was higher than patients with prior normal karyotype of conception products (71% vs. 44%) [14].

The suffering that the couple goes through experiencing abortion episodes without knowing the etiological factor can by itself justify the investigation of the existence of genetic alterations as a cause of the events.

3.2 Parental genetic analysis

In about 5% of all couples suffering two or more fetal losses, one partner carries a balanced chromosomal rearrangement, which represents approximately eightfold increase compared to the general population [15]. Guiding this couple for genetic counseling is important, as the likelihood of a healthy child born will depend on the type of rearrangement found and the chromosomes involved—for example, gestational losses are more present in carriers of balanced translocations and inversions than in carriers of Robertsonian translocations [16]. Even with one spouse carrying a chromosomal rearrangement, the cumulative rate of live birth, even in natural conception, is significant—63.4% despite the increased risk for miscarriage [17].

As for the existing guidelines regarding parental cytogenetic investigation, ESHRE determines that such assessment should not be performed routinely, but in specific cases after individual risk assessment [2]. ASRM, however, recommends routine parental karyotyping as information obtained may assist in counseling on the prognosis of future pregnancies, including guidance for performing preimplantation genetic testing (PGT), amniocentesis, or chorionic villus analysis [3].

Couples with structural cytogenetic changes have an increased number of gametes with chromosomal imbalances, so it would be expected that the implantation of embryos selected by PGT increases the rate of live births. However, in spouses carrying chromosomal rearrangement with RPL, the rate of live births, time to subsequent conception, and miscarriage rates were similar in both naturally conceived and in vitro fertilization associated with preimplantation diagnosis (IVF-PGT) [18]. Other papers showed discordant results. Similar live birth rate and time to new pregnancy were reported; however, the miscarriage rate was significantly lower in the IVF-PGT group [19]. Thus, there is no consensus showing the benefit of such strategy in this population, and no randomized controlled trials have been conducted to this date to validate possible benefits.

4. Thrombophilias

Thrombophilias are inherited and/or acquired conditions that predispose individuals to thrombosis, with varied prevalence in the general population [20]. The most common hereditary thrombophilias are methylenetetrahydrofolate reductase (MTHFR) gene polymorphism 4–16%, factor V Leiden mutation 1691G → A (heterozygote, 1–15%; homozygote, <1%), prothrombin mutation 20210G → A (heterozygote, 2–5%; homozygote, <1%), antithrombin deficiency (0.02%), protein C deficiency (0.2–0.4%), protein S deficiency (0.03–0.13%) [21], and serpin gene polymorphism. On the other hand, acquired thrombophilia is mainly represented by the antiphospholipid antibody syndrome (APS) 2% [20]. Successful pregnancy requires an adequate endovascular implantation and remodeling measured by trophoblast, and these prothrombotic conditions would be the target of investigation and intervention with anticoagulant therapy to prevent miscarriage [21].

4.1 Inherited thrombophilias

The screening of inherited thrombophilias even in patients with a thrombosis context is still questioned [2]. The factor V Leiden mutation (1691G→ A) and the prothrombin mutation (20210G→ A) were related to recurrent miscarriage [22]; however, the lack of evidence that the treatment changes the gestational outcome leads to questioning the relevance of investigating such mutations. Other thrombophilias, such as protein C deficiency, protein S deficiency, and antithrombin deficiency, although associated with thromboembolic event, were not associated with RPL [2, 3, 20, 22]. MTHFR gene polymorphisms are no longer considered risk factors for thrombophilias [2].

The association between RPL and inherited thrombophilias is weak or absent [2]. Thus, thrombophilic screening should be restricted to patients with family history of thrombophilias or previous thrombotic event [1, 2]. There is no recommendation to screen inherited thrombophilias in patients with RPL without other risk factors [1, 2, 21, 23]. Screening tests may be influenced by physiological/pathophysiological changes in the pregnancy-puerperal period, thrombotic event, or use of anticoagulants [21]. It should be performed within 6 weeks or more after delivery, miscarriage, or thrombotic event or early if necessary [2, 21].

The use of anticoagulant therapy with low-molecular-weight heparin and/or aspirin has no benefit in preventing early (<10 weeks) or late (≥10 weeks) RPL [24]. Thus, ineffectiveness of the treatment, the risk exposure, and the increased cost do not justify treatment with anticoagulants in patients with inherited thrombophilias and RPL without other risk factors for thrombosis [2, 20].

4.2 Acquired thrombophilias

APS is indicated in patients with RPL, as well as in patients with adverse gestational outcome or episode of thrombosis without apparent cause [25]. The diagnosis of APS is based on the combination of at least one clinical criterion, which includes thrombotic events and/or gestational morbidity, and a laboratory criterion, which includes three antibodies: lupus anticoagulant, anticardiolipin, and anti-β2 glycoprotein 1 (anti-β2GP1) [25].

In the cases of late gestational loss, lupus anticoagulant was more closely related to RPL than any of the other antibodies [26, 27]. Anticardiolipin (IgG and IgM) has been associated with early and late gestational loss [26, 27]. The relationship between anti-β2GP1 and late gestational loss seems to be controversial [26, 27]. ESHRE recommends for patients with two losses, consecutive or not, to conduct a research for lupus anticoagulant antibodies and anticardiolipin, and the research should consider anti-β2GP1.

The use of combined therapy, low-molecular-weight heparin at prophylactic dose, and low aspirin dose (75–100 mg/day) increases the live birth rate in patients with APS and RPL from 10% to 70–80% [28]. In treatment failure, the use of heparin in therapeutic dose may be used, although there is no benefit evidence [28]. Other treatment regimens with limited evidence are the use of hydroxychloroquine or low dose of prednisolone in the first trimester [28]. The use of immunoglobulin is questioned because studies are limited and show no increase in live birth rate [28].

5. Immunological factors

To be successful in pregnancy, the maternal organism needs to undergo immunological changes that allow and assist in the trophoblastic invasion of the embryo. During pregnancy, the maternal immune system faces a dilemma: it needs to protect the mother against infection while accepting the semi-allogeneic fetus [29]. Leukocytes are important components of the endometrium, and their concentration increases in the middle of the secretory phase in which embryonic implantation is expected and continues to increase during early pregnancy [30]. The progesterone plays a key role in this balance by creating an appropriate environment for embryonic implantation and development [28]. This change in maternal endometrial immunology becomes essential for early pregnancy implantation and success. Changes in this phase can lead to implantation failure, miscarriage, and other unfavorable obstetric outcomes such as preeclampsia.

5.1 Natural killer (NK) cell

The uterine natural killer (uNK) cells are the most commonly found leukocytes in the maternal endometrium. Two phenotypes are observed—CD56bright and CD16dim—unlike peripheral blood where CD56dim and CD16+ are the largest population [31]. There is a variability of their own concentration during the menstrual cycle. There are a significant increase of NK cells in the endometrium 6 to 7 days after the peak of luteinizing hormone (LH), which persists throughout the early pregnancy. This increase suggests an important role of these cells in embryonic implantation, but the exact function is still unknown [30].

5.1.1 Killer immunoglobulin-like receptors (KIR)

The placental formation is regulated by the interaction between the killer immunoglobulin-like receptors (KIR) and the surface human leukocyte antigens on the embryo trophoblastic cells (HLA-C). The embryo presents maternal and paternal HLA-C, and both haplotypes are presented to NK cells that, in turn, will recognize the human leukocyte antigen (HLA) foreign to their organism. There are two types of HLA-C: C1 and C2 which are a strong ligand to the receptor. On the other hand, there are two KIR haplotypes: A, which is inhibitory, and B, which is stimulating. The receptors can then be AA, AB, or BB. The presence of haplotype B confers pregnancy protection, and its absence (in the cases of KIR AA) increases the risk of gestational complications.

Studies have shown that when maternal KIR is homozygous for haplotype A (KIR AA), there is an increased risk of gestational complications if the embryo carries paternal HLA-C2 [32, 33]. In the future, these studies may be applicable to couples who will undergo IVF. Further studies on the subject are still needed, and these tests are not quoted to be traced by societal guidelines.

5.2 Macrophages

The macrophages represent 20–30% of leukocytes in the maternal endometrium and are the second largest group behind only NK cells. Macrophages differ in specific phenotypes to perform different biological functions and can be divided into two subgroups: M1 and M2. M1 macrophages are pro-inflammatory and antimicrobial, whereas M2 have anti-inflammatory function [34]. For maternal and fetal tolerance to occur, more macrophages are polarized into the M2 subtype with immunosuppressive properties necessary for normal pregnancy to occur [35]. When polarization of these cells does not occur correctly favoring the M1 subgroup, improper remodeling of the arteries and trophoblastic invasion occurs, leading to a higher incidence of miscarriage, preeclampsia, and premature birth [35].

5.3 Regulatory T cells

Regulatory T cells (Treg) are a subpopulation of T cells that play an essential role in maintaining maternal immune tolerance. These cells are activated by the presented antigens and from that moment secrete cytokines that will determine the differentiation of T cell subtypes, thus modulating the immune response. Depending on the released cytokines, T cells may differentiate into Treg cells expressing interleukin 10 and transforming growth factor β (TGFβ) responsible for immune tolerance to the conceptus or Th17 expressing interleukins 17, 21, and 22 responsible for autoimmunity and gestational loss. Treg cells will then regulate the response to foreign antigens when an aggressive response is not appropriate, having the ability to inhibit type 1 helper (Th1) cells. There is evidence in the cases of recurrent gestational loss of unknown cause to increase Th17 and to decrease Treg cells, leading to an inadequate immune response [29].

6. Anatomical factors

Uterine anatomical abnormalities, both acquired and congenital, are associated with RPL. It is estimated that uterine factors may account for 10–50% of RPL [36].

6.1 Congenital uterine anomalies

6.1.1 Congenital Müllerian duct anomalies

Congenital uterine anomalies (CUA) arise from defects along any stage of the Müller duct development process during embryonic development, whether in formation, fusion, or reabsorption. The frequency of CUA has been reported between 1.8 and 37.6% in women with a history of RLP. This variation is due to the different diagnostic methods and criteria [37]. Septate uterus is the most common anomaly in patients with a history of abortion. Arched, septate, and bicornuate uterus account for up to 85% of anomalies [38].

In a meta-analysis it was observed that patients with septate or bicornuate uterus had a higher rate of miscarriage in the first and second trimester than a control group [39]. In another meta-analysis, the evaluation of uterine abnormality subtypes resulting from fusion defect showed that women with unicornuate and bicornuate uterus were more likely to have first-trimester abortion compared to those with normal uterus [40].

ASRM's original classification system for congenital uterine anomalies has been modified and adapted and is still the most widely used today [41]. In 2012, ESHRE/ESGE published a classification system aiming to replace the subjective criteria of ASRM's classification by the absolute morphometric criteria [42]. Based on this classification, up to 58% of women previously diagnosed with ASRM arched uterus would be reclassified as having a partial septate uterus. There would be a potential increase in the number of surgical corrections for uterine anomaly, without any evidence showing that such a practice would be beneficial [43]. Therefore, caution is needed in using this new classification until further prospective, randomized, controlled, long-term studies are available to associate the severity of uterine cavity distortion with reproductive results.

Given the suspicion, it is necessary to use diagnostic methods that can clearly visualize the external contour of the uterus and endometrial cavity. Both 3D ultrasound with inversion mode (3D US) and magnetic resonance imaging (MRI) can be used for this purpose, with good correlation between them [44]. The disadvantages of MRI are that it is a more expensive and less available method than ultrasound.

In a comparative study of different diagnostic modalities, higher accuracy of 3D hysterosonography compared with 3D US and 2D hysterosonography was observed, although the differences between these imaging techniques did not reach statistical significance in the diagnosis of arched, bicornuate, and septate uterus [45].

The uterine septum is the most common abnormality related to RPL [36] and the only remediable one. Despite the lack of randomized and controlled prospective studies comparing surgery to expectant treatment, limited studies indicate that hysteroscopy septal resection is associated with a reduction in subsequent abortion rates and an improvement in live birth rates in patients with RPL [41]. After hysteroscopic resection of the septum, an interval of at least 2 months should be expected for complete healing of the endometrial cavity before a new pregnancy [41].

In general, CUA may be associated with renal abnormalities in approximately 11–30% of individuals [41]; for this reason there is a need for urinary tract investigation in these cases.

6.1.2 Cervical incompetence

Cervical incompetence (CI) is the inability of the cervix to keep the intrauterine fetus in the absence of uterine contractions or labor (painless cervical dilatation) due to a functional or structural defect. It is a recognized cause of RPL in the second trimester, but the true incidence is unknown, as the diagnosis is essentially clinical [2].

The CI can be congenital or acquired. The most common congenital cause is a defect in the embryological development of the Müllerian ducts. The most common acquired cause is cervical trauma, such as cervical lacerations during childbirth, cervical conization, or forced cervical dilation during uterine procedures [46].

The diagnosis is usually based on a history of miscarriage in the second trimester, preceded by spontaneous rupture of membranes or painless cervical dilation. There are currently no objective tests capable of identifying women with cervical weakness in the nonpregnant state [2].

Transvaginal ultrasound may be used in at-risk patients during pregnancy. CI might be suspected when there is a short cervical length, less than or equal to 25 mm, or funneling, protrusion of the membrane into a dilated internal orifice but with closed external orifice [46].

Many surgical and nonsurgical modalities have been proposed to treat cervical incompetence. Among nonsurgical activities, restriction of activities and bed rest were not effective in the treatment of cervical incompetence. Its isolated use is discouraged. The use of vaginal pessary is another option, but the evidence is still limited. Surgical approaches include transvaginal and transabdominal cervical cerclage [46].

6.2 Acquired anatomical factors

Acquired anatomical factors commonly associated with RPL include uterine fibroids, endometrial polyps, and uterine synechiae. They usually develop after puberty due to physical or hormonal stimuli and are present in about 12% of patients with RPL [47].

6.2.1 Uterine fibroids

Fibroid is reported in 8,2% of women with RPL [48]. Submucosal fibroids deform the endometrial cavity, thus affecting implantation and embryonic development [47]. Hysteroscopy is considered the gold standard for the diagnosis of submucosal fibroids, but this pathology can be identified through other imaging exams, such as ultrasound mapping [2]. The evaluation of the uterine cavity is strongly recommended for all women with RPL, since the removal of submucosal fibroids in infertile patients seems to reduce the chance of miscarriage [2, 49]. Regarding fibroids that do not distort the uterine cavity, there is no evidence indicating that myomectomy may reduce the chances of an abortion [2, 49].

6.2.2 Uterine polyps

There seems to be a higher prevalence of endometrial polyps in women with gestational loss (2.4%), but with no well-defined clinical importance [2, 47]. Hysteroscopy is considered the gold standard exam for the diagnosis and treatment of endometrial polyps but can also be identified through other imaging exams, such as ultrasound with color Doppler [2]. Although there is no evidence of the benefit of polypectomy in women with RPL, hysteroscopic removal should be considered when the polyp is larger than 1 cm when no other known etiology is found [2, 47]. ASRM reports that research for uterine polyps in women with gestational loss is controversial as there is no conclusive evidence that surgical treatment reduces the risk of gestational loss [49].

6.2.3 Uterine synechiae/Asherman syndrome

The prevalence of uterine synechiae ranges from 0.5 to 28% in patients with RPL [47]. Women with RPL are more likely to have uterine synechiae as they often undergo curettage or manual vacuum aspiration. The probable pathophysiology of abortion occurs due to a reduction in the amount of functional endometrium which may interfere with the invasion and normal development of the placenta [47]. The gold standard exam for the diagnosis of synechiae is hysteroscopy and should be the exam of choice in the cases of suspicion [2]. ESHRE concludes that there is insufficient evidence to recommend adhesiolysis in women with RPL as there are only small observational studies. ESHRE reinforces that treatment should focus on preventing recurrence of adhesions [2, 3]. However, ASRM points out that surgical correction of significant uterine cavity defects should be considered [3]. Nonsurgical experimental techniques for the treatment of uterine synechiae and endometrial fibrosis, such as stem cell therapy, should be further studied before being indicated in clinical practice [2].

7. Endocrine factors

Hormones play a key role in placentation, and their changes may result in the risk of miscarriage [2].

7.1 Luteal phase insufficiency

It is a condition of insufficient exposure to progesterone to maintain a secretory endometrium that will lead to normal embryo implantation and growth [50]. The diagnostic criteria for luteal insufficiency are not well established which makes it difficult to conduct studies that can demonstrate the causal link between luteal phase insufficiency and RPL. Thus, luteal phase failure testing is not recommended for patients with RPL [2, 3]. The use of progesterone or human chorionic gonadotropin (hCG) for its treatment is divergent in the literature [2, 3].

7.2 Thyroid disorders

Studies relating subclinical hypothyroidism, defined as thyroid-stimulating hormone (TSH) > 2.5 mU/L and normal free thyroxine, and increased risk of RPL, have low levels of evidence [2]. The anti-thyroid peroxidase antibodies' (anti-TPO) presence in patients with RPL, even euthyroid, is an important gestational prognostic factor [51]. Thus, a TSH and anti-TPO dosage is recommended for women with RPL. And, in detecting abnormal levels of the above exams, it recommends that T4 levels should be evaluated [2].

Patients with clinical hypothyroidism should be treated with levothyroxine [2, 3]. In women with RPL and subclinical hypothyroidism, the benefit of treatment should be evaluated as the evidences are conflicting [2, 3]. In addition, euthyroid women with positive anti-TPO should not be treated with levothyroxine [2, 52].

7.3 Polycystic ovary syndrome and disorders of insulin metabolism

Several abnormalities observed in patients with polycystic ovary syndrome (PCOS) have been independently associated with RPL, including insulin resistance, hyperinsulinemia, hyperandrogenemia, hyperprolactinemia, and obesity.

There is a higher prevalence of insulin resistance among women with RPL than controls [53]. However, no study has confirmed the cause-effect relationship between insulin resistance and RPL. Thus, there is insufficient evidence to recommend assessment of PCOS, fast insulin and fast glucose, and insulin and glycemia nor the use of metformin in pregnancy to prevent gestational loss in women with RPL and defects in glucose metabolism [2].

The presence of an independent link between hyperandrogenemia and RPL remains controversial. Therefore, researching androgen levels is not recommended in women with RPL [2].

7.4 Prolactin disorders

Most studies fail to establish a direct link between RPL and serum prolactin concentration. Thus, prolactin test is not routinely recommended in the absence of clinical signs of hyperprolactinemia [2]. But if hyperprolactinemia is detected, treatment with dopaminergic agonists may be considered in women to increase live birth rates [2, 3].Since hyperprolactinemia is an easily treatable cause, most centers routinely test serum prolactin levels.

7.5 Vitamin D

There are few studies evaluating the association between vitamin D deficiency and RPL [2]. One of them showed increased prevalence of hypovitaminosis D in women with RPL, but it was unable to demonstrate cause-effect relationship [2, 54]. Thus, based on the significant prevalence of hypovitaminosis D in women with RPL and possible association with obstetric and fetal complications, the preconception counseling in these women may include prophylactic vitamin D supplementation [2].

8. Chronic endometritis

Chronic endometritis (CE) is defined as a persistent inflammation of the endometrial mucosa caused by the presence of bacterial pathogens in the uterine cavity [55]. Its prevalence in patients with RPL is approximately 12–13% [56]. The influence of CE on reproductive capacity is controversial, but many authors suggest that CE may negatively affect embryonic implantation [56]. Some studies suggest an infectious etiology with positive cultures in 75% of women with histologically confirmed CE, with the most common bacteria being *Escherichia coli*, *Enterococcus faecalis*, and *Streptococcus agalactiae* (77.5%) [57]. Most patients are asymptomatic, with pain on uterine or cervical mobilization being the most common clinical presentation [58, 59].

CE is histopathologically diagnosed as a lymphoplasmacytic infiltrate in the endometrial stroma [58, 59]. Immunohistochemistry for the marker present in CD138 plasma cells is used to improve diagnostic accuracy [60]. A diagnostic video hysteroscopy can help identify CE, with direct visualization of the endometrial cavity, which usually presents with mucosal edema, focal or diffuse endometrial hyperemia, or micropolyps. The sensitivity, specificity, and positive and negative predictive values of hysteroscopy in diagnosing CE were 86.36, 87.30, 70.37, and 94.82%, respectively [61].

Up to a few years ago, the uterine cavity was thought of as a sterile environment. Recently, there has been discussed that an imbalance of the uterine microbiota might compromise embryonic implantation or induce an abortion. Endometrial biopsy for next-generation sequencing (NGS) microbiota evaluation and etiological agent research can now be done through commercial kits [55]. However, further studies are needed to evaluate diagnostic efficacy and therapy on the reproductive outcomes.

Some studies suggest that treatment is related to increased live birth rates and reduced abortion rates [62]. There are several therapeutic options; the main ones mentioned in the literature refer to the use of doxycycline alone (100 mg, 12/12 hours orally, for 14 days) or the combination of metronidazole (250 mg, 12/12 hours orally, for 14 days) and ciprofloxacin (250 mg orally 12/12 hours for 14 days) [59].

9. Male factors

There is a growing acceptance of male etiological factors for RPL. Its screening consists of detailed sperm analysis. Excessive sperm DNA fragmentation is an important constraint to conception. Two meta-analyses have shown the association of gestational losses with high rates of sperm DNA fragmentation [63, 64]. The available tests for sperm DNA fragmentation index are the sperm chromatin structure assay (SCSA), the terminal deoxynucleotidyl transferase (TdT)-mediated dUTP nick end labeling (TUNEL), the Sperm Chromatin Dispersion test, and the comet assay.

Some clinical conditions are related to increased fragmentation of sperm DNA. High seminal plasma leukocyte concentration, systemic infections, varicocele, and smoking, among others, were related to spermatic DNA damage [65]. A Cochrane meta-analysis suggests that the use of antioxidants, including vitamins C and E, may have benefits for subfertile men with no apparent cause, improving sperm DNA fragmentation [66]. The generally recommended dose is 1 gram of vitamin C and 1000 IU of vitamin E per day for at least 2 months [67]. However, this effect is not yet established in patients with RPL. ESHRE determines that sperm DNA fragmentation research should be considered for explanatory purposes for RPL [2].

For intracytoplasmic sperm injection (ICSI)-indicated couples, laboratory techniques may be performed to select sperm with lower DNA fragmentation rate, such as physiological intracytoplasmic sperm injection (PICSI) and intracytoplasmic morphologically selected injection (IMSI). However, the use of testicular sperm seems to improve fertilization, pregnancy, and live birth rates when compared to PICS and IMSI techniques [68]. Nevertheless, further studies are needed to identify the best method for selecting sperm to reduce abortion rates.

The morphological analysis of sperm is another point to consider in cases of RPL. The presence of spermatozoa with structural anomalies may be associated with aneuploidy, resulting in aneuploid embryos that usually do not implant or are aborted. This is especially true in cases of globozoospermia and macrospermia, forms of monomorphic teratospermia—when all sperms have the same anomaly [69]. Infertility is generally associated with these cases, and the prognosis of IVF is reserved. Thus, when associated with abortion, IVF followed by embryonic biopsy for preimplantation genetic testing for aneuploidies (PGT-A) may be an option.

10. Conclusion

Recurrent spontaneous abortion is an entity with a multifactorial etiology, and in approximately 50% of cases, we did not identify the cause of the loss. This explains the large number of controversies regarding the investigation and treatment of the pathologies that lead to repeated losses.

Despite so much controversy, there are some points on which experts agree. Psychological support for couples is essential and is associated with a better prognosis in subsequent pregnancy. Undergoing through periodic consultations and ultrasounds especially during the period of previous losses reduces the stress of these couples. The woman's age and number of previous losses are the most important factors in predicting the couple's chance of having a live baby in the next pregnancy.

There is a need for consensus among human reproduction societies on the tests that must be ordered and diagnostic criteria for all specialists to evaluate couples evenly. In this way, we will be able to evaluate the effectiveness of each available treatment, avoiding further financial burns, emotional disorders, and iatrogenesis for these couples.

Conflict of interest

The authors have no conflicts of interest that are relevant to this report.

Author details

Vinicius M. Lopes*, Murilo C. Souza-Oliveira, Amanda Evelyn C. Goulart, Eduardo S. Pimentel, Natalia I. Zavattiero Tierno, Tatianna Q. F. Ribeiro, Cristina T. Medina, Valéria L. Mathias Castro, Leilane G. Noleto Lima, Anna Luiza M. Souza and Jean Pierre B. Brasileiro
VERHUM Institute, Brasilia-DF, Brazil

*Address all correspondence to: vinicius@verhum.com.br

References

[1] Practice Committee of American Society for Reproductive Medicine. Definitions of infertility and recurrent pregnancy loss: A committee opinion. Fertility and Sterility. 2013;**99**(1):63. DOI: 10.1016/j.fertnstert.2012.09.023

[2] The EGGoRPL. Bender Atik R, Christiansen OB, Elson J, Kolte AM, Lewis S, et al. ESHRE guideline: Recurrent pregnancy loss. Human Reproduction Open. 2018;**2018**(2):hoy004. DOI: 10.1093/hropen/hoy004

[3] Practice Committee of the American Society for Reproductive M. Evaluation and treatment of recurrent pregnancy loss: A committee opinion. Fertility and Sterility. 2012;**98**(5):1103-1111. DOI: 10.1016/j.fertnstert.2012.06.048

[4] Broughton DE, Moley KH. Obesity and female infertility: Potential mediators of obesity's impact. Fertile and Sterility. 2017;**107**(4):840-847. DOI: 10.1016/j.fertnstert.2017.01.017

[5] Boots CE, Bernardi LA, Stephenson MD. Frequency of euploid miscarriage is increased in obese women with recurrent early pregnancy loss. Fertility and Sterility. 2014;**102**(2):455-459. DOI: 10.1016/j.fertnstert.2014.05.005

[6] Denison FC, Aedla NR, Keag O, Hor K, Reynolds RM, Milne A, et al. Care of Women with obesity in pregnancy. Green-top guideline No. 72. British journal of obstetrics and gynaecology. 2019;**126**(3):e62-e106. DOI: 10.1111/1471-0528.15386

[7] Pfeifer S, Butts S, Fossum G, Gracia C, La Barbera A, Mersereau J, et al. Optimizing natural fertility: A committee opinion. Fertility and Sterility. 2013;**107**(1):52-58. DOI: 10.1016/j.fertnstert.2016.09.029

[8] Ajayi OO, Charles-Davies MA, Arinola OG. Progesterone, selected heavy metals and micronutrients in pregnant Nigerian women with a history of recurrent spontaneous abortion. African Health Sciences. 2012;**12**:153-159. DOI: 10.4314/ahs.v12i2.12

[9] Pathak R, Mustafa M, Ahmed RS, Tripathi AK, Guleria K, Banerjee BD. Association between recurrent miscarriages and organochlorine pesticide levels. Clinical Biochemistry. 2010;**43**:131-135. DOI: 10.1016/j.clinbiochem.2009.09.019

[10] Kolte AM, Olsen LR, Mikkelsen EM, Christiansen OB, Nielsen HS. Depression and emotional stress is [sic] highly prevalent among women with recurrent pregnancy loss. Human Reproduction. 2015;**30**:777-782. DOI: 10.1093/humrep/dev014

[11] Ogasawara M, Aoki K, Okada S, Suzumori K. Embryonic karyotype of abortuses in relation to the number of previous miscarriages. Fertility and Sterility. 2000;**73**(2):300-304. DOI: 10.1016/s0015-0282(99)00495-1

[12] Popescu F, Jaslow CR, Kutteh WH. Recurrent pregnancy loss evaluation combined with 24-chromosome microarray of miscarriage tissue provides a probable or definite cause of pregnancy loss in over 90% of patients. Human Reproduction. 2018;**33**(4):579-587. DOI: 10.1093/humrep/dey021

[13] Khalife D, Ghazeeri G, Kutteh W. Review of current guidelines for recurrent pregnancy loss: New strategies for optimal evaluation of women who may be superfertile. Seminars in Perinatology. 2019;**43**(2):105-115. DOI: 10.1053/j.semperi.2018.12.008

[14] Sugiura-Ogasawara M, Ozaki Y, Katano K, Suzumori N, Kitaori T, Mizutani E. Abnormal

embryonic karyotype is the most frequent cause of recurrent miscarriage. Human Reproduction. 2012;**27**(8):2297-2303. DOI: 10.1093/humrep/des179

[15] Sudhir N, Kaur T, Beri A, Kaur A. Cytogenetic analysis in couples with recurrent miscarriages: A retrospective study from Punjab, North India. Journal of Genetics. 2016;**95**:887-894. DOI: 10.1007/s12041-016-0713-3

[16] Franssen MTM, Korevaar JC, Van der Veen F, Leschot NJ, Bossuyt PMM, Goddijn M. Reproductive outcome after chromosome analysis in couples with two or more miscarriages: Index [corrected]-control study. BMJ. 2006;**332**(7544):759-763. DOI: 10.1136/bmj.38735.459144.2F

[17] Kabessa M, Harlev A, Friger M, Sergienko R, Litwak B, Koifman A, et al. Pregnancy outcomes among patients with recurrent pregnancy loss and chromosomal aberration (CA) without PGD. Journal of Perinatal Medicine. 2018 Sep 25;**46**(7):764-770. DOI: 10.1515/jpm-2016-0408

[18] Iews M, Tan J, Taskin O, Alfaraj S, AbdelHafez FF, Abdellah AH, et al. Does preimplantation genetic diagnosis improve reproductive outcome in couples with recurrent pregnancy loss owing to structural chromosomal rearrangement? A systematic review. Reproductive Biomedicine Online. 2018;**36**(6):677-685. DOI: 10.1016/j.rbmo.2018.03.005

[19] Ikuma S, Sato T, Sugiura-Ogasawara M, Nagayoshi M, Tanaka A, Takeda S. Preimplantation genetic diagnosis and natural conception: A comparison of live birth rates in patients with recurrent pregnancy loss associated with translocation. PLoS One. 2015;**10**(6):17. DOI: 10.1371/journal.pone.0129958

[20] Stevens SM, Woller SC, Bauer KA, Kasthuri R, Cushman M, Streiff M, et al. Guidance for the evaluation and treatment of hereditary and acquired thrombophilia. Journal of Thrombosis and Thrombolysis. 2016;**41**(1):154-164. DOI: 10.1007/s11239-015-1316-1

[21] ACOG. Practice bulletin No. 200: Early pregnancy loss. Obstetrics and Gynecology. 2018;**132**(5):e197-e207. DOI: 10.1097/AOG.0000000000002899

[22] Bradley LA, Palomaki GE, Bienstock J, Varga E, Scott JA. Can factor V Leiden and prothrombin G20210A testing in women with recurrent pregnancy loss result in improved pregnancy outcomes? Results from a targeted evidence-based review. Genetics in Medicine. 2012;**14**:39-50. DOI: 10.1038/gim.0b013e31822e575b

[23] Royal College of Obstetricians and Gynaecologists (RCOG). The Investigation and Treatment of Couples with Recurrent First-trimester and Second-trimester Miscarriage. Green-top Guideline No. 17. 2011. Available from: https://www.rcog.org.uk/globalassets/documents/guidelines/gtg_17.pdf

[24] Skeith L, Carrier M, Kaaja R, Martinelli I, Petroff D, Schleussner E, et al. A meta-analysis of low-molecular-weight heparin to prevent pregnancy loss in women with inherited thrombophilia. Blood. 2016;**127**:1650-1655. DOI: 10.1182/blood-2015-12-626739

[25] Miyakis S, Lockshin MD, Atsumi T, Branch DW, Brey RL, Cervera R, et al. International consensus statement on an update of the classification criteria for definite antiphospholipid syndrome (APS). Journal of Thrombosis and Haemostasis. 2006;**4**(2):295-306. DOI: 10.1111/j.1538-7836.2006.01753.x

[26] Opatrny L, David M, Kahn SR, Shrier I, Rey E. Association between antiphospholipid antibodies and recurrent fetal loss in women without

autoimmune disease: A meta-analysis. The Journal of Rheumatology. 2006;**33**(11):2214-2221

[27] Xu J, Chen D, Duan X, Li L, Tang Y, Peng B. The association between antiphospholipid antibodies and late fetal loss: A systematic review and meta-analysis. Acta Obstetricia et Gynecologica Scandinavica. 27 May 2019. DOI: 10.1111/aogs.13665. [Epub ahead of print]

[28] Tektonidou MG, Andreoli L, Limper M, Amoura Z, Cervera R, Costedoat-Chalumeau N, et al. EULAR recommendations for the management of antiphospholipid syndrome in adults. Annals of the Rheumatic Diseases. 2019;**78**(10):1296-1304. DOI: 10.1136/annrheumdis-2019-215213. [Epub 15 May 2019]

[29] Figueiredo AS, Schumacher A. The helper type 17/regulatory T cell paradigm in pregnancy. Immunology. 2016;**148**(1):13-21. DOI: 10.1111/imm.12595

[30] Bulmer JN, Williams PJ, Lash GE. Immune cells in the placental bed. The International Journal of Developmental Biology. 2010;**54**(2-3):281-294. DOI: 10.1387/ijdb.082763jb

[31] Chen X, Mariee N, Jiang L, Liu Y, Wang CC, Li TC, et al. Measurement of uterine natural killer cell percentage in the periimplantation endometrium from fertile women and women with recurrent reproductive failure: Establishment of a reference range. American Journal of Obstetrics and Gynecology. 2017;**217**(6):680. DOI: 10.1016/j.ajog.2017.09.010

[32] Alecsandru D, Garrido N, Vicario JL, Barrio A, Aparicio P, Requena A, et al. Maternal KIR haplotype influences live birth rate after double embryo transfer in IVF cycles in patients with recurrent miscarriages and implantation failure. Human Reproduction. *2014*;**29**(12):2637-2643. DOI: 10.1093/humrep/deu251

[33] Alecsandru D, Guerrero A, Aparicio P, Romero M, Barrio A, Pellicer A, et al. Treatment strategies to increase the live birth rate in patients with KIR-HLA-C mismatch: A retrospective cohort study. In: Annual Meeting of European Society of Human Reproduction and Embryology, 35., June/2019, Vienna-Austria. SCIENTIFIC PROGRAMME – Oral communications. Trial registration number: 1812-MAD-101-DA

[34] Porta C, Riboldi E, Ippolito A, Sica A. Molecular and epigenetic basis of macrophage polarized activation. Seminar in immunology 2015;**27**(4): 237-248. DOI: 10.1016/j.smim.2015.10.003

[35] Yao Y, Xu XH, Jin L. Macrophage polarization in physiological and pathological pregnancy. Frontiers in Immunology. 2019;**10**:792. DOI: 10.3389/fimmu.2019.00792.eCollection 2019

[36] Turocy JM, Rackow BW. Uterine factor in recurrent pregnancy loss. Seminars in Perinatology. 2019;**43**(2):74-79. DOI: 10.1053/j.semperi.2018.12.003. [Epub 20 Dec 2018]

[37] Sugiura-Ogasawara M, Ozaki Y, Katano K, Suzumori N, Mizutani E. Uterine anomaly and recurrent pregnancy loss. Seminars in Reproductive Medicine. 2011;**29**(06):514-521. DOI: 10.1055/s-0031-1293205

[38] Chan YY, Jayaprakasan K, Zamora J, Thornton JG, Raine-Fenning N, Coomarasamy A. The prevalence of congenital uterine anomalies in unselected and high-risk populations: A systematic review. *Human Reproduction Update*. 2011;**17**:761-771. DOI: 10.1093/humupd/dmr028

[39] Venetis CA, Papadopoulos SP, Campo R, Gordts S, Tarlatzis BC, Grimbizis GF. Clinical implications of congenital uterine anomalies: A meta-analysis of comparative studies. Reproductive Biomedicine Online. 2014;**29**(6):665-683. DOI: 10.1016/j.rbmo.2014.09.006.

[40] Chan YY, Jayaprakasan K, Tan A, Thornton JG, Coomarasamy A, Raine-Fenning NJ. Reproductive outcomes in women with congenital uterine anomalies: A systematic review. Ultrasound in Obstetrics & Gynecology. 2011;**38**(4):371-382. DOI: 10.1002/uog.10056

[41] Pfeifer S, Butts S, Dumesic D, Gracia C, Vernon M, Fossum G, et al. Uterine septum: a guideline. Fertile and Sterility. 2016;**106**(3):530-540. DOI: 10.1016/j.fertnstert.2016.05.014

[42] Grimbizis GF, Campo R. Clinical approach for the classification of congenital uterine malformations. Gynecological Surgery. 2012;**9**(2):119-129. DOI: 10.1007/s10397-011-0724-2

[43] Knez J, Saridogan E, Van Den Bosch T, Mavrelos D, Ambler G, Jurkovic D. ESHRE/ESGE female genital tract anomalies classification system—The potential impact of discarding arcuate uterus on clinical practice. Human Reproduction. 2018;**33**(4):600-606. DOI: 10.1093/humrep/dey043

[44] Bermejo C, Martínez Ten P, Cantarero R, Diaz D, Pérez Pedregosa J, Barrón E, et al. Three-dimensional ultrasound in the diagnosis of Mullerian duct anomalies and concordance with magnetic resonance imaging. Ultrasound in Obstetrics & Gynecology. 2010;**35**(5):593-601. DOI: 10.1002/uog.7551

[45] Ludwin A, Pityński K, Ludwin I, Banas T, Knafel A. Two- and three-dimensional ultrasonography and Sonohysterography versus hysteroscopy with laparoscopy in the differential diagnosis of Septate, Bicornuate, and Arcuate uteri. Journal of Minimally Invasive Gynecology. 2013;**20**(1):90-99. DOI: 10.1016/j.jmig.2012.09.011

[46] Thakur M, Mahajan K. Cervical Incompetence. StatPearls [Internet]. Treasure Island (FL): StatPearls Publishing; 2019. Available from: https://www.ncbi.nlm.nih.gov/books/NBK525954/

[47] Jaslow CR. Uterine factors. Obstetrics and Gynecology Clinics of North America. 2014;**41**:57-86. DOI: 10.1016/j.ogc.2013.10.002

[48] Saravelos SH, Yan J, Rehmani H, Li TC. The prevalence and impact of fibroids and their treatment on the outcome of pregnancy in women with recurrent miscarriage. Human Reproduction. 2011;**26**:3274-3279. DOI: 10.1093/humrep/der293

[49] Practice Committee of the American Society for Reproductive Medicine. Removal of myomas in asymptomatic patients to improve fertility and/or reduce miscarriage rate: A committee: A guideline. Fertility and Sterility. 2017;**108**:416-425. DOI: 10.1016/j.fertnstert.2017.06.034

[50] Palomba S, Santagni S, La Sala GB. Progesterone administration for luteal phase deficiency in human reproduction: An old or new issue? Journal of Ovarian Research. 2015;**8**:77. DOI: 10.1186/s13048-015-0205-8

[51] Thangaratinam S, Tan A, Knox E, Kilby MD, Franklyn J, Coomarasamy A. Association between thyroid autoantibodies and miscarriage and preterm birth: Meta-analysis of evidence. BMJ. 2011;**342**:d2616. DOI: 10.1136/bmj.d2616

[52] Huang C, Liang P, Diao L, Liu C, Chen X, Li G, et al. Thyroid

autoimmunity is associated with decreased cytotoxicity T cells in women with repeated implantation failure. International Journal of Environmental Research and Public Health. 2015;**12**(9):10352-10361. DOI: 10.3390/ijerph120910352

[53] Craig LB, Ke RW, Kutteh WH. Increased prevalence of insulin resistance in women with a history of recurrent pregnancy loss. Fertility and Sterility. 2002;**78**(3):487-490. DOI: 10.1016/s0015-0282(02)03247-8

[54] Ota K, Dambaeva S, Han AR, Beaman K, Gilman-Sachs A, Kwak-Kim J. Vitamin D deficiency may be a risk factor for recurrent pregnancy losses by increasing cellular immunity and autoimmunity. Human Reproduction. 2014;**29**:208-219. DOI: 10.1093/humrep/det424

[55] Moreno I, Cicinelli E, Garcia-Grau I, Gonzalez M, Bau D, Vilella F, et al. The diagnosis of chronic endometritis in infertile asymptomatic women: A comparative study of histology, microbial cultures, hysteroscopy, and molecular microbiology. American Journal of Obstetrics and Gynecology. 2018;**218**(6):602.e1-602.e16. DOI: 10.1016/j.ajog.2018.02.012. [Epub 2018 Feb 23]

[56] Chen YQ, Fang RL, Luo YN, Luo CQ. Analysis of the diagnostic value of CD138 for chronic endometritis, the risk factors for the pathogenesis of chronic endometritis and the effect of chronic endometritis on pregnancy: A cohort study. BMC Women's Health. 2016;**16**(1):60. DOI: 10.1186/s12905-016-0341-3

[57] Cicinelli E, Matteo M, Tinelli R, Lepera A, Alfonso R, Indraccolo U, et al. Prevalence of chronic endometritis in repeated unexplained implantation failure and the IVF success rate after antibiotic therapy. Human Reproduction. 2015;**30**(2):323-330. DOI: 10.1093/humrep/deu292

[58] Bouet PE, El Hachem H, Monceau E, Gariépy G, Kadoch IJ, Sylvestre C. Chronic endometritis in women with recurrent pregnancy loss and recurrent implantation failure: Prevalence and role of office hysteroscopy and immunohistochemistry in diagnosis. Fertility and Sterility. 2016;**105**(1):106-110. DOI: 10.1016/j.fertnstert.2015.09.025

[59] Kitaya K, Matsubayashi H, Takaya Y, Nishiyama R, Yamaguchi K, Takeuchi T, et al. Live birth rate following oral antibiotic treatment for chronic endometritis in infertile women with repeated implantation failure. American Journal of Reproductive Immunology. 2017;**78**(5);e12719. https://doi.org/10.1111/aji.12719

[60] de Ziegler D, Pirtea P, Galliano D, Cicinelli E. Optimal uterine anatomy and physiology necessary for normal implantation and placentation. Fertility and Sterility. 2016;**105**(4):844-854. DOI: 10.1016/j.fertnstert.2016.02.023

[61] Zargar M, Ghafourian M, Nikbakht R, Mir Hosseini V, Moradi Choghakabodi P. Evaluating chronic Endometritis in women with recurrent implantation failure and recurrent pregnancy loss by hysteroscopy and immunohistochemistry. Journal of Minimally Invasive Gynecology. 2019;**pii**:S1553-4650(19)30116-5. DOI: 10.1016/j.jmig.2019.02.016

[62] McQueen DB, Perfetto CO, Hazard FK, Lathi RB. Pregnancy outcomes in women with chronic endometritis and recurrent pregnancy loss. Fertility and Sterility. 2015;**104**(4):927-931. DOI: 10.1016/j.fertnstert.2015.06.044

[63] Robinson L, Gallos ID, Conner SJ, Rajkhowa M, Miller D, Lewis S, et al. The effect of sperm DNA fragmentation

on miscarriage rates: A systematic review and meta-analysis. Human Reproduction. 2012;**27**(10):2908-2917. DOI: 10.1093/humrep/des261

[64] McQueen DB, Zhang J, Robins JC. Sperm DNA fragmentation and recurrent pregnancy loss: A systematic review and meta-analysis. Fertility and Sterility. 2019;**112**(1):54-60.e3. DOI: 10.1016/j.fertnstert.2019.03.003

[65] Wright C, Milne S, Leeson H. Sperm DNA damage caused by oxidative stress: Modifiable clinical, lifestyle and nutritional factors in male infertility. Reproductive Biomedicine Online. 2014;**28**(6):684-703. DOI: 10.1016/j.rbmo.2014.02.004

[66] Showell MG, Mackenzie-Proctor R, Brown J, Yazdani A, Stankiewicz MT, Hart RJ. Antioxidants for male subfertility. Cochrane Database of Systematic Reviews. 2014;**12**:CD007411. DOI: 10.1002/14651858.CD007411.pub3

[67] Greco E, Iacobelli M, Rienzi L, Ubaldi F, Ferrero S, Tesarik J. Reduction of the incidence of sperm DNA fragmentation by oral antioxidant treatment. Journal of Andrology. 2005;**26**:349-353. DOI: 10.2164/jandrol.04146

[68] Bradley CK, McArthur SJ, Gee AJ, Weiss KA, Schmidt U, Toogood L. Intervention improves assisted conception intracytoplasmic sperm injection outcomes for patients with high levels of sperm DNA fragmentation: A retrospective analysis. Andrology. 2016;**4**:903-910. DOI: 10.1111/andr.12215

[69] De Braekeleer M, Nguyen MH, Morel F, Perrin A. Genetic aspects of monomorphic teratozoospermia: A review. Journal of Assisted Reproduction and Genetics. 2015;**32**(4):615-623. DOI: 10.1007/s10815-015-0433-2

Chapter 11

In Vitro Maturation and Fertilization of Oocytes: From Laboratory Bench to Clinical Practice

Adrian Ellenbogen, Einat Shalom Paz, Medeia Michaeli, Anna Smirnova and Yona Barak

Abstract

Retrieval of immature oocytes from non-stimulated ovaries, followed by in vitro maturation (IVM), was initially proposed in order to avoid side effects of gonadotropin administration. The goal is to eradicate or significantly decrease the risk of ovarian hyperstimulation syndrome (OHSS) in patients with polycystic ovary syndrome (PCOS) and to reduce drug cost and burden of patients. This technology was also proposed for treatment of normal ovulatory women, fertility preservation, or infrequent conditions as failure of oocyte to mature or repeated development of poor-quality embryos. There is no downregulation, and only a small amount of hormones are injected if at all. In vitro maturation of the oocyte procedure obtained up to 35% clinical pregnancy rate in young women, compared with in vitro fertilization (IVF) in many programs. The obstetric and perinatal outcomes of IVM cycles are comparable with IVF/ICSI cycles; therefore it may gradually substitute IVF in certain cases, as the technique continues to develop and pregnancy rates continue to increase. IVM holds great promises as an alternative to assisted reproductive technologies and may be the procedure of choice not only for infertile patients but also for obtaining oocytes for donation or fertility preservation.

Keywords: in vitro fertilization, in vitro oocyte maturation, oocytes, fertilized ovum, pregnancy outcome, pregnancy rates, reproductive techniques

1. Introduction

The concept of in vitro maturation of oocytes (IVM) was firstly mentioned in literature by Pincus and Enzmann, initially in 1935 [1]. They conducted experiments in which ova, taken from tubes at various intervals after fertile matting, were cultured in vitro. Thirty-four years later, Eppig and Schroeder [2] designed the possibility to use IVM rather than protocols of hormonal stimulation currently in use. These authors mentioned "it may be possible to recover immature oocytes from several antral follicles, excluding the dominant preovulatory follicle, and mature them in proper culture." At that time it was impossible to accomplish that assignment due to technical reasons. However, 2 years later, Cha et al. [3] mentioned, "this is an engineering problem with the ultrasound equipment that will be resolved in the future." Recently, Cha et al. were the first to succeed with IVM in human using immature oocytes retrieved from antral follicles. Trounson et al. [4] were the first who put IVM firmly in the clinical realm, obtaining a live birth from oocytes, recovered from untreated polycystic ovarian patient who underwent in vitro maturation.

In vitro maturation of oocytes have potential advantages over conventional IVF: a simple protocol with decreased or no hormonal stimulation before oocyte retrieval, lower cost of the treatment cycle, and reduced psychological impact. Moreover, and not of less of importance, the risk of OHSS is entirely avoided. Despite these benefits, however, there are still many debatable problems surrounding this treatment. Until one can say that IVM could be an alternative to conventional IVF treatment, these advantages have to be weighed against the pregnancy and delivery rates, children outcome, and possible risks.

There are several basic differences between routine in vitro fertilization (IVF) and IVM. These differences might be related to the size of aspirated follicles, the nuclear and cytoplasmic maturity of the oocytes, and the laboratory procedures. In order to achieve proper fertilization and embryo development, Gougeon and Testart in [5] pointed out that the follicles at the time of the collection for IVM procedures should be in the early antral to antral stage (0.2–14 mm) vs. preovulatory stage (0.16–20 mm) for IVF. After retrieval, majority of the oocytes are immature (MI, GV). However, only few will proceed in vitro to metaphase II (MII) in culture media, some after 6 h, but most of them after 24–48 h and only then will be able to undergo successful fertilization after ICSI. This is in comparison with conventional IVF, where most of the retrieved oocytes are mature, and fertilization might occur immediately after ICSI.

There are many controversial areas of debate, especially regarding the process of oocyte maturation in vitro: (a) nuclear maturation—the process that reverses meiotic arrest at prophase I (GV), driving the progression to MII. This process is followed by the expansion of cumulus granulosa cells and loss of intercellular communications between the cumulus cells and also between cumulus and the surface of the oocyte (a visible laboratory course); (b) cytoplasmic maturation—metabolic and structural modifications within the oocyte that prepares the ovum for activation, fertilization, and embryonic development (an invisible laboratory process) [2, 4, 5]; it should, therefore, be kept in mind that IVM may not be free of possible future complications and counseling of the patients thoroughly before commencing the treatment is essential.

2. Guidelines for IVM treatment

2.1 Ultrasound monitoring

Follicle monitoring follow-up is mainly performed using ultrasound scans of the ovaries and endometrium. However, in contrast to IVF, in IVM cycles, there is no need for serum hormonal level (estradiol, progesterone) follow-up.

First ultrasound should be performed on days 2–3 of the menstrual (or induced) cycle in order to record the number and size of all follicles along with endometrial thickness and a second scan on days 6–8, to determine the presence and size of the largest follicle in each ovary. A third scan should be completed on day of hCG trigger, to measure the endometrial thickness (**Figure 1**).

2.2 FSH priming

Fadini et al. [6] reported that 77.4% of retrieved immature oocytes underwent maturation in vitro followed by 29.8% pregnancy rate vs. 48.4 and 15.2% in primed and non-primed IVM cycles, respectively. Mikkelsen et al. [7] pointed that priming

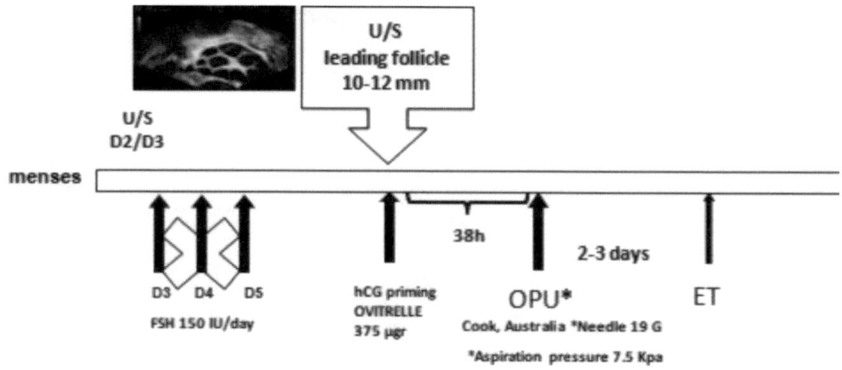

Figure 1.
In vitro maturation oocytes: clinical protocol.

with r-FSH for 2–3 days before the harvesting of immature oocytes from patients with polycystic ovarian syndrome (PCOS) may improve the maturational potential of the oocytes and the implantation rate. Similar results were described by other investigators in PCOS patients [8–11].

2.3 Human chorionic gonadotropin (hCG)/GnRh-agonist priming and retrieval interval

The beneficial effect of hCG priming in IVM cycles and extension of the period of time from 35 to 36 h (routinely administrated in IVF cycles) to 38 h from hCG administration was demonstrated by Son et al. [12]. This hCG priming promotes GV oocytes to reach MI stage and increases the maturation rate of immature oocytes in vitro. Gonadotropin-releasing hormone agonist (GnRH-a) has been used recently in triggering oocyte maturation. In this approach, small follicles were stimulated with gonadotropins for 3–5 days. GnRH-a administration was performed, to trigger ovulation, when the largest follicles were 10–12 mm in diameter. Many immature oocytes, which underwent maturation in vitro, were then harvested, fertilized, and subsequently developed into blastocysts that resulted in live births [13]. This interesting observation might have a great importance in follicular cytoplasmic maturation due to the FSH surge obtained after GnRH triggering. The FSH surge might promote formation of LH receptors on the granulosa cells enhancing LH activity, induce plasminogen activator activity causing dissociation of oocytes from somatic cells of the follicle (therefore more immature oocytes could be obtained), and maintain the opening of gap junction between cumulus cells and oocyte which contributes to oocyte maturation [14–17].

2.4 Timing of collection: at what follicle size?

Son et al. [18] conducted a study in which patients were triggered when the leading follicle was <10 mm, 10–14 mm, or >14 mm. In the group with a leading follicle >14 mm, only one pregnancy was obtained. The authors of the current paper administer, therefore, hCG trigger once a leading follicle of 10–12 mm is developed.

2.5 Endometrial preparation and luteal support

In IVM, estradiol levels are physiological, and oocyte collection is done before the endometrium is fully estrogenized. After aspiration, there is an insufficient support from the corpus luteum for endometrial receptivity. It was demonstrated

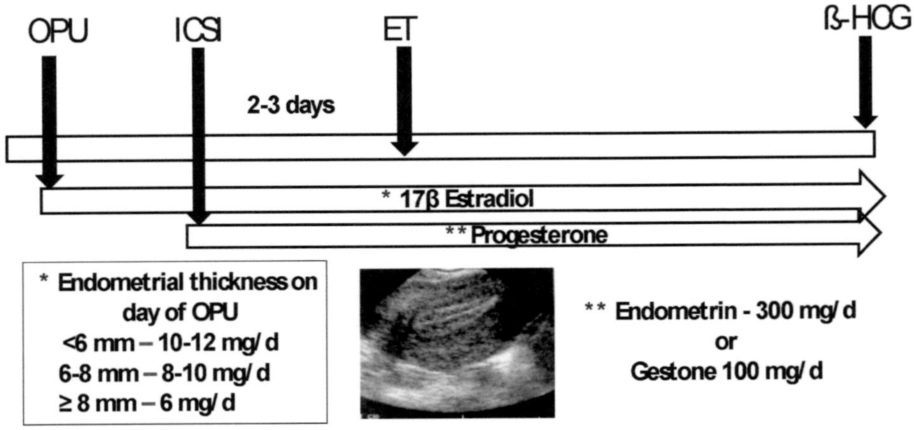

Figure 2.
Endometrial support.

that endometrial thickness is an important predictor of IVM outcome [19]. Thus, endometrial preparation is an important factor for IVM success rates. The protocol for endometrial preparation, which the authors currently use, is similar to that originally described by Trounson et al. [19] and modified by Elizur et al. [20], depending upon the endometrial thickness at day of hCG administration: when endometrial thickness is less than 6 mm, 6–8 mm, or higher than 8 mm, supplementation with 10–12 mg/day, 8–10 mg/day, and 6 mg/day 17-beta estradiol is given, respectively, starting at the day of oocyte retrieval. This approach mimics the natural estrogen rise from the dominant follicle in a natural cycle. In terms of progesterone, supplementation usually begins on the day of oocyte aspiration (as this is the progesterone rise in a natural cycle) using vaginal micronized progesterone (Endometrin, Florish Ltd. Industrial Park Misgav, Israel, Ferring Pharmaceuticals Ltd.) 300 mg daily until pregnancy test is performed (**Figure 2**).

2.6 Oocyte retrieval by transvaginal ultrasound

An high-resolution ultrasound device is obligatory. The oocyte retrieval is done with a single-channel needle 19 G (Swemed, Reduced Single Lumen, Vitrolife, Göteborg, Sweden AB), using a reduced aspiration pressure of 7.5 kPa. This is essential to minimize damage to the immature oocytes.

Usually general anesthesia/sedation is provided. However, local anesthesia with lidocaine 1%, 5 cc injected into the lateral fornixes, could be sufficient.

Oocytes from each ovary are aspirated in separate flask containing 15 ml of flushing medium (Origio, Denmark) and placed on a heated block. Collected cumulus oocyte complexes (OCCs) were classified immediately after OPU (Day 0).

Oocyte cumulus complexes could be classified in one of five groups: (1) expanded cumulus, slack and fluffy multilayer of granulosa cells; (2) full cumulus, multilayer of strictly compact and cubical granulosa cells; (3) full corona, thin layer of strictly compact and cubical granulosa cells; (4) partial cumulus, oocytes surrounded partially with cumulus cells; (5) nude, oocytes without cumulus cells (**Figure 3**). This classification may serve as a prognostic indication of the future maturation and fertilization rate of the immature collected oocytes.

Each complex was then separately cultured in IVM medium (Sage, Cooper Surgical Company, Trumbull, CT, USA) supplemented with FSH + LH (Menogon, Ferring GmbH, Kiel, Germany) with a final concentration of 75 mIU/ml (maturation medium). Oocyte maturation was assessed after 6 (a) and 24–30 h (b),

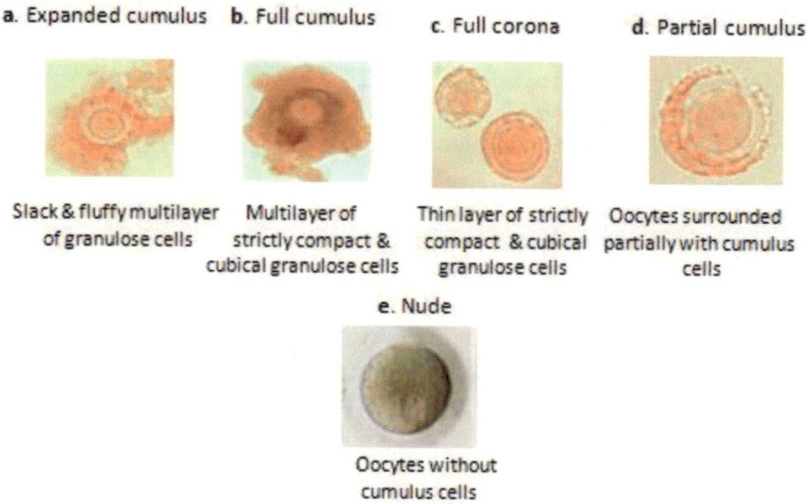

Figure 3.
Classification of collected cumulus complexes.

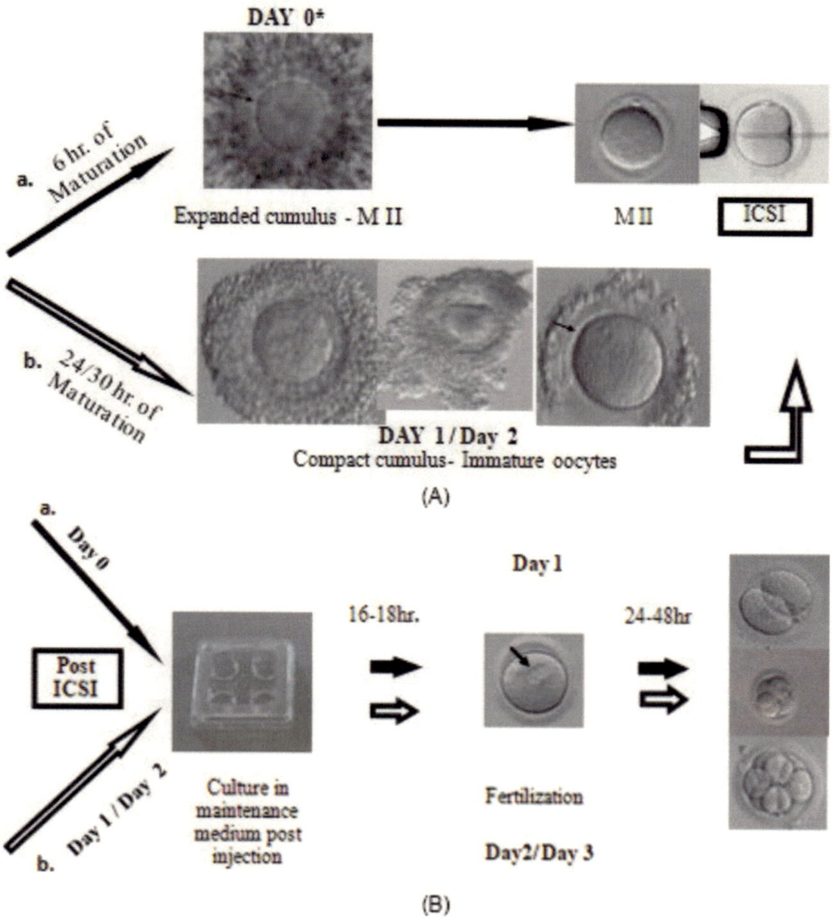

Figure 4.
*(A) In vitro maturation procedure. *Day 0 = day of OPU; [a]MII oocytes detected in maturation medium 6 h after OPU (solid fill arrows); [b]MII oocytes detected in maturation medium 24–30 h after OPU (open arrows) and (B) in vitro maturation procedure. *Day 0 = day of OPU; [a]MII oocytes detected in maturation medium 6 h after OPU (solid fill arrows); [b]MII oocytes detected in maturation medium 24–48 h after OPU (open arrows).*

according to oocyte cumulus complex classification. This was followed by oocyte intracytoplasmic sperm injection (ICSI) for the injection of a single sperm cell into the MII oocytes on the day of OPU or 1–2 days afterward, according to oocyte maturation (**Figure 4A** (a and b) and **B** (a and b)). Two to three embryos were transferred 48–78 h post ICSI. Supplementary embryos were vitrified.

3. Definitions of IVM in human

The biological definition of oocyte IVM is to aspirate GV oocytes from antral follicles and culture them for in vitro maturation to a MII stage. Apart from routine IVF, the clinical definition of an IVM cycle should include an understanding that it involves the retrieval of oocytes from small and intermediate-sized follicles in an ovary before the largest follicle has surpassed 13 mm in mean diameter [21]. However, since modifications of the IVM technique are commonly employed, it is suggested, though, to designating the cycle when an oocyte trigger is given. When oocyte triggering is not performed, the cycle should be designated as IVM without triggering. When the addition of gonadotropin stimulation is given for few days in the early follicular phase, the cycle should be designated as IVM with short gonadotropin stimulation or modified natural cycle IVF with early triggering combined with IVM (if hCG or GnRh-agonist triggering was delivered) [21].

4. Indications for IVM

The indications for IVM include normal ovulatory women (mechanical factor or male infertility), PCOS patients or susceptible to develop ovarian hyperstimulation (OHSS), contraindication to hormonal administration, patients with estrogen-sensitive cancers, or those who require rapid fertility preservation before undergoing potentially gonadotoxic treatments. Other occasional indications may include fertilization failure; poor ovarian response [22]; rescue of oocytes, which have failed to mature in stimulated cycles [23]; or unexplained primarily poor-quality embryos [24].

4.1 IVM in women with normal ovulatory cycles

In early studies, Mikkelsen et al. [7, 25, 26] reported a 17–18% pregnancy rates resulting from in vitro matured oocytes. These pregnancy rates were disappointingly low in comparison with regular IVF results obtained in that time. A constant improvement in pregnancy rate up to 30% was achieved during the last decade, mainly due to application of FSH/hCG priming in IVM protocol [6] and proper patient selection [27]. It seems that in normal ovulatory patients IVM may be an intriguing alternative to conventional IVF techniques resulting in comparable pregnancy rates. It removes the side effects of pituitary suppression and gonadotropin stimulation, especially OHSS; reduces the costs of the entire procedure, both in terms of time consumption and patient/society costs for drugs; and reduces psychological impact.

4.2 PCOS patients

PCOS patients are likely to develop OHSS with conventional IVF treatments. Substituting IVM in PCOS patients eliminates the risk of OHSS and lowers the cost of the treatment. From the early 2000s until nowadays, studies have demonstrated a reassuring pregnancy and delivery rate in PCOS patients undergoing

IVM treatments of 21.9–29.9% [28–31]. Recent studies reported up to 32–44% pregnancy and 22–29% delivery rates [32, 33], compared with IVF pregnancy rate results of 38–45% [33–35]. Junk and Yeap transferred a single blastocyst embryo obtained after IVM in patients with PCOS. A live birth rate of 42.4% per oocyte collection and 45.2% per embryo transfer were obtained [34]. Vitek et al. [35] have recently described implantation, pregnancy, and delivery rates of 17.5, 40, and 40%, respectively, in 20 estrogens suppressed in vitro maturation cycles. In a latest retrospective study comparing results of 61 IVM vs. 53 antagonist protocol cycles in young patients with PCOS, a comparable pregnancy and delivery rates of 30% vs. 40% and 21.3% vs. 28.8%, respectively, was obtained [36]. Those recent reports are encouraging, as in Europe the pregnancy and delivery rates in this group of patients undergoing ICSI was 35.5% and 24.3%, respectively [37]. de Ziegler et al. [38] opposed the need of IVM in the gonadotropin-releasing hormone (GnRH) antagonist era. However, his conclusion is based on outdated publication [28, 39, 40], with poor results in terms of pregnancy and delivery rates in IVM. However, to update, it is ascertained that such data has already improved. GnRH-agonist (GnRH-a) used as a trigger to control the risk of OHSS may cause higher pregnancy losses due to luteal phase defects [41]. In order to overcome this complication in antagonist protocol/agonist trigger, the dual-trigger approach (GnRH-a + low hCG) was proposed; 2.9% of OHSS complications developed [42]. GnRH trigger combined with intensive luteal support in OHSS high-risk patients can facilitate fresh embryo transfer; however, the occurrence of late OHSS was not totally eliminated [43]. Applying the policy of ovarian stimulation with a dual-trigger approach and freezing all of the oocytes or embryos for future use [44] do not, necessarily, eliminate totally OHSS. In a few patients after dual trigger and freeze all, severe OHSS was reported [45]. It seems that in PCOS patient, IVM is a simple, less stressful, and economical protocol of treatment. The puncture is simple and safe, and it may improve the disrupted endocrine environment and induce a spontaneous recovery of ovulation in women with PCOS [46]. It can also avoid short-term complications, such as OHSS, and elude massive hormonal stimulation and long-term complications, such as hormone-dependent neoplasms including breast and ovarian cancer.

4.3 Fertilization failure

Repeated IVF failure is a highly upsetting condition for patients who have apparently normal ovarian stimulation and follicular development, which underwent numerous unsuccessful IVF cycles with no embryos for transfer. Often, these patients are referred to surrogacy or egg donation program, which is also a psychological and economic burden for the couples [47]. Failures following IVF treatment might occur due to many reasons, such as formation of low-quality embryos, maturation arrest of oocytes [48], uncertain diagnosis of oocyte factor, or empty follicle syndrome. Thus, IVM was also proposed for treating patients with poor ovarian response; moreover it might serve the last choice to achieve pregnancy in IVF [22]. Other indications can be applying IVM in rare conditions, such as to rescue oocytes which have failed to mature in stimulated cycles [49] or cases with unexplained primarily poor-quality embryos. Hourvitz et al. [23] examined efficacy of IVM in seven patients with three or more conventional IVF failures due to abnormal oocyte development due to empty follicle syndrome, oocyte maturation arrest, or failure of fertilization. Four women received minimal ovarian stimulation with FSH. Oocytes were obtained in all patients: mean maturation rate was 39.6%, and mean fertilization rate is 45.8%. Embryo transfer was performed in four women; two patients with previous empty follicle syndrome conceived and delivered.

4.4 Fertility preservation

The emerging technology of IVM has recently become another option for fertility preservation. This process can be done without hormonal stimulation [50]. In the cases of cancer patients, who must be started on immediate chemotherapy, IVM might be the only option to preserve fertility by collecting oocytes during the follicular phase, within up to 13 days from cancer diagnosis, and cryopreservation [51, 52]. To shorten the period of time until cancer treatment, studies by Maman et al. [53] reported on luteal phase minimal ovarian stimulation with a reasonable number of harvested oocytes. Therefore, in the cases of cancer patients, especially in whom hormonal treatment is contraindicated and in those who must start chemotherapy without postponement, IVM might be the only choice to preserve fertility [53]. Recently, one successful pregnancy resulting from cryopreserved embryos obtained from IVM oocytes after oophorectomy in an ovarian cancer patient was reported [54]. Other studies have raised the possibility to preserve fertility even in pediatric patients.

Preserving in vitro matured oocytes from antral follicles found in harvested ovarian tissue is an experimental technique that offers a possible advantage over ovarian tissue cryopreservation. Using a mature, frozen, and later thawed oocyte for fertilization might serve as a safer option for fertility preservation than re-implantation of ovarian cortex tissue, due to the risk of malignant cell reseeding [55]. Caravani et al. followed a total of 84 chemotherapy-naïve patients ages < 1–18 years old, who were referred for fertility preservation. Thirty-three children were premenarche and 51 postmenarche. IVM was performed in the pre- and postmenarche groups and in subgroups of very young (up to age 5 years) and older (5–10 years) premenarche patients. The study concluded that IVM is feasible in the prepubertal age group. However, the success of in vitro maturation of those oocytes was correlated with the patient's age (more oocytes were obtained from the post pubertal vs. prepubertal); no mature oocytes are cryopreserved for girls under the age of five [55]. Additionally, it was found that fertilization potential of oocytes was negatively affected after vitrification of IVM oocytes [56]. This implies that vitrification/warming itself could also induce some detrimental effects on IVM oocytes. Actually, present vitrification methods have been adapted to use good-quality in vivo matured oocytes from young women. Therefore, studies to improve survival and further embryological developmental competence of the oocytes retrieved from IVM program are urgently required in order to successfully apply them to IVM fertility preservation program for cancer patients [57].

5. Pregnancy results

Two thousand healthy infants have been born following immature oocyte retrieval and IVM [58].

5.1 Obstetric and fetal complications

Soderstrom-Anttila et al. presented comparable complications and malformations for babies born after IVM and IVF [31]. Buckett et al. commented on a normal pregnancy course for IVM patients compared to routine IVF [59]. Fadini et al. performed a retrospective cohort study involving 196 babies born from IVM cycles compared with 194 children born from conventional ICSI cycles, which were performed during the same period of time. In single births, gestational age at delivery was comparable, but birth weight was significantly higher ($P = 0.009$) in children from IVM cycles (3091 ± 669 vs. 3269 ± 619 g). In a separate analysis of the IVM group, comparing singleton births derived with certainty from oocytes matured in vitro (n = 71) or in vivo (n = 74), no statistically significant differences were observed in terms of birth weight (3311 ± 637 vs. 3194 ± 574 g, respectively) and gestational age (38.9 ± 2.4 vs. 38.4 ± 2.1 weeks, respectively). In twin births, gestational age was lower in IVM cycles, while weight at birth was comparable (ICSI, 2432 ± 540 g; IVM, 2311 ± 577 g). In single births, major and minor abnormalities were 2 (1.4%) and 6 (4.1%) in the ICSI group and 0 (0.0%) and 8 (5.2%) in the IVM category, respectively. In twin children, major and minor abnormalities were 1 (2.2%) and 2 (4.3%) in ICSI babies and 0 (0.0%) and 2 (4.6%) in IVM cycles, respectively [60].

Obstetric outcome and congenital anomalies of 1421 babies (960 singletons, 442 twins, 15 triplets, and 4 quadruplets) born from 1187 IVM pregnancies were recently summarized by Chian et al. Reassuring results were obtained. The incidence of congenital malformation was 2% in singletons and 1% in twins [61].

6. Future concerns

In vitro maturation as a part of assisted reproductive technologies, may not, yet, be free of possible unidentified future problems. Epigenetic modifications necessary for normal development are established during oocyte growth. In vitro maturation, therefore, may modify the normal maturation of the oocytes [62]. Moreover, the capability of reprogramming the male chromatin after fertilization is dependent upon the maturity of the oocyte. It is questionable, whether this process might be affected by IVM [63]. It was postulated that IVM oocytes were more likely to have abnormal chromosomal configurations and disorganized meiotic spindle microtubules [64]. This finding may be a probable explanation for the reduced developmental potential of oocytes matured in vitro compared to those matured in vivo. However, despite the great achievements obtained in treating infertile couples by standard IVF during the last 34 years, it has become apparent in recent years that ovarian stimulation may itself have disadvantageous effects on oogenesis, with production of aneuploidy [65], reduced embryo quality, and lower endometrial receptivity and might even contribute to perinatal effects [66]. Moreover, human and animal data have demonstrated the potential changes in the implantation process that may occur following superovulation [67]:

1. Changing endometrial gene expression.

2. Causing immunologic changes to the endometrium.

3. Affecting endometrial-embryo interaction causing impairment on fetal development and growth.

4. Increasing the risk of abnormal placentation, leading to increased rates of low birth weight.

7. Improving IVM outcome

There is no doubt that efforts should be made to improve IVM outcome. An adequate learning curve taking into consideration clinical decisions, retrieval procedure, laboratory knowledge, and experience is required [33, 68].

Improving culture condition to optimum must be determined, for instance, adding epidermal growth factor family molecules, such as amphiregulin and epiregulin to the culture media which augmented oocyte maturation [69], or brain-derived neurotrophic factor (BDNF) and glial-cell-derived neurotrophic factor (GDNF), which recently were reported to improve maturation rates in human oocytes [70], or addition of dibutyryl cyclic adenosine 3′,5′-monophosphate (cAMP) to mouse oocytes in vitro to arrest germinal vesicle break down, in order to combine it with the cytoplasmic maturation [71].

8. Conclusions

The results of the process of IVM may be comparable and may have advantages over standard IVF. It is a simple procedure without pituitary downregulation. For stimulation of IVM cycle, a very small amount of hormones are administered if at all. Treatment time is short with low side effects (no OHSS), resulting in a reduced psychosocial impact.

The method of IVM holds great promise as an alternative to assisted reproductive technologies and may be the procedure of choice not only for infertile patients but also to obtain oocytes for donation or fertility preservation. Improving embryonic-endometrial synchrony through pharmaceutical or other manipulation of endometrial/uterine receptivity will hopefully improve IVM success rates. Appropriate counseling of the patients about the benefits and difficulties of the process should be done routinely [72].

9. Summary points

In vitro maturation of oocytes is a simple and less stressful process of treatment.

Main indication: PCOS patients, selected cases with fertilization failure, and fertility preservation.

Pregnancy rates are comparable.

Author details

Adrian Ellenbogen[1,2,3]*, Einat Shalom Paz[2], Medeia Michaeli[4], Anna Smirnova[5] and Yona Barak[6,7]

1 Rapport School of Medicine, Technion—Israel Institute of Technology, Haifa, Israel

2 IVF Unit, Hillel Yaffe Medical Center, Hadera, Israel

3 Meuhedet Female Health Center, Bnai Brak, Israel

4 IVF Laboratory, Hillel Yaffe Medical Center, Hadera, Israel

5 IVF & Reproductive Genetics Centre, Moscow, Russian Federation

6 Dr Yona Barak Laboratories Ltd., Israel

7 Alpha Scientists in Reproductive Medicine, Israel

*Address all correspondence to: ellenbogen55@gmail.com

References

[1] Pincus G, Enzmann EV. The comparative behavior of mammalian eggs in vivo and in vitro: I. The activation of ovarian eggs. The Journal of Experimental Medicine. 1935;**62**:665-675

[2] Eppig JJ, Schroeder AC. Capacity of mouse oocytes from preantral follicles to undergo embryogenesis and development to live young after growth, maturation, and fertilization in vitro. Biology of Reproduction. 1989;**41**:268-276

[3] Cha KY, Koo JJ, Ko JJ, Choi DH, Han SY, Yoon TK. Pregnancy after in vitro fertilization of human follicular oocytes collected from nonstimulated cycles, their culture in vitro and their transfer in a donor oocyte program. Fertility and Sterility. 1991;**55**:109-113

[4] Trounson A, Wood C, Kausche A. In vitro maturation and the fertilization and developmental competence of oocytes recovered from untreated polycystic ovarian patients. Fertility and Sterility. 1994;**62**:353-362

[5] Gougeon A, Testart J. Germinal vesicle breakdown in oocytes of human atretic follicles during the menstrual cycle. Journal of Reproduction and Fertility. 1986;**78**:389-401

[6] Fadini R, Dal Canto MB, Mignini Renzini M, Brambillasca F, Comi R, Fumagalli D, et al. Effect of different gonadotrophin priming on IVM of oocytes from women with normal ovaries: A prospective randomized study. Reproductive Biomedicine Online. 2009;**19**:343-351

[7] Mikkelsen AL, Lindenberg S. Benefit of FSH priming of women with PCOS to the in vitro maturation procedure and the outcome: A randomized prospective study. Reproduction. 2001;**122**:587-592

[8] Son WY, Tan SL. Laboratory and embryological aspects of hCG-primed in vitro maturation cycles for patients with polycystic ovaries. Human Reproduction Update. 2010;**16**:675-689. DOI: 10.1093/humupd/dmq014 [Epub: 26 May 2010]

[9] Chian RC, Buckett WM, Tulandi T, Tan SL. Prospective randomized study of human chorionic gonadotrophin priming before immature oocyte retrieval from unstimulated women with polycystic ovarian syndrome. Human Reproduction. 2000;**15**:165-170

[10] Chian RC, Cao YX. In vitro maturation of immature human oocytes for clinical application. Methods in Molecular Biology. 2014;**1154**:271-288. DOI: 10.1007/978-1-4939-0659-8_12

[11] Choi MH, Lee SH, Kim HO, Cha SH, Kim JY, Yang KM, et al. Comparison of assisted reproductive technology outcomes in infertile women with polycystic ovary syndrome: In vitro maturation, GnRH agonist, and GnRH antagonist cycles. Clinical and Experimental Reproductive Medicine. 2012;**39**:166-171. DOI: 10.1007/978-1-4939-0659-8_12

[12] Son WY, Chung JT, Chian RC, Herrero B, Demirtas E, Elizur S, et al. A 38 h interval between hCG priming and oocyte retrieval increases in vivo and in vitro oocyte maturation rate in programmed IVM cycles. Human Reproduction. 2008;**23**:2010-2016

[13] Dahan MH, Zhang L, Chen HY, Tan SL. Early short stimulation modified natural cycle IVF with GnRH agonist trigger and in vitro maturation in a woman with polycystic ovary syndrome: A case report. Journal of Obstetrics and Gynaecology Canada. 2016;**38**(5):465-469. DOI: 10.1016/j.jogc.2016.02.002 [Epub: 14 April 2016]

[14] Galway AB, Lapolt PS, Tsafriri A, Dargan CM, Boime I, Hsueh AJ. Recombinant follicle-stimulating hormone induces ovulation and tissue plasminogen activator expression in hypophysectomized rats. Endocrinology. 1990;**127**(6):3023-3028

[15] Atef A, François P, Christian V, Marc-André S. The potential role of gap junction communication between cumulus cells and bovine oocytes during in vitro maturation. Molecular Reproduction and Development. 2005;**71**(3):358-367

[16] Christenson LK, Stouffer RL. Follicle-stimulating hormone and luteinizing hormone/chorionic gonadotropin stimulation of vascular endothelial growth factor production by macaque granulosa cells from pre- and periovulatory follicles. The Journal of Clinical Endocrinology and Metabolism. 1997;**82**(7):2135-2142

[17] Reich R, Miskin R, Tsafriri A. Follicular plasminogen activator: Involvement in ovulation. Endocrinology. 1985;**116**(2):516-521

[18] Son WY, Chung JT, Herrero B, Dean N, Demirtas E, Holzer H, et al. Selection of the optimal day for oocyte retrieval based on the diameter of the dominant follicle in hCG-primed in vitro maturation cycles. Human Reproduction. 2008;**23**:2680-2685

[19] Reinblatt SL, Son WY, Shalom-Paz E, Holzer H. Controversies in IVM. Journal of Assisted Reproduction and Genetics. 2011;**28**:525-530. DOI: 10.1007/s10815-011-9575-z [Epub: 10 May 2011]

[20] Elizur SE, Son WY, Yap R, Gidoni Y, Levin D, Demirtas E, et al. Comparison of low-dose human menopausal gonadotropin and micronized 17beta-estradiol supplementation in in vitro maturation cycles with thin endometrial lining. Fertility and Sterility. 2009;**92**:907-912. DOI: 10.1016/j.fertnstert.2008.07.1750 [Epub: 30 October 2008]

[21] Dahan MH, Tan SL, Chung J, Son WY. Clinical definition paper on in vitro maturation of human oocytes. Human Reproduction. 2016;**31**(7):1383-1386. DOI: 10.1093/humrep/dew109 [Epub: 09 May 2016]

[22] Liu J, Lu G, Qian Y, Mao Y, Ding W. Pregnancies and births achieved from in vitro matured oocytes retrieved from poor responders undergoing stimulation in in vitro fertilization cycles. Fertility and Sterility. 2003;**80**:447-449

[23] Hourvitz A, Maman E, Brengauz M, Machtinger R, Dor J. In vitro maturation for patients with repeated in vitro fertilization failure due to "oocyte maturation abnormalities". Fertility and Sterility. 2010;**94**:496-501. DOI: 10.1016/j.fertnstert.2009.03.040 [Epub: 08 July 2009]

[24] Tan SL. In vitro maturation: Clinical and biological aspects. Journal de Gynecologie, Obstetrique et Biologie de la Reproduction. 2003;**32**:S52-S56

[25] Mikkelsen AL, Smith SD, Lindenberg S. In-vitro maturation of human oocytes from regularly menstruating women may be successful without follicle stimulating hormone priming. Human Reproduction. 1999;**14**:1847-1851

[26] Mikkelsen AL, Smith S, Lindenberg S. Possible factors affecting the development of oocytes in in-vitro maturation. Human Reproduction. 2000;**15**(Suppl 5):11-17

[27] Fadini R, Mignini Renzini M, Dal Canto M, Epis A, Crippa M, Caliari I, et al. Oocyte in vitro maturation in normo-ovulatory women. Fertility and Sterility. 2013;**99**:1162-1169. DOI:

10.1016/j.fertnstert.2013.01.138 [Epub: 20 February 2013]

[28] Child TJ, Phillips SJ, Abdul-Jalil AK, Gulekli B, Tan SL. A comparison of in vitro maturation and in vitro fertilization for women with polycystic ovaries. Obstetrics and Gynecology. 2002;**100**:665-670

[29] Child TJ, Sylvestre C, Pirwany I, Tan SL. Basal serum levels of FSH and estradiol in ovulatory and anovulatory women undergoing treatment by in-vitro maturation of immature oocytes. Human Reproduction. 2002;**17**:1997-2002

[30] Ellenbogen A, Atamny R, Fainaru O, Meidan E, Rotfarb N, Michaeli M. In vitro maturation of oocytes: A novel method of treatment of patients with polycystic ovarian syndrome undergoing in vitro fertilization. Harefuah. 2011;**150**:833-836, 876

[31] Soderstrom-Anttila V, Makinen S, TuuriT,SuikkariAM.Favourablepregnancy results with insemination of in vitro matured oocytes from unstimulated patients. Human Reproduction. 2005;**20**:1534-1540

[32] Shalom-Paz E, Almog B, Wiser A, Levin I, Reinblatt S, Das M, et al. Priming in vitro maturation cycles with gonadotropins: Salvage treatment for nonresponding patients. Fertility and Sterility. 2011;**96**:340-343. DOI: 10.1016/j.fertnstert.2011.06.003 [Epub: 30 Junuary 2011]

[33] Shalom-Paz E, Holzer H, Son W, Levin I, Tan SL, Almog B. PCOS patients can benefit from in vitro maturation (IVM) of oocytes. European Journal of Obstetrics, Gynecology, and Reproductive Biology. 2012;**165**:53-56. DOI: 10.1016/j.ejogrb.2012.07.001 [Epub: 21 July 2012]

[34] Junk SM, Yeap D. Improved implantation and ongoing pregnancy rates after single-embryo transfer with an optimized protocol for in vitro oocyte maturation in women with polycystic ovaries and polycystic ovary syndrome. Fertility and Sterility. 2012;**98**:888-892. DOI: 10.1016/j.fertnstert.2012.06.055 [Epub: 24 July 2012]

[35] Vitek WS, Witmyer J, Carson SA, Robins JC. Estrogen-suppressed in vitro maturation: A novel approach to in vitro maturation. Fertility and Sterility. 2013;**99**:1886-1890. DOI: 10.1016/j.fertnstert.2013.01.148 [Epub: 18 March 2013]

[36] Shavit T, Ellenbogen A, Michaeli M, Kartchovsky E, Ruzov O, Shalom-Paz E. In-vitro maturation of oocytes vs in-vitro fertilization with a gonadotropin-releasing hormone antagonist for women with polycystic ovarian syndrome: Can superiority be defined? European Journal of Obstetrics, Gynecology, and Reproductive Biology. 2014;**179**:46-50. DOI: 10.1016/j.ejogrb.2014.05.013 [Epub: 02 June 2014]

[37] Ferraretti AP, Goossens V, Kupka M, Bhattacharya S, de Mouzon J, Castilla JA, et al. Assisted reproductive technology in Europe, 2009: European IVF-Monitoring (EIM) Consortium for the European Society of Human Reproduction and Embryology (ESHRE). Human Reproduction. 2013;**28**:2318-2331. DOI: 10.1093/humrep/det278 [Epub: 09 July 2013]

[38] de Ziegler D, Streuli I, Gayet V, Frydman N, Bajouh O, Chapron C. Retrieving oocytes from small non-stimulated follicles in polycystic ovary syndrome (PCOS): In vitro maturation (IVM) is not indicated in the new GnRH antagonist era. Fertility and Sterility. 2012;**98**:290-293. DOI: 10.1016/j.fertnstert.2012.06.043

[39] Chian RC, Gulekli B, Buckett WM, Tan SL. Pregnancy and delivery after

cryopreservation of zygotes produced by in-vitro matured oocytes retrieved from a woman with polycystic ovarian syndrome. Human Reproduction. 2001;**16**:1700-1702

[40] Le Du A, Kadoch IJ, Bourcigaux N, Doumerc S, Bourrier MC, Chevalier N, et al. In vitro oocyte maturation for the treatment of infertility associated with polycystic ovarian syndrome: The French experience. Human Reproduction. 2005;**20**:420-424

[41] Humaidan P, Bredkjaer HE, Bungum L, Bungum M, Grondahl ML, Westergaard L, et al. GnRH agonist (buserelin) or hCG for ovulation induction in GnRH antagonist IVF/ICSI cycles: A prospective randomized study. Human Reproduction. 2005;**20**:1213-1220

[42] Griffin D, Benadiva C, Kummer N, Budinetz T, Nulsen J, Engmann L. Dual trigger of oocyte maturation with gonadotropin-releasing hormone agonist and low-dose human chorionic gonadotropin to optimize live birth rates in high responders. Fertility and Sterility. 2012;**97**:1316-1320. DOI: 10.1016/j.fertnstert.2014.04.028 [Epub: 17 May 2014]

[43] Iliodromiti S, Lan VT, Tuong HM, Tuan PH, Humaidan P, Nelson SM. Impact of GnRH agonist triggering and intensive luteal steroid support on live-birth rates and ovarian hyperstimulation syndrome: A retrospective cohort study. Journal of Ovarian Research. 2013;**6**:93. DOI: 10.1186/1757-2215-6-93

[44] Devroey P, Polyzos NP, Blockeel C. An OHSS-free clinic by segmentation of IVF treatment. Human Reproduction. 2011;**26**:2593-2597. DOI: 10.1093/humrep/der251 [Epub: 09 August 2011]

[45] Fatemi HM, Popovic-Todorovic B, Humaidan P, Kol S, Banker M, Devroey P, et al. Severe ovarian hyperstimulation syndrome after gonadotropin-releasing hormone (GnRH) agonist trigger and "freeze-all" approach in GnRH antagonist protocol. Fertility and Sterility. 2014;**101**:1008-1011. DOI: 10.1016/j.fertnstert.2014.01.019 [Epub: 15 February 2014]

[46] Ortega-Hrepich C, Polyzos NP, Anckaert E, Guzman L, Tournaye H, Smitz J, et al. The effect of ovarian puncture on the endocrine profile of PCOS patients who undergo IVM. Reproductive Biology and Endocrinology. 2014;**12**:18. DOI: 10.1186/1477-7827-12-18

[47] Smirnova A, Anshina M, Sergeev S, Ellenbogen A. Live birth after *in vitro* maturation of oocytes in a patient with repeated fertilization failure in IVF: A case report. Obstetrics & Gynecology. 2016;**6**(6):1-3. DOI: 10.4172/2161-0932.1000390

[48] Levran D, Farhi J, Nahum H, Glezerman M, Weissman A. Maturation arrest of human oocytes as a cause of infertility: Case report. Human Reproduction. 2002;**17**:1604-1609

[49] Tan SL, Child TJ. In-vitro maturation of oocytes from unstimulated polycystic ovaries. Reproductive Biomedicine Online. 2002;**4**(Suppl 1):18-23

[50] Sonigo C, Grynberg M. In vitro oocyte maturation for female fertility preservation. Gynécologie, Obstétrique & Fertilité. 2014;**42**:657-660. DOI: 10.1016/j.gyobfe.2014.07.009 [Epub: 19 August 2014]

[51] Huang JY, Chian RC, Gilbert L, Fleiszer D, Holzer H, Dermitas E, et al. Retrieval of immature oocytes from unstimulated ovaries followed by in vitro maturation and vitrification: A novel strategy of fertility preservation for breast cancer patients. American Journal of Surgery. 2010;**200**:177-183. DOI: 10.1016/j.amjsurg.2009.04.004

[52] Shalom-Paz E, Almog B, Shehata F, Huang J, Holzer H, Chian RC, et al. Fertility preservation for breast-cancer patients using IVM followed by oocyte or embryo vitrification. Reproductive Biomedicine Online. 2010;**21**:566-571. DOI: 10.1016/j.rbmo.2010.05.003 [Epub: 13 May 2010]

[53] Maman E, Meirow D, Brengauz M, Raanani H, Dor J, Hourvitz A. Luteal phase oocyte retrieval and in vitro maturation is an optional procedure for urgent fertility preservation. Fertility and Sterility. 2011;**95**:64-67. DOI: 10.1016/j.fertnstert.2010.06.005 [Epub: 18 July 2010]

[54] Prasath EB, Chan ML, Wong WH, Lim CJ, Tharmalingam MD, Hendricks M, et al. First pregnancy and live birth resulting from cryopreserved embryos obtained from in vitro matured oocytes after oophorectomy in an ovarian cancer patient. Human Reproduction. 2014;**29**:276-278. DOI: 10.1093/humrep/det420 [Epub: 09 December 2013]

[55] Karavani G, Schachter-Safrai N, Revel A, Mordechai-Daniel T, Bauman D, Imbar T. In vitro maturation rates in young premenarche patients. Fertility and Sterility. 2019;**112**(2): 315-322. DOI: 10.1016/j.fertnstert.2019.03.026 [Epub: 02 May 2019]

[56] Cohen Y, St-Onge-St-Hilaire A, Tannus S, Younes G, Dahan MH, Buckett W, et al. Decreased pregnancy and live birth rates after vitrification of *in vitro* matured oocytes. Journal of Assisted Reproduction and Genetics. 2018;**35**:1683-1689. DOI: 10.1007/s10815-018-1216-3

[57] Son WY, Henderson S, Cohen Y, Dahan M, Buckett W. Immature oocyte for fertility preservation. Frontiers in Endocrinology. 2019;**10**:464. DOI: 10.3389/fendo.2019.00464

[58] Chian RC. In vitro maturation of immature oocytes for clinical application: Past, today and tomorrow. In: Poncelet C, Sifer C, editors. Physiologie, pathologie, et therapie de la reproduction chez l'human. XXIII ed. Paris, France: Springer-Verlag; 2011. pp. 461-471

[59] Buckett WM, Chian RC, Holzer H, Dean N, Usher R, Tan SL. Obstetric outcomes and congenital abnormalities after in vitro maturation, in vitro fertilization, and intracytoplasmic sperm injection. Obstetrics and Gynecology. 2007;**110**:885-891

[60] Fadini R, Mignini Renzini M, Guarnieri T, Dal Canto M, De Ponti E, Sutcliffe A, et al. Comparison of the obstetric and perinatal outcomes of children conceived from in vitro or in vivo matured oocytes in in vitro maturation treatments with births from conventional ICSI cycles. Human Reproduction. 2012;**27**:3601-3608. DOI: 10.1093/humrep/des359 [Epub: 04 October 2012]

[61] Chian RC, Xu CL, Huang JY, Ata B. Obstetric outcomes and congenital abnormalities in infants conceived with oocytes matured in vitro. Facts Views & Vision in Obgyn. 2014;**6**:15-18

[62] Bao S, Obata Y, Carroll J, Domeki I, Kono T. Epigenetic modifications necessary for normal development are established during oocyte growth in mice. Biology of Reproduction. 2000;**62**:616-621

[63] Gioia L, Barboni B, Turriani M, Capacchietti G, Pistilli MG, Berardinelli P, et al. The capability of reprogramming the male chromatin after fertilization is dependent on the quality of oocyte maturation. Reproduction. 2005;**130**:29-39

[64] Li Y, Feng HL, Cao YJ, Zheng GJ, Yang Y, Mullen S, et al. Confocal microscopic analysis of the spindle and chromosome configurations of human oocytes matured in vitro. Fertility and Sterility. 2006;**85**:827-832

[65] Baart EB, Martini E, Eijkemans MJ, Van Opstal D, Beckers NG, Verhoeff A, et al. Milder ovarian stimulation for in-vitro fertilization reduces aneuploidy in the human preimplantation embryo: A randomized controlled trial. Human Reproduction. 2007;**22**:980-988

[66] Santos MA, Teklenburg G, Macklon NS, Van Opstal D, Schuring-Blom GH, Krijtenburg PJ, et al. The fate of the mosaic embryo: Chromosomal constitution and development of Day 4, 5 and 8 human embryos. Human Reproduction. 2010;**25**:1916-1926. DOI: 10.1093/humrep/deq139 [Epub: 02 June 2010]

[67] Weinerman R, Mainigi M. Why we should transfer frozen instead of fresh embryos: The translational rationale. Fertility and Sterility. 2014;**102**:10-18. DOI: 10.1016/j.fertnstert.2014.05.019 [Epub: 02 June 2014]

[68] Faundez R, Sikorska O, Rokicki T, Karwacka A, Dworniak T, Barak Y. In vitro maturation in women with PCOS. Fertility and Sterility Supplement. 2008;**90**:S214. DOI: 10.1016/j.fertnstert.2008.07.51269

[69] Ben-Ami I, Komsky A, Bern O, Kasterstein E, Komarovsky D, Ron-El R. In vitro maturation of human germinal vesicle-stage oocytes: Role of epidermal growth factor-like growth factors in the culture medium. Human Reproduction. 2011;**26**:76-81. DOI: 10.1093/humrep/deq290 [Epub: 20 October 2010]

[70] Zhao P, Qiao J, Huang S, Zhang Y, Liu S, Yan LY, et al. Gonadotrophin-induced paracrine regulation of human oocyte maturation by BDNF and GDNF secreted by granulosa cells. Human Reproduction. 2011;**26**:695-702. DOI: 10.1093/humrep/deq390 [Epub: 12 January 2011]

[71] Chen J, Hudson E, Chi MM, Chang AS, Moley KH, Hardie DG, et al. AMPK regulation of mouse oocyte meiotic resumption in vitro. Developmental Biology. 2006;**291**:227-238

[72] Ellenbogen A, Shavit T, Shalom-Paz E. IVM results are comparable and may have advantages over standard IVF. Facts Views & Vision in Obgyn. 2014;**6**:77-80

Section 3

Ethics and Laws

Chapter 12

Bioethics of Assisted Reproductive Technology

Justo Aznar and Julio Tudela

Abstract

There is no doubt that for a couple who are having difficulties in conceiving, having a child is an objective good. However, it is also indisputable that assisted reproduction techniques raise clear ethical issues. In order to begin this bioethical reflection, it should be clearly established that the early embryo, which can be manipulated or destroyed using these techniques, is a living being of our species. We believe this is unquestionable from a biological point of view, and it therefore deserves our full respect. The bioethical assessment of assisted reproduction techniques includes analysis of the embryo losses caused by their selection and manipulation through preimplantation genetic diagnosis, 'social freezing' or the possible lack of rigour in the information provided by the clinics involved, to which must be added the higher morbidity reported in babies born as a result of these procedures.

Keywords: assisted reproduction, in vitro fertilisation, ICSI, bioethical considerations, loss of human embryos

1. Introduction

There is no doubt that for a couple who are having difficulties in conceiving, having a child is an objective boon. In an attempt to achieve this goal, many will avail assisted reproductive technology (ART) or natural family planning methods [1–3].

ART refers to a number of techniques, primarily: (a) in vitro fertilisation (IVF), in which the fertilisation of an egg by sperm takes place in a laboratory setting; (b) intracytoplasmic sperm injection (ICSI), in which a single sperm is introduced into the egg to be fertilised, also in a laboratory setting; (c) artificial insemination, which involves artificially delivering semen to the female genital tract—the semen may be from the woman's own partner or a donor; and (d) gamete intrafallopian tube transfer (GIFT), which involves removing eggs laparoscopically after controlled ovarian hyperstimulation, followed by introduction of the mixture of the couple's eggs and sperm into the fallopian tube so that fertilisation occurs in the body, unlike IVF and ICSI, in which it takes place 'in vitro' although several modifications of these techniques have been proposed [4].

2. Efficacy of ART

One important aspect to consider is the efficacy of these techniques, which is generally calculated based on two parameters: the pregnancy rate (PR) and the live birth rate (LBR) per ovarian stimulation cycle.

IntechOpen

Based on data published by the European Society of Human Reproduction and Embryology (ESHRE) in 2014 [5–18], the PR and LBR following IVF in Europe between 1997 and 2010 varied between 22.28 and 29.2% for the PR, with a mean rate of 26.41%, and between 13.07 and 22.4% for the LBR, with a mean rate of 18.81%.

When ICSI was used, these same rates varied between 23.37 and 29.9% for the PR, with a mean rate of 27.22%, and between 12.68 and 21.10% for the LBR, with a mean rate of 18.31% [6].

ARTs have wide social acceptance today. Following the birth of the first girl, Louise Brown, by IVF in 1978, more than 200,000 children are now born annually worldwide using these techniques [19], i.e. more than 3% of all children born [14], with the total number of births estimated at over 5 million [20].

3. Ethical assessment of ARTs

Nevertheless, regardless of the medical and social benefits they offer, it is also a reality that ARTs may present bioethical issues that are worth considering. These may be moral or ethical. Moral implications are related with the fact that they involve the instrumental manipulation of fertilisation, disregarding its natural environment, the sexual act, and the implications that may arise from this. Ethical implications entail the bioethical problems related to the medical aspects of these techniques, which are the concerns that we shall analyse in this chapter.

These ethical concerns include those related to:

1. Children born by these techniques.

2. Couples who use IVF.

3. The surplus human embryos that are frozen, as well as the problems that may arise from the treatment given to such embryos.

4. The loss of embryos that occurs in IVF.

5. The embryo selection that is carried out using preimplantation genetic diagnosis (PGD) to transfer only the best quality embryos.

6. Gamete donation, especially the right to privacy of donors and of children to know their parents.

7. The production of saviour siblings.

8. The possible use of these techniques for social purposes, unrelated to the woman's own fertility, such as 'gestational surrogacy' and 'social freezing'.

9. The possible hyperinflated success rates in advertisement of assisted reproduction clinics may present to attract customers.

4. Medical problems in children born by ART

Children born by ART have a higher percentage of adverse medical effects than those conceived naturally [21–29], which gives rise to unanswered bioethical questions.

Thus, these children have higher rates of prematurity and low birth weight [30] as well as an increased risk of birth defects [31–33], especially cardiac malformations [34, 35] and chromosomal abnormalities [36], than children conceived naturally. Another study nonetheless failed to confirm these differences when children were stratified according to the age of their mothers, parity and gestational age [37].

Although some evidence has suggested that these types of medical disorders extend to early childhood [38] and even longer term [30], a recent article assessing whether the negative side effects are maintained until 25–30 years after birth found that these abnormalities are not detected in adulthood [39].

In addition to the disorders mentioned above, children born by ART may also show an increase in acquired medical problems, such as: impaired psychomotor development, cerebral palsy, autism and even asthma [38, 40, 41].

Another issue that has also arisen is whether the increased risk of these negative side effects occurs equally in children born by IVF or by ICSI. Most researchers' opinions are that there seem to be no differences between both techniques [42–45], although others have found a greater number of problems when ICSI is used as compared to IVF [25].

With respect to the cause of the problems in children born by ART, this seems to be multifactorial, and it may basically be due to the technique itself (the manipulation of gametes, the practice of PGD, the culture medium and the time that embryos have been frozen), ovarian hyperstimulation of the mother [46, 47] and also due to paternal subfertility [21]. In particular, it may be related to the greater number of multiple pregnancies that occur in ART [48–52], since multiple pregnancies are known to be accompanied by more foetal congenital abnormalities [49, 53–55], although these are also found in singleton pregnancies using ART [21, 23, 28, 47, 56].

It has recently been suggested that the medical problems found in children born by ART could also be related to epigenetic modifications, which may occur during maturation of the gametes, fertilisation or in the early stages of embryonic development [21, 22, 28, 30, 57, 58].

5. Medical problems in mothers who use ART

A majority of adverse medical events that occur in women who use ART seem due to the greater number of multiple pregnancies that occur in them [49–52, 59] since, as has already been mentioned, obstetric problems are known to be more common in multiple compared to singleton pregnancies [49, 53–55].

Nevertheless, ART-conceived singleton pregnancies also present a higher risk of adverse events in mothers, such as antepartum haemorrhage, hypertension during pregnancy, premature rupture of membranes or gestational diabetes, than naturally conceived singleton pregnancies [60].

6. Ethical problems related to frozen surplus embryos from ART and how their untoward situation can be resolved

As already mentioned, the efficacy of IVF is low. In order to improve this, a large number of embryos are typically produced, usually between 10 and 12, of which 1 or 2 are transferred and the rest frozen. This practice inevitably means that the number of frozen human embryos is gradually increasing.

Knowing what to do with these frozen embryos raises objective bioethical problems. In our view, there are four solutions for these embryos: (a) leave them frozen indefinitely; (b) use them for biomedical experimentation; (c) thaw them and let them die; and (d) adoption.

Of these four solutions, the most widely employed is the second—using them for biomedical experiments—but this solution clearly poses obvious bioethical problems, since it entails the inevitable destruction of the embryos used.

The solution that presents least ethical problems is the adoption of such embryos by the biological parents, but this is not always possible. What occurs most frequently is the adoption by a couple biologically unrelated to the embryo in question.

The ethics of this type of adoption can be considered from three aspects: (a) from moral philosophy; (b) from secular ethics; and (c) from the point of view of the morality of the monotheistic religions [61].

6.1 Frozen embryo adoption in the light of moral philosophy

They are very few studies that address the moral licitness or illicitness of frozen human embryo adoption in the light of moral philosophy. In our view, this has been addressed in most depth by Antonio Pessina [62].

In his opinion, 'two lines of argument can be raised when evaluating frozen embryo adoption. In the first, it is assumed that human life is an absolute value, immeasurable, and as such is not comparable to any other. In the second, it is recognized that human life is a basic value, because it is a necessary condition to uphold other human goods, but not sufficient to achieve the specific ends of man, which means that the value of human life can be deferred to other values, for example, by giving one's life for another'.

If we accept the first principle, 'there would be no objection to the adoption of frozen embryos; it could even be presented as morally positive and not only licit'. If the second line of argument is accepted, 'the life of the human embryo should be defended only by proportionate, ordinary and morally legitimate means, in this sense the only possibility being to invite the biological mother to have her child's frozen embryo implanted and to carry the pregnancy to term. Other options could be considered disproportionate and extraordinary, which could lead to the violation of other fundamental values related to the dignity of the human person and of human procreation'.

In conclusion, Pessina declares himself morally opposed to frozen embryo adoption.

6.2 Frozen embryo adoption from the perspective of secular ethics

From secular ethics, there does not appear to be any difficulty for frozen embryo adoption. In fact, it is even considered to be a positive solution for these embryos, since, according to it, if the embryos are not used by the parents for reproductive purposes, their adoption is ethically more defensible than any other fate that may be given them. Undertaking a reproductive process to try to have a child born is in their opinion the best solution, since the aim is to help build families, i.e. to help infertile couples to have a child, and also to protect a primary good of the embryo, its life. Consequently, many experts or lay institutions see in frozen embryo adoption an alternative for the fate of such embryos that is ethically better than using them for biomedical research, destroying them or leaving them stored indefinitely [61].

6.3 Frozen embryo adoption from the perspective of the monotheistic religions

In relation to Islam, Sunni Muslims are not in favour of considering third-party gamete donation as morally acceptable nor, by analogy, frozen embryo adoption; however, Shiite Muslims are more agreeable to morally accepting this practice [61].

In relation to Judaism, it is difficult to find specific texts that refer to the moral assessment of frozen embryo adoption [61]. There are, however, texts on third-party gamete donation [63] so, again by analogy, that assessment could be extrapolated to frozen embryo adoption. In practice, though, most Orthodox rabbis are hesitant about the moral licitness of frozen embryo adoption [61].

Evangelists consider frozen embryo adoption as analogous to gestational surrogacy [64].

In relation to Catholicism [65], there are two documents in the Magisterium of the Catholic Church that address the issue of embryo adoption: the Instruction *Donum Vitae*, published by the Congregation for the Doctrine of the Faith in 1978 [66], and *Dignitas Personae*, published on 8 September 2008, by the same Congregation [67]. The Instruction *Dignitas Personae* is the last document of the Magisterium of the Catholic Church in which the topic of embryo adoption is explicitly addressed. Proposals to *use these embryos for research* or *for the treatment of disease* are obviously unacceptable because they treat the embryos as mere 'biological material' and result in their destruction. The proposal that these embryos could be put at the disposal of infertile couples as a *treatment for infertility* is also ethically unacceptable for the same reasons that make artificial heterologous procreation and any form of surrogacy illicit [67].

7. Human embryo loss in IVF

Among the negative bioethical aspects of IVF, possibly the most significant is the high number of embryos—human lives—that are lost.

We have attempted to calculate this figure [68] based on previous data from a published article [61]. This study in question evaluated 572 ovarian stimulation cycles that yielded 7213 oocytes, i.e. 12.6 oocytes per cycle. A total of 2252 embryos were produced and 326 live babies were born (226 from fresh embryos and 64 from frozen embryos). Based on these figures, the number of live babies born for every 100 embryos was 14.47; or to put it another way, for every 100 embryos produced, 85.53 embryos were lost, i.e. 6.9 embryos were lost for every live baby born.

Another more recent study by the same group [69] analysed 191 ovarian stimulation cycles performed on 53 female donors. The donors were classified into two groups: 28 were highly successful donors, and 23 were classified as standard. The highly successful donor group yielded a total of 2470 oocytes from 130 ovarian stimulation cycles. This produced 779 embryos; 342 were transferred as fresh embryos and 437 were cryopreserved. A total of 125 live babies were born. The standard donor group yielded 1044 oocytes from 61 ovarian stimulation cycles. This produced 336 embryos; 131 embryos were transferred and 205 were cryopreserved. The total number of live babies born was 26. Based on these figures, a total of 1115 embryos were produced and a total of 151 live babies were born. Consequently, the number of live babies born per 100 embryos was 13.54; in other words, the number of embryos lost for every 100 embryos produced was 86.46. Thus, for every live baby born, 7.38 embryos were lost.

Accordingly, based on the above data, if approximately 6 or 7 embryos are lost for every child born by IVF, and since 1978, the year in which Louise Brown was born, around 5 million children have been born [20], we can estimate that, so far, around 30 million human lives may have been lost worldwide as a result of the use of IVF [68]. This leads one to say—while admitting that it is a very strong assertion—that IVF is a medical practice that, for the time being, generates more death than life. The natural cycle itself is associated with follicle recruitment followed by dominance and selection, while the nondominant follicles undergo atresia in the same cycle. The controlled ovarian stimulation has an advantage of opening the follicular window and rescuing this cohort of follicles who would have undergone atresia if the FSH window was not kept open and multiple follicles salvaged. The current scenario is practical nonavailability of embryos for embryo donation to aspiring couples where female partners are undergoing endometrial preparation for transfer for Donor embryos. Though there are concerns for discarded embryos, the fertility clinics are in practise at a deficiency of embryos that can be transferred. The ethics of embryo transfer should be discussed in a clinically practical rational scenario.

8. Use of preimplantation genetic diagnosis in IVF: ethical assessment

PGD is a laboratory method especially directed to the genetic study of embryos before they are transferred and, therefore, before implantation in the uterus. The aim of this procedure is to determine if the embryos have a genetic or chromosomal abnormality, or if they are carriers of a genetic risk factor of disease, especially in those couples in which at least one of the partners presents a high risk of having a genetic condition that they could transmit to their offspring [70]. Another common indication in the field of assisted reproduction is aneuploidy screening to ensure the implantation of euploid embryos [70]. Similarly, PGD is currently and increasingly often being used to try to prevent diseases that can appear in adulthood [71]. In general, it may be said that PGD is used in IVF to improve its efficacy.

The technique essentially involves in vitro culture of the embryos to be examined, so that when these reach an adequate number of cells, a single cell can then be extracted for study.

There different biopsy methods are used for PGD at present [72]. The most common is the biopsy of one or two blastomeres on Day 3 of embryonic development, during the screening or cell segmentation phase. However, the ESHRE recommends extracting six or more cells in the embryos [72, 73], because more cells can be biopsied in this phase with less risk of damaging the embryo [72].

As regards its use for improving IVF outcomes, this seems controversial, since many authors obtain positive outcomes using it, while others have been unable to detect such an improvement. Furthermore, Mastenbroek concludes that, not only does it fail to improve IVF outcomes, but it lowers the LBR in women of advanced maternal age, with no beneficial effects in the rest of the women [74].

When assessing this practice bioethically, the main difficulties are: (1) that it treats the human embryo as experimental material, objectifying it, which is absolutely incompatible with its intrinsic dignity, and (2) practising embryo selection for health reasons is a clearly eugenic practice.

Nevertheless, there are authors who not only are not opposed to the use of PGD, but also encourage its use, due to the benefit that it may bring for children by trying to prevent them from being born with a genetic or chromosomal disease or who have the risk of having one of these diseases in the future. In fact, some even advocate the positive duty of parents to use PGD when they consider that its use may be beneficial for their children [75, 76].

To circumvent the ethical difficulties of the use of PGD, and to maintain its hypothetical advantages, it has been proposed to analyse one of the two polar bodies of the oocyte, to thus determine whether said oocyte is a carrier of its mother's disease before the zygote is formed. In this way, only the healthy eggs would be fertilised [72, 77, 78], although this technique has the limitation that it could only be used in women.

It is also known that the oocyte is surrounded by several cell layers and that those layers play a key role in its normal function, ovulation, fertilisation and embryo development. However, the study of gene expression of these cell layers could be the basis of a non-invasive method for predicting oocyte quality, serving as a biomarker for selecting oocytes and embryos, as an alternative to the use of PGD [79]. Another alternative constitutes trophectoderm biopsy in human blastocysts, where extraembryonic material can be obtained by this technique for preimplantation diagnosis of genetic disorders [80].

9. Ethical problems arising from donor gametes in IVF, especially the right to privacy of donors and of children to know their parents

From a bioethical point of view, in our opinion, there are a number of issues with respect to whether the donation of gametes, both eggs and sperm, should be anonymous or not. We consider these four the most important: (a) to know whether the good of the child should prevail in the overall assessment of the process, as we believe it should; (b) to determine whether the privacy of the donors should be ensured; (c) to assess whether the interests of assisted reproduction clinics should be safeguarded; and (d) to establish whether even the good of society should be ensured.

9.1 Good of the child

With regard to children, it seems obvious that they have the right to know their biological origin, i.e. to know who their parents are. This is not only for emotional reasons, which must also be considered, but mainly for medical ones, since it cannot be ruled out that it may be necessary during the child's life to know who his parents are, if he has a genetic disease that needs to be identified, in order to be diagnosed and treated.

Moreover, this policy is in accordance with the first major document developed by the United Nations in 1989, on the 'Rights of the Child', which, in Article 7, defines that one of those rights is the right of the child to know his or her parents.

9.2 Good of the donors

In relation to donors, there is a trend towards suppressing anonymity in gamete donation, which may be a negative factor for donors. This is because, if the parent-child relationship can be established, it could lead to parental obligations for the donors that they may not want to assume. This is especially so if we also take into account that there are websites specialising in genetic matters that can match people who were born through gamete donation, so it can be determined if they have a genetic relationship [81].

9.3 Good of the assisted reproduction clinics

There is no doubt that suppressing anonymity in gamete donation can dramatically reduce the number of donors who attend those clinics, as has already happened in the United Kingdom, which is undoubtedly an added difficulty for these practices. In addition, it is also possible that if anonymity is suppressed, it will particularly affect younger donors, which could be detrimental to IVF procedures, since gametes from older donors are usually of lower quality.

9.4 Good of society

One risk of anonymous donation is that a donor can make a donation repeatedly and in different places, in the absence of real control over the process. This could facilitate marital consanguinity, which is certainly a not insignificant public health problem.

It has also been argued that in a society immersed in a clear demographic winter, reducing births by IVF (given the high number of these) could negatively impact it.

To prevent any difficulties that anonymous donation might have, the creation of an 'Assisted Human Reproduction Information System' (SIRHA) has been proposed. This would collect data on all donations made, identifying donors through a European code, and thus avoiding the problems posed by multiple donations from the same donor.

Certainly, the solution to this problem is controversial, so it would probably be positive to consider the one already proposed by Penningsin 1997 with his 'double track' policy, an option that would allow donors to participate in an anonymous or non-anonymous programme. However, and also in our opinion, while this proposal could guarantee the hypothetical rights of assisted reproduction clinics, donors and the couples who use these techniques, does it guarantee the right of children to know their parents if the latter choose the option of anonymous donor? [82].

10. Use of IVF for the production of saviour siblings

Saviour siblings are children produced by IVF who are used as donors of haematopoietic material to treat a sick sibling. Their use entails objective medical, social and ethical issues.

A first ethical aspect to consider is the low efficacy of use. Thus, initial studies by Verlinsky found that 33 embryos were used to produce only one saviour sibling, i.e. its efficacy was 3% [83]. In another paper by the same group, the percentage was 2.5% [84] and in another, approximately 1% [85]. Even in a larger study, in which data were collected from the Reproductive Genetics Institute in Chicago itself and other leading assisted reproduction centres in Australia, Belgium, Turkey and the United States, the efficacy was 1.15% [86].

Obviously, the low efficacy of this technique overshadows the bioethical judgement it merits. But in addition, in order to establish such a judgement, it must also be considered that: (1) with the production of saviour siblings, the child produced is being instrumentalised; (2) to achieve this end requires the use of means that inevitably necessitate the destruction of human embryos, in part, as a consequence of the technique itself and, in part, due to the eugenic selection by PGD to find a 'histocompatible sibling' who is suitable as a donor; and (3) there are alternative techniques to obtain the desired good ethically: the use of umbilical cord blood stored in public or private banks may be an alternative in the near future, from both a medical and bioethical point of view, to treat children who require transplantation of haematopoietic material and who do not have an immunologically compatible family member who can act as a donor. That is to say, in all likelihood, saviour siblings will have ceased to be useful before their production becomes widespread.

11. Possibility of using IVF for social purposes other than women's fertility

11.1 Gestational surrogacy

'Surrogate motherhood is an assisted procreation practice by which a woman gestates an embryo with which she has no biological relationship on behalf of a contracting couple or individual, having to relinquish the child to them after its birth. This practice normally entails a financial remuneration for the pregnant woman; when this is not the case, it is called altruistic surrogacy. From a medical perspective, potential problems for the surrogate and for children born through this practice should be taken into account, especially the existence of possible disabilities in the child. The bioethical aspects are of most interest because the practice of surrogacy objectifies the expectant mother, by using her body for a purpose other than her own good, treating her as a commodity, as a thing. The same is true for the child because it makes him a disposable object, something that can be instrumentalized, similarly objectifying him' [87].

However, it could be argued that acceptance of the pregnancy by the surrogate could be justified as an expression of their personal autonomy, although in the vast majority of cases, it is reasonable to admit that their autonomy is expressed against a background of desperation and vulnerability, so it is difficult to accept this practice uncritically.

This practice, however, presents objective bioethical difficulties for the surrogate. First of all, commercial surrogacy objectifies the woman, by using her body for an end other than her own good, by treating her as a commodity, as something that can be bought and sold, like a thing, which is incompatible with the dignity of women and their rights.

Secondly, it is not ethically admissible because of the social injustice that non-altruistic surrogacy entails, given that only those contracting parents or individuals who are financially well off can benefit from it, i.e. it could become exploitation of economically weak women by economically strong couples or individuals.

Third, surrogacy ruptures what has come to be called the 'mother-child bond', which can be defined as the emotional relationship developed by the mother towards her child during pregnancy. This emotional and biological relationship between mother and child strengthens throughout pregnancy and is important for the normal development of the child [88]. It seems that this 'bond' is largely biological [89], so it also affects altruistic surrogacy.

Fourth, in our ethical assessment of surrogacy there is a further difficulty, due to the selection processes to which potential surrogates are often subjected. These clearly and directly undermine their dignity, since very strict personal requirements are commonly insisted upon to guarantee the quality of the 'product' that the woman may gestate.

Fifth, it should also be taken into account whether future surrogate mothers are always informed of the problems that their pregnancy may entail, i.e. if they are guaranteed to sign an informed consent, which, it seems, is not always the case [90].

It also presents objective bioethical issues related to the children, because a child is always a gift that is given to parents, never a right of parents to acquire it. If this right to a child were prioritised, he or she would be denied the consideration of absolute good in and of himself. He would become a disposable object, something instrumentalisable, i.e. he would be treated as an object. Not all that one wishes acquires the category of right. Desires for parenthood have as their limits the dignity of children and the protection of their fundamental rights. Defending the right of parents to have a child—with no ethical limitations whatsoever—could violate the rights of the child, although it should be established that the right to a child should not be confused with the right to parenthood, because no one can prevent the autonomous decision to have children.

Whatever the reasons put forward to defend the right of parents to a child, no action justifies violation of the fundamental right of children not to be treated as an object. If children were an object of desire of parents, their life would have no more value than that which the parents wished to give it, which is clearly unacceptable.

A further bioethical issue that arises in relation to gestational surrogacy is the consideration that it is not ethically acceptable whenever it is paid, but it is acceptable when it is altruistic surrogacy. In our view, the latter is not admissible either, because it also objectifies the child by demanding quality standards, which if they are not met may affect their fundamental rights, and even their life.

11.2 Social freezing

As we discussed in a previously published paper [91], 'when eggs or ovarian tissue are not frozen for medical causes, the process is called "social freezing". In this case, there are two fundamental reasons why a woman might choose to undergo this procedure: the first is that she has not found a partner who she considers suitable for a matter as important as creating a family, and the second is for professional reasons. In the latter case, the woman considers that becoming pregnant at a young age—usually before age 35—could harm her professional career, prompting her to freeze her eggs for use at a later date. The biological reasons that underlie social freezing are that women's fertility declines with age, especially due to a decrease in ovarian function, owing to a reduction in the number of eggs'.

11.3 Ethical assessment

Aside from the aforementioned biomedical and social problems, social freezing unquestionably presents ethical concerns. In our opinion [91], 'the main one is that, although not explicit, it implicitly objectifies the woman by prompting her to make a decision that is disguised a good for her when, as reported, this practice entails objective negative medical consequences for the user and also for her child'. According to Martinelli et al., '"Social egg freezing" is a paradigmatic demonstration of how the medicalization of women's bodies can be used to mask social and cultural anxieties about aging'.

However, 'we believe there is another ethical difficulty, derived from the fact that it is hard to guarantee the autonomy of women to make such a decision if they are not provided with adequate information on the risks and benefits entailed in social freezing, something that is not always easily verifiable, as previously mentioned' [91].

'Another ethical problem that social freezing may pose is the possible social inequality between groups of women who work in economically powerful companies, which can bear the costs of social freezing for their employees and those who work in companies that cannot do so. Another question therefore arises: to avoid social injustice, should social freezing be supported with public funds? We believe the answer should be that, given the myriad of objective medical problems that exist—some of vital importance—and that have to be treated with these funds, would it not be creating a problem of distributive justice? Finally, it should also be pointed out that social freezing implies that fertile women, capable of conceiving and carrying a child naturally, renounce this, substituting natural conception for IVF.

This not only reduces the possibilities of eventually becoming pregnant but also, as mentioned, increases the health risks for mother and child. It must be carefully considered whether the advantage of using young eggs compensates for the risks derived from the processes required in social freezing' [91].

12. Possible misleading advertising that assisted reproduction clinics may present to attract clients

The main vehicle used by assisted reproduction clinics to attract new customers is to advertise their efficacy, expressed in terms of pregnancy rates and live births achieved per ovarian stimulation cycle.

However, an ethical issue that may occur is if the data presented by these clinics are correct or are manipulated to improve their efficacy, i.e. whether there is 'misleading advertising' aimed at bringing in more clients.

We evaluated this issue in a recent paper [92], the most relevant aspects of which are presented below.

Based on data published by the ESHRE in 2014, the PR and LBR following IVF in Europe between 1997 and 2010 varied between 22.28 and 29.2% for the PR, with a mean rate of 26.41%, and between 13.07 and 22.4% for the LBR, with a mean rate of 18.81%.

When ICSI was used, these same rates varied between 23.37 and 29.9% for the PR, with a mean rate of 27.22%, and between 12.68 and 21.10% for the LBR, with a mean rate of 18.31%.

The aforementioned data refer to the PR and LBR per ovarian stimulation cycle. However, these data do not seem to be the most appropriate to evaluate the efficacy of assisted reproduction clinics, because normally women who attend them undergo more than one cycle (usually three) to increase the efficacy of the technique, in terms of having the desired child. We therefore feel that it is better to use the 'cumulative pregnancy rate' (CPR) or the 'cumulative live birth rate' (CLBR), understood as the success rates that are achieved after all ovarian stimulation cycles that the woman undergoes.

After analysing data from the 13 studies that we consider most representative, the mean CLBR is 26.6%, after one cycle; 38.3% after two cycles; 57.4% after three cycles and 66.0% in cases of more than three cycles, with a mean rate of 56.3% [92].

The CLBR varies by country of course, and thus the lowest in Europe is Italy, with 18.3% and the highest in Poland, with 36.5%. This rate is 24.7% in Russia, 38.1% in Canada and 41.8% in the United States, the country with the highest rate in the world.

To compare the data referred to above with the data published by private assisted reproduction clinics on their websites, we analysed the data presented by 123 private clinics [92]. Surprisingly, none of the clinics we looked at provides data on the CLBR. These rates ranged between 28.0 and 72.2%, with a mean of 47.2%. The same rates for women under 35 years of age varied between 39.0 and 82.4%, with a mean of 59.0%; for women between the ages of 35 and 39 years of age, it ranged from 27.0 to 77.8%, with a mean of 47.4%; and for women older than 40 years of age, it varied between 12.0 and 48.6%, with a mean rate of 30.7%.

When the data provided by the 169 assisted reproduction clinics on their websites were compared with the data reported by the same clinics to various scientific societies, it was found that the mean PR per stimulation cycle was 47.2% when autologous oocytes were used and 65.0% with donor oocytes, according to their websites. However, the rates per ovarian stimulation cycle of these same clinics presented by the Fertility Society were 30.55% for IVF and 32.59% for ICSI, which means that the figures provided by the 169 assisted reproduction clinics on their websites are 49.5% higher than reported by the same clinics to the relevant scientific societies when autologous oocytes are used and 108.9% higher when donor oocytes are used.

Another rather startling aspect is that 16 of these clinics claim on their websites to guarantee that a pregnancy will be achieved in 100% of cases.

In conclusion, it may be said that many countries, assisted reproduction clinics present data on their websites that are not consistent with those obtained from the scientific societies. It is also notable that those clinics do not present data on LBRs, which is the rate that best matches the real likelihood that assisted reproduction treatments will eventually lead to the goal of parenthood [92].

13. Final conclusion

As we mentioned at the beginning of this chapter, having a child for a couple who wishes to have one and has difficulty in doing so, turning to assisted reproduction, is certainly an objective good, which has contributed to the wide social acceptance of such techniques.

Nevertheless, this good should be balanced by the bioethical difficulties these techniques present, and that we have analysed in depth in this chapter.

We therefore believe that it should be an important bioethical objective that in assisted reproduction clinics, prospective clients are informed of the risks and adverse effects of ARTs, as well as providing reasonable accurate data on the chances of success of the techniques we have analysed here. Thus, having been well informed, they can make a well-founded, well-informed personal or couple's decision, because ultimately, personal freedom is what should decide the option taken. Respect for the bioethical principle of patient autonomy requires it and counselling needs to be informative and nondirective.

Author details

Justo Aznar* and Julio Tudela

Life Sciences Institute, Catholic University of Valencia, Spain

*Address all correspondence to: justo.aznar@ucv.es

References

[1] Aznar J, Tudela J. The Biological Status of the Early Human Embryo: When Does Human Life Begin? In Etheredge F. Conception: An Icon of the Beginnning. EnRoute: St. Louis; 2019

[2] Aznar J. Respect for human life in assisted procreation techniques. Medicina e Morale. 2013;**5**:935-945

[3] Aznar J, Tudela J, Aznar J. Analysis of the truth advertising on the efficacy provided by assisted reproduction techniques. Acta Bioethica. 2017;**23**:311-325

[4] Niederberger C, Pellicer A, Simón C, Kathrins M, Goldstein M, Sigman M, et al. 25 historic papers: An ASRM 75th birthday gift from fertility and sterility. Fertility and Sterility. 2019;**112**:e2-e27

[5] Nygren KG, Andersen AN. Assisted reproductive technology in Europe, 1997. Results generated from European registers by ESHRE. Human Reproduction. 2001;**16**:384-391

[6] Nygren KG. Andersen AN, European IVF-monitoring programme (EIM). Assisted reproductive technology in Europe, 1998. Results generated from European registers by ESHRE. Human Reproduction. 2001;**16**:2459-2471

[7] Nygren KG, Andersen AN. Assisted reproductive technology in Europe, 1999. Results generated from European registers by ESHRE. Human Reproduction. 2002;**17**:3260-3274

[8] Nyboe Andersen A, Gianaroli L, Nygren KG, European IVF-monitoring programme; European Society of Human Reproduction and Embryology. Assisted reproductive technology in Europe, 2000. Results generated from European registers by ESHRE. Human Reproduction. 2004;**19**:490-403

[9] Andersen AN, Gianaroli L, Felberbaum R, de Mouzon J, Nygren KG, European IVF-Monitoring Programme (EIM). Assisted reproductive technology in Europe, 2001. Results generated from European registers by ESHRE. Human Reproduction. 2005;**20**:1158-1176

[10] European IVF-monitoring programme (EIM) for the European Society of Human Reproduction and Embryology (ESHRE), Andersen AN, Gianaroli L, Felberbaum R, de Mouzon J, Nygren KG. Assisted reproductive technology in Europe, 2002. Results generated from European registers by ESHRE. Human Reproduction. 2006;**21**:1680-1697

[11] Andersen A, Goossens V, Gianaroli L, Felberbaum R, De Mouzon J, Nygren K. Assisted reproductive technology in Europe, 2003. Results generated from European registers by ESHRE. Human Reproduction. 2007;**22**:1513-1525

[12] Andersen A, Goossens V, Ferraretti A, Bhattacharya S, Felberbaum R, de Mouzon J, et al. Assisted reproductive technology in Europe, 2004: Results generated from European registers by ESHRE. Human Reproduction. 2008;**23**:756-771

[13] Andersen A, Goossens V, Bhattacharya S, Ferraretti A, Kupka M, de Mouzon J, et al. Assisted reproductive technology and intrauterine inseminations in Europe, 2005: Results generated from European registers by ESHRE: ESHRE. The European IVF monitoring Programme (EIM), for the European Society of Human Reproduction and Embryology (ESHRE). Human Reproduction. 2009;**24**:1267-1212

[14] De Mouzon J, Goossens V, Bhattacharya S, Castilla J, Ferraretti A,

Korsak V, et al. Assisted reproductive technology in Europe, 2006: Results generated from European registers by ESHRE. Human Reproduction. 2010;**25**:1851-1862

[15] De Mouzon J, Goossens V, Bhattacharya S, Castilla J, Ferraretti A, Korsak V, et al. Assisted reproductive technology in Europe, 2007: Results generated from European registers by ESHRE. Human Reproduction. 2012;**27**:954-966

[16] Ferraretti A, Goossens V, De Mouzon J, Bhattacharya S, Castilla J, Korsak V, et al. Assisted reproductive technology in Europe, 2008: Results generated from European registers by ESHRE. Human Reproduction. 2012;**27**:2571-2584

[17] Ferraretti A, Goossens V, Kupka M, Bhattacharya S, de Mouzon J, Castilla J, et al. Assisted reproductive technology in Europe, 2009: Results generated from European registers by ESHRE. Human Reproduction. 2013;**28**:2318-2331

[18] Kupka MS, Ferraretti AP, de Mouzon J, Erb K, D'Hooghe T, Castilla JA, et al. Assisted reproductive technology in Europe, 2010: Results generated from European registers by ESHRE. Human Reproduction. 2014;**29**:2099-2113

[19] Nygren KG, Sullivan E, Zegers-Hochschild F, Mansour R, Ishihara O, Adamson G, et al. International Committee for Monitoring assisted Reproductive Technology (ICMART) world report: Assisted reproductive technology 2003. Fertility and Sterility. 2011;**95**:2209-2222

[20] Kissin DM, Jamieson DJ, Barfield WD. Monitoring health outcomes of assisted reproductive technology. The New England Journal of Medicine. 2014;**371**:91-93

[21] Pinborg A, Wennerholm UB, Romundstad LB, Loft A, Aittomaki K, Söderström-Anttila V, et al. Why do singletons conceived after assisted reproduction technology have adverse perinatal outcome? Systematic review and meta-analysis. Human Reproduction Update. 2013;**19**:87-104

[22] Henningsen AK, Pinborg A, Lidegaard O, Vestergaard C, Forman JL, Andersen AN. Perinatal outcome of singleton siblings born after assisted reproductive technology and spontaneous conception: Danish national sibling cohort study. Fertility and Sterility. 2011;**95**:959-963

[23] Pandey S, Shetty A, Hamilton M, Bhattacharya S, Maheshwari A. Obstetric and perinatal outcomes in singleton pregnancies resulting from IVF/ICSI: A systematic review and meta-analyses. Human Reproduction Update. 2012;**18**:485-503

[24] Helmerhorst FM, Perquin DA, Donker E, Keirse MJ. Perinatal outcome of singletons and twins after assisted conception: A systematic review of controlled studies. British Medical Journal. 2004;**328**:261

[25] Davies MJ, Moore VM, Willson KJ, Van Essen P, Priest K, Scott H, et al. Reproductive technologies and the risk of birth defects. The New England Journal of Medicine. 2012;**366**:1803-1813

[26] McDonald SD, Han Z, Mulla S, Murphy KE, Beyene J, Ohlsson A, et al. Preterm birth and low birth weight among in vitro fertilization singletons: A systematic review and meta-analyses. The European Journal of Obstetrics & Gynecology and Reproductive Biology. 2009;**146**:13

[27] Buckett WM, Chian RC, Holzer H, Dean N, Usher R, Tan SL, et al. Obstetric outcomes and congenital abnormalities after in vitro

maturation, in vitro fertilization, and intracytoplasmic sperm injection. Obstetrics and Gynecology. 2007;**110**:885-891

[28] Cheng M, Heilbronn LK. The health outcomes of human ofspring conceived by assisted reproductive technologies (ART). Journal of Developmental Origins of Health and Disease. 2017;**8**:388-302

[29] Goisis A, Remes H, Martikainene P, Klemetti R, Myrskylä M. Medically assisted reproduction and birth outcomes: A within-family analysis using Finnish population registers. Lancet. 2019;**393**:1225-1232

[30] Berntsen S, Söderström-Anttila V, Wennerholm UB, Laivuori H, Loft A, Oldereid NB, et al. The health of children conceived by ART: 'The chicken or the egg?'. Human Reproduction Update. 2019;**25**:137-158

[31] Kelley-Quon LI, Tseng C, Janzen C, Shew SB. Congenital malformations associated with assisted reproductive technology: A California statewide analysis. Journal of Pediatric Surgery. 2013;**48**:1218-1224

[32] Seggers J, de Walle H, Bergman J, Groen H, Hadderd-Algra M, Bos M, et al. Congenital anomalies in offspring of subfertile couples: A registry-based study in the northern Netherlands. Fertility and Sterility. 2015;**103**:1001-1010

[33] Mozafari Kermani R, Farhangniya M, Shahzadeh Fazeli S, Bagheri P, Ashrafi M, Vosough Taqi Dizaj A. Congenital malformations in singleton infants infants conceived by assisted reproductive technologies and singleton infants by natural conception in Tehran, Iran. International Journal of Fertility & Sterility. 2018;**11**:304-308

[34] Olson CK, Keppler-Noreuil K, Romitti P, Budelier W, Ryan G, Sparks A, et al. In vitro fertilization is associated with an increase in major birth defects. Fertility and Sterility. 2005;**84**:1308-1315

[35] Giorgione V, Parazzini F, Fesslova V, Cipriani S, Candiani M, Inversetti A, et al. Congenital heart defects in IVF/ICSI pregnancy: Systematic review and meta-analysis. Ultrasound in Obstetrics & Gynecology. 2018;**51**:33-32

[36] Zheng Z, Chen L, Yang T, Yu H, Wang H, Qin J. Multiple pregnancies achieved with IVF/ICSI and risk of specific congenital malformations: A meta-analysis of cohort studies. Reproductive Biomedicine Online. 2018;**36**:472-482

[37] Anthony S, Buitendijk SE, Dorrepaal CA, Lindner K, Braat DD, den Ouden AL. Congenital malformations in 4224 children conceived after IVF. Human Reproduction. 2002;**17**:2089-2095

[38] Klemetti R, Sevón T, Gissler M, Hemminki E. Health of children born after ovulation induction. Fertility and Sterility. 2010;**93**:1157-1168

[39] Novakovic B, Lewis S, Halliday J, Kennedy J, Burgner DP, Czajko A, et al. Assisted reproductive technologies are associated with limited epigenetic variation at birth that largely resolves by adulthood. Nature Communications. 2019;**10**(1):3922

[40] Hvidtjørn D, Schieve L, Schendel D, Jacobsson B, Svaerke C, Thorsen P. Cerebral palsy, autism spectrum disorders, and developmental delay in children born after assisted conception: A systematic review and meta-analysis. Archives of Pediatrics & Adolescent Medicine. 2009;**163**:72-83

[41] Sandin S, Nygren KG, Iliadou A, Hultman CM, Reichenberg A. Autism and mental retardation among offspring born after in vitro fertilization. Journal

of the American Medical Association. 2013;**310**:75-84

[42] Bonduelle M, Liebaers I, Deketelaere V, Derde MP, Camus M, Devroey P, et al. Neonatal data on a cohort of 2889 infants born after ICSI (1991-1999) and of 2995 infants born after IVF (1983-1999). Human Reproduction. 2002;**17**:671-694

[43] Wen J, Jiang J, Ding C, Dai J, Liu Y, Xia Y, et al. Birth defects in children conceived by in vitro fertilization and intracytoplasmic sperm injection: A meta-analysis. Fertility and Sterility. 2012;**97**:1331-1337.e1-4

[44] Hansen M, Kurinczuk JJ, Milne E, de Klerk N, Bower C. Assisted reproductive technology and birth defects: A systematic review and meta-analysis. Human Reproduction Update. 2013;**19**:330-353

[45] Hoorsan H, Mirmiran P, Chaichian S, Moradi Y, Hoorsan R, Jesmi F. Congenital malformations in infants of mothers undergoing assisted reproductive technologies: A systematic review and meta-analysis study. Journal of Preventive Medicine and Public Health. 2017;**50**:347-360

[46] Nakashima A, Araki R, Tani H, Ishihara O, Kuwahara A, Irahara M, et al. Implications of assisted reproductive technologies on term singleton birth weight: An analysis of 25,777 children in the national assisted reproduction registry of Japan. Fertility and Sterility. 2013;**99**:450-455

[47] Kamath MS, Kirubakaran R, Mascarenhas M, Sunkara SK. Perinatal outcomes after stimulated versus natural cycle IVF: A systematic review and meta-analysis. Reproductive Biomedicine Online. 2018;**36**:94-101

[48] Land JA, Evers JL. Risks and complications in assisted reproduction techniques: Report of an ESHRE consensus meeting. Human Reproduction. 2003;**18**:455-457

[49] Moini A, Shiva M, Arabipoor A, Hosseini R, Chehrazi M, Sadeghi M. Obstetric and neonatal outcomes of twin pregnancies conceived by assisted reproductive technology compared with twin pregnancies conceived spontaneously: A prospective follow-up study. European Journal of Obstetrics, Gynecology, and Reproductive Biology. 2012;**165**:29-32

[50] Vasario E, Borgarello V, Bossotti C, Libanori E, Biolcati M, Arduino S, et al. IVF twins have similar obstetric and neonatal outcome as spontaneously conceived twins: A prospective follow-up study. Reproductive Biomedicine Online. 2010;**21**:422-428

[51] Pinborg A, Lidegaard Ø, la Cour Freiesleben N, Andersen AN. Consequences of vanishing twins in IVF/ICSI pregnancies. Human Reproduction. 2005;**20**:2821-2829

[52] Pinborg A, Lidegaard O, Nl F, Andersen AN. Vanishing twins: A predictor of small-for-gestational age in IVF singletons. Human Reproduction. 2007;**22**:2707-2714

[53] Centers for Disease Control and Prevention (CDC). Contribution of assisted reproductive technology and ovulation-inducing drugs to triplet and higher-order multiple births—United States, 1980-1997. Morbidity and Mortality Weekly Report. 2000;**49**:535-538

[54] Henningsen AA, Gissler M, Skjaerven R, Bergh C, Tiitinen A, Romundstad LB, et al. Trends in perinatal health after assisted reproduction: A Nordic study from the CoNARTaS group. Human Reproduction. 2015;**30**:710-716

[55] Farhi A, Reichman B, Boyko V, Hourvitz A, Ron-El R, Lerner-Geva L.

Maternal and neonatal health outcomes following assisted reproduction. Reproductive Biomedicine Online. 2013;**26**:454-461

[56] McDonald SD, Han Z, Mulla S, Murphy KE, Beyene J, Ohlsson A, et al. Preterm birth and low birth weignt among in vitro fertilization singletons: A systematic review and meta-analyses. European Journal of Obstetrics, Gynecology, and Reproductive Biology. 2009;**146**:138-148

[57] Jiang Z, Wang Y, Lin J, Xu J, Ding G, Huang H. Genetic and epigenetic risks of assisted reproduction. Best Practice & Research. Clinical Obstetrics & Gynaecology. 2017;**44**:90-04

[58] Sutcliffe AG, Ludwig M. Outcome of assisted reproduction. Lancet. 2007;**370**:351-359

[59] Qin J, Wang H, Sheng X, Liang D, Tan H, Xia J. Pregnancy-related complications and adverse pregnancy outcomes in multiple pregnancies resulting from assisted reproductive technology: A meta-analysis of cohort studies. Fertility and Sterility. 2015;**103**:1492-1495

[60] Pastore LM, Williams CD. Perinatal outcomes in singletons following in vitro fertilization: A meta-analysis. Obstetrics and Gynecology. 2004;**104**:411

[61] Aznar J, Martínez M, Navarro P. Valoración de la adopción de embriones humanos congelados desde el punto de vista de la filosofía moral, la ética laica y dos religiones monoteístas. Acta Bioethica. 2016;**22**:187-194

[62] Pessina A. La cosiddetta adozione pre natale. Questione etiche. (Texto pro-manuscripto. Per concessione dell'autore)

[63] Klein JU. Religious Views: The Impact of Traditional Theological Opinion on the Practice of Third-Party Reproduction. In Sauer MV. Principles of Oocyte and Embryo Donation. London: Springer-Verlag; 2013

[64] Rae SB, Cox PM. Bioethics: A Christian Approach in a Pluralistic Age Grand Rapids. Michigan: Wm. B. Eerdmans Publishing Company; 1999

[65] Aznar J, Martínez M, Navarro P. Moral assessment of frozen human embryo adoption in the light of the magisterium of the Catholic Church. Acta Bioethica. 2017;**23**:137-149

[66] Congregation for the Doctrine of the Faith. Instruction Donum Vitae. 1987

[67] Congregation for the Doctrine of the Faith. Instruction Dignitas Personae on certain Bioethical questions. 2008

[68] Aznar J, Mínguez JA. Loss of human embryos secondary to in vitro fertilization. Medicina e Morale. 2012;**4**:613-616

[69] Martin JR, Bromer JG, Sakkas D, Patrizio P. Live babies born per oocyte retrieved in a subpopulation of oocyte donors with repetitive reproductive success. Fertility and Sterility. 2010;**94**:2064-2068

[70] Coco R. Reprogenetics: Preimplantational genetics diagnosis. Genetics and Molecular Biology. 2014;**37**:271-274

[71] Ethics Committee of American Society for Reproductive Medicine. Use of preimplantation genetic diagnosis for serious adult onset conditions: A committee opinion. Fertility and Sterility. 2013;**100**:54-57

[72] Collins SC. Preimplantation genetic diagnosis: Technical advances and expanding applications. Current

Opinion in Obstetrics & Gynecology. 2013;**25**:201-206

[73] Harton GL, Magli MC, Lundin K, Montag M, Lemmen J, Harper JC, et al. ESHRE PGD consortium/embryology special interest group--best practice guidelines for polar body and embryo biopsy for preimplantation genetic diagnosis/screening (PGD/PGS). Human Reproduction. 2011;**26**:41-46

[74] Mastenbroek S, Twisk M, van Echten-Arends J, Sikkema-Raddatz B, Korevaar JC, Verhoeve HR, et al. In vitro fertilization with preimplantation genetic screening. The New England Journal of Medicine. 2007;**357**:9-17

[75] Savulescu J, Kahane G. The moral obligation to create children with the best chance of the best life. Bioethics. 2009;**23**:274-290

[76] Malek J, Daar J. The case for a parental duty to use preimplantation genetic diagnosis for medical benefit. The American Journal of Bioethics. 2012;**12**:3-11

[77] Verlinsky Y, Ginsberg N, Lifchez A, Valle J, Moise J, Strom CM. Analysis of the first polar body: Preconception genetic diagnosis. Human Reproduction. 1990;**5**:826-829

[78] Montag M, van der Ven K, Rösing B, van der Ven H. Polar body biopsy: A viable alternative to preimplantation genetic diagnosis and screening. Reproductive Biomedicine Online. 2009;**18**(Suppl 1):6-11

[79] Hamamah S, I26 Alternatives to PGD. Non-invasive assessment of oocytes and embryos. Reproductive BioMedicine Online. 2013;**26** (Suppl 1):S10-S11

[80] Dokras A, Sargent I, Ross C, Gardner R, Barlow D. Trophectoderm biopsy in human blastocysts. Human Reproduction. 1900;**5**(7):821-825

[81] Pennings G. Genetic databases and the future of donor anonymity. Human Reproduction. 2019;**34**:786-790

[82] Pennings G. The 'double track' policy for donor anonymity. Human Reproduction. 1997;**12**:2839-2844

[83] Valerio M. Sólo cinco 'bebés salvadores' han nacido en España desde 2006. El Mundo Salud. Nov 2, 2015

[84] Verlinsky Y, Rechitsky S, Sharapova T, et al. Preimplantation HLA testing. Journal of the American Medical Association. 2004;**291**:2079-2085

[85] Kuliev A, Rechitsky S, Verlinsky O, Tur-Kaspa I, Kalakoutis G, et al. Preimplantation diagnosis and HLA typing for haemoglobin disorders. Reproductive Biomedicine Online. 2005;**11**:362-370

[86] Kuliev A, Rechitsky S, Tur-Kaspa I, Verlinsky Y. Preimplantation genetics: Improving access to stem cell therapy. Annals of the New York Academy of Sciences. 2005;**1054**:223-227

[87] Aznar J, Martínez PM. Gestational surrogacy: Current view. The Linacre Quarterly. 2019;**86**:56-57

[88] Lorenceau ES, Mazzucca L, Tisseron S, Pizitz TD. A cross-cultural study on surrogate mother's empathy and maternal-foetal attachment. Women and Birth. 2015;**28**:154-159

[89] Vilella F, Moreno-Moya JM, Balaguer N, Grasso A, Herrero M, Martínez S, et al. Hsa-miR-30d, secreted by the human endometrium, is taken up by the pre-implantation embryo and might modify its transcriptome. Development. 2015;**142**:3210-3221

[90] Tanderup M, Reddy S, Patel T, Nielsen BB. Informed consent in medical decision-making in commercial gestation surrogacy: A mixed methods study in New Dehli,

India. Acta Obstetricia et Gynecologica Scandinavica. 2015;**94**:465-472

[91] Aznar J, Tudela J. Social freezing: Analysis of an ethical dilema. The Ethics in Medicine. 2019;**35**:161-170

[92] Aznar J, Tudela J, Aznar J. Analysis of the truth in advertising on the efficacy provided by assisted reproduction clinics. Acta Bioethica. 2017;**23**:311-325

Section 4

Human Contraception

Chapter 13

Human Contraceptives: Current Status, Sperm Antigen Inhibitors and an Insight into PCSK4

Dahril Dahril, Widi Nugroho and Aulanni'am Aulanni'am

Abstract

Rapid growth of global human population has been implicating to food shortage, social problems and environmental degradation. Contraceptive devices have long been applied as a major method to reduce natality. Current application of this technology relies upon hormonal administration, condom, withdrawal and recently hormonal vaccino-contraceptive. Discoveries of antisperm proteins have been directing current researches toward developments of antisperm antibody (ASA) contraceptions. Actions of ASA are targeting antigens either on the head or on the tail of sperm. Antibodies targeting head antigens aimed at blocking gamete fusion, ZP penetration and/or acrosome reaction. Molecules working on sperm tails are aimed to block sperm motility or energy production. PCSK4 is one sperm antigen firstly expressed on the human sperm acrosome during its initial development on the round spermatid and retains on the acrosome until sperm is matured. It is known to contribute to the post-capacitational hyperactivation of sperm essential for zona penetration. Rat models injected with rabbit-anti human PCSK4 developed incompetent sperm and allowance of these male rats to fertile female rats resulted significant reduction of conception rate. Apart from antibody, synthetic inhibitors of PCSK4 have also been developed. Future developments of ASA contraception are discussed.

Keywords: contraception, ASA, PCSK4, synthetic peptide

1. Introduction

The world population had grown enormously during the period of 40 years since 1960 to 2000, doubled from 3 to 6.1 billion peoples [1–3]. In 2010, it became 6.9 billion and was estimated to reach 9.3 billion in 2050 or to increase by 35% from that in 2010 [2, 4, 5]. The growth seems slower after 2000 and the global population growth in the next decades until 2050 was estimated to be slower by three times compared to those during the period of 1960–2000 [1–5].

Despite a slower growth, negative impacts of high human population on environment as well as on human have been remaining high. In one hand, the need to provide more foods to feed more peoples has triggered environment degradation through the use of chemical fertilisers, practices of intensified farming and farming mechanisations, to boost the amount of yields and frequency of harvests [6]. Moreover, increased land uses for housings and agricultures have led further environment degradation in tropical regions through deforestation [7]. On the other hand, population growth along with poverty was reported to link to further serious social problems and terrorism in some communities [8]. Therefore, efforts to further effectively suppress the world population growth needs updated strategies that fits with current issues.

A method that globally has been used as a measure to control birth is contraceptive practice. Contraception includes all means to prevent pregnancy resulted from an intercourse. Contraceptions currently used widely among women are hormonal (pills, blotch and injectable forms), natural (near ovulation abstinence and before ejaculation withdrawal), intravaginal or intrauterine (vaginal rings, diaphragm, spermicides or intrauterine devices) and sterilisation, while popular men contraceptives are withdrawal method (*coitus interruptus*), condom and vasectomy [9].

More than 6.5 billion of global population have used at least one contraception method, with the increase of new users are of 75 million couples annually [3]. The largest number of contraceptive users are women while male contraceptions are practiced only by 30% of couples worldwide [3, 9–11]. Existing women contraceptive methods however, pose discomforts as well as adverse effects. For example, pills have to be taken daily. Interruptions due to some practical reasons such as forgets have been commonly heard and would risk its infectivity. Moreover, the hormonal pill contraception in selective cases might risk occurrence of venous thrombosis and breast cancer [12]. Intra uterine devices are thought to be effective for long term usage but some users reported side effects such as bleeding, discomforts, infection and pain [13].

Likewise, current male contraceptives utilisation have been known to cause several side effects which might have attributed to the low utilisation among men. Condom uses cause sexual discomforts and low rate failures have been reported (5–15%) [3]. In addition, the application of steroid male contraceptive such as testosterone enanthate (TE) was reported to cause obesity, testicular atrophy in 25% of cases and reduced level of high density lipoprotein (HDL) in 10% of cases [14].

Vasectomy, the *vas deferens* ligation, is by far the most effective and economical male contraceptive method and as many as 7% (40–60 million) of worldwide couples practice this method [12]. One advantage of vasectomy is, that it can be reversed by *vasovasostomy* surgery to restore fertility with the rate of pregnancy after the reversal was between of 30–60% but, the rate decreased when the *vasovasostomy* was performed 8 years after vasectomy was conducted [3]. Fertility restoration and pregnancy rate after vasectomy reversal are influenced by, among others, the interval of vasectomy to reversal surgery, the presence of azoospermia, presence of sperm granuloma, the age of female partner and the same female partner [15].

Some studies reported the association of vasectomy and prostatic cancers but, studies claimed as such were mainly conducted before year 2000, while more recent studies indicated the opposites [16]. A cohort study involved 2 million samples of Danish men, reported only weak statistical association between prostatic cancers and vasectomy [17]. Likewise, a systematic review of 53 epidemiological studies with total samples of more than 2 millions men indicated that the role of vasectomy in the development of prostatic cancers was weak if any, and further analysis after controlling potential bias indicated that the association did not exist, statistically [16]. Other population based study reported no association between vasectomy and prostatic cancer [18]. Besides these unclear statistical associations, there have not been biological evidence supporting the causal role of vasectomy to prostatic cancers [16]. These indicate that being vasectomised are safe from risk of contracting prostatic cancers. However, vasectomised men experienced post operational discomforts such as pain, infection, scrotal area swelling and granulomatous inflammation of *vas deferens* [3].

Those limitations of existing contraceptive methods indicate the need to develop new procedures. The latest should be effective in preventing pregnancy but ideally acting specifically to reproductive organs, easy in application, eliminating side effects, and reversible. The aim of this chapter is to describe the current knowledge in regard to antisperm antibody (ASA) contraception and the characteristics of proprotein convertase subtilisin/kexin type 4 (PCSK4) as an ASA contraceptive candidate as well as to shed light into the direction of future ASA developmental researches.

2. Novel immune-contraceptive methods and the discovery of ASA

With the continued human population growth, its consequential problems and limitation of present contraceptive approaches, alternatives methods of contraception have been reported and immune-contraceptive modes has become one popular theme. Immuno-contraception is a mean of contraception conducted by administering immunogenic substance into human body to induce antibody formation against particular antigens involved in the conception process [19]. Immuno-contraceptive agents target at least one of three reproductive physiology pathways i.e. preventing gamete production (target antigens: FSH, LH, GnRH), stopping embryonic development (target antigen: hCG), or inhibiting gamete function (target antigens: Zona Pellucida, spermatozoa) [9].

Vaccine candidates to prevent gamete production have been studied. Heterologous ovine LH based vaccine was reported to cause muscle wastage, reduced testicular weight and alopecia in monkey [20]. Vaccines against LH were known to elicit steroidal side effect and hormonal depression in humans therefore, cannot be used for the species [21]. Vaccine against FSH in men inhibited spermatogenesis to oligospermia but not azoospermia, thus only partially affected fertility [21]. A vaccine against GnRH has been proven to reduce serum testosterone to castration level and has undergone phase II clinical trial to treat prostate carcinoma [22]. However, its use for contraception in humans is currently not practical due to feared side effects, such as loss of body hair, atrophy of prostate and impotency after chronic exposure [21, 23]. In contrast, clinical trials on hCG based vaccine have been conducted in women from several countries including India, Brazil, Finland, Sweden and Chile under the International Committee on Contraception Research of Population Council, New York. These trials indicated that the vaccine has no apparent side effects [24]. The vaccine has prepared to enter a further phase of clinical trial in India [24].

Inhibition of gamete function, such as debilitating the function of sperm using ASA, has also been seen as one promising alternative of immuno-contraceptive approach [21, 25–27]. ASA were discovered in 2–30% of either infertile men or in their women partners and in 70% of men following vasectomy [21, 25, 28, 29]. ASA might become a potential method of immuno-contraceptive in mammals, provided that they fulfil a few criteria: (1) Antigens are expressed only in sperm, therefore the risk of side effect of cross reaction with other somatic cells will be omitted. (2) Antigens are expressed on the outer surface of sperm cell membrane, making them highly exposed to antibody recognition. (3) Sperm antigens play roles in fertilisation process so that the inactivation will impair sperm fertilizability [30].

It has been reported that ASA or other sperm antigen inhibitors could influence fertilisation process through at least one of four ways: (1) blocking gamete fusion, (2) preventing sperm-zona pellucida binding and penetration, (3) inhibiting acrosome reaction or (4) immobilising sperm [31–48].

2.1 ASA that block gamete fusion

Zona-free hamster-egg system was used for sperm-egg fusion which is an important step of fertilisation process [39]. Using this system, several mammalian sperm antigens have been studied for their role in sperm-oocyte membrane fusion including acrosomal protein equatorin (EQT), A disintegrin and metalloproteases (ADAMs) family proteins, DE, sperm acrosomal membrane-associated protein 32 (SAMP32), SAMP14, cluster of differentiation 46 (CD46), human equatorial segment protein (hESP) and Izumo [31–39].

The EQT is found in various mammalian sperm, including human [40]. Equatorin protein is first detected on the budding acrosomal membrane of round spermatids, retaining on acrosome during its remodelling in elongating spermatids and translocating to the equatorial region of acrosome during the acrosome reaction [40, 41]. Anti-equatorin antibody was reported to block sperm–oocyte fusion *in-vitro* [37]. In other *in-vivo* study, antibody-containing and control solutions were injected directly into the right and left oviductal ampullae, respectively. The results revealed that the rates of pregnancy in mice injected with antibody-antiequatorin-containing solution were significantly lower than that in the control group [37].

The ADAMs (also known as fertilin β) were believed to play some role in fertilisation of mammalian gametes [31, 42]. Sperm from mice lacking ADAM2 were incapable of binding to egg membrane, migrating inside female reproductive tract and binding to the zona pellucida [43]. In human, many ADAMs proteins are expressed in many different organs, while many other ADAM genes presents only as pseudogenes [42]. However, only three human ADAMs (ADAMs 2, 20 and 30) are specifically expressed in testicular tissues. Courtesy of Human Protein Atlas, www.proteinatlas.org [49]. ADAM2 are expressed in abundant in early and round spermatid, ADAM20 presents in abundant in late and elongated spermatids and ADAM 30 are expressed in cells along seminiferous duct. Courtesy of Human Protein Atlas, www.proteinatlas.org [49]. However, ADAM2 and ADAM20 are not detected either in the human sperm [44] or in ovarian tissue. Courtesy of Human Protein Atlas, www.proteinatlas.org [49]. These imply that these two human ADAMs could be important in sperm maturation but might not be important in human fertilisation process. Further, although aforementioned mice study indicated the role of ADAMs in gamete fusion, the role of human ADAM30 in fertilisation process remains unclear.

Epididymal glycoprotein DE (37 kDa) of rat is secreted by the epithelium of the proximal epididymis and attached to the head of spermatozoa during its transit in the epididymis. It participates in the gamete fusion process by binding its ligand on the ovum surface [33]. Immunisation of male rats with DE induced specific antibodies and produced a significant reduction in the animal fertility until as low as 0–33% as shown by an *in-vitro* study. The antibody did not interfere with the synthesis or secretion of DE, with its attachment to the sperm membrane, or with changes in sperm motility, viability, or ability to undergo capacitation and acrosome reaction but, antibody against DE debilitated sperm ability to fuse with zona free-egg [33].

The SAMP32, also called sperm acrosome-associated 1 (SPACA1), was expressed in the inner membrane of equatorial segment of human sperm acrosome and other acrosomal segments [34, 45]. An anti-rSAMP32 was demonstrated to block fusion of capacitated human sperm with zona-free hamster eggs *in-vitro* [34]. A study to monitor the outcomes of *in-vitro* fertilisation (IVF) confirmed that the rate of zygotes developed into blastocysts were much lower when the sperms weakly expressed SAMP32 on their acrosome, than sperms with high expression of SAMP32 [45]. These studies indicate that SAMP32 could prevent conception through at least one of two mechanisms i.e. inhibiting gamete fusion or interfering zygote development.

Another member of SAMPs family, SAMP14 was shown to be specifically expressed in the testis. The protein is localised on outer and inner acrosomal membranes and in the acrosomal matrix of human sperm. However, it retains on the inner acrosomal membrane after the acrosome reaction. SAMP14 might have a role in gamete interaction, as antibodies anti-recombinant SAMP14 inhibited the binding and the fusion of human sperm to zona free hamster eggs *in-vitro* [35].

Human CD46 is a protein involved in immune response against external antigenic exposure [40]. Human CD46 or Membrane Cofactor Protein (MCP) are also known to anchor membrane of sperm and involved in fertilisation process. Antibodies against MCP significantly inhibited human sperm binding to hamster oocytes, *in-vitro* [36].

The other family of MCP, the CD52 sperm antigen has been detected on the mature sperm and seminal plasma; Antibody anti-CD52 showed sperm immobilisation properties *in-vitro*. As anti-CD52 is reported to cross react with CD46, CD55 and CD59 cofactor proteins [46] and because substances are expressed in many somatic tissues as humoral immunity agents, their use as contraceptive agent could compromise immune system.

hESP is known to localise to the equatorial segment of human sperm. ESP first appears in the early phase of acrosomal biogenesis in round spermatids, persists during acrosomal maturation and isolated to the edge of the mature acrosome [47]. Antisera to recombinant human ESP inhibited both binding of oolemma and fusion of human sperm in the hamster egg penetration assay. ESP immunoreacted with 27% of 15 antisperm antibody (ASA)-positive serum samples from infertile male patients and 40% of 5 ASA-positive female sera indicating the possible role of ESP in some cases of infertility [38].

Both mouse and human Izumo proteins are detectable on sperm surface only after the acrosome reaction. Thus, it was suggested that Izumo is hidden under plasma membrane and exposed only after the acrosome reaction occurs. When an antibody anti-human Izumo was added to the mixture of mouse sperm and hamster egg, no fusion was observed, whereas the fusion was observed in the control assay [39]. Izumo1 was hypothesized to act at a molecule designated as Juno, as its receptor on mouse eggs and in other mammals [48].

2.2 ASA that prevent sperm-zona pellucida binding and penetration

A notable sperm antigen that acts in sperm-zona pellucida interaction in mammals is fertilisation antigen-1 (FA-1) [50]. Immunofluorescent reactivity of FA-1 was detected in acrosome region of human sperm [51]. This protein is known to react strongly with 55 kDa Zona Pellucida protein-3 (ZP3) [52]. Zona pellucida pre-incubated with human sperm FA-1 failed to bind to sperm, indicated that FA-1 blocked sperm binding to zona pellucida. Similar blockage was also observed when the antibody against FA-1 was pre-incubated with sperm before insemination, indicating that the FA-1 is localised on the sperm [50].

In an in-vivo study, female mice injected intradermally with a sperm-specific FA-1 DNA vaccine caused a long-term systemic and local immunity resulting in anti-fertility effects. The effects were further enhanced when the vaccine was mixed with YLP12 DNA vaccine and oligodeoxynucleotide (ODN) [53]. Further study suggested that almost half of infertile women studied had circulating antibodies against human FA-1 antigen and YLP12 peptide sequence [54]. The development of FA-1 based for male contraceptive vaccine warrants further studies.

2.3. ASA that inhibit acrosome reaction (YLP-12 peptide)

Most of mammalian sperm are incapable of fertilising eggs when ejaculated and fertilisation occurs only after an exocytotic process called the acrosome reaction [39]. The halts of acrosome reaction thus, might potentially debilitate the competence of sperm to fertilise egg.

Two sperm antigens have been studied for this property and for their potential to base a development of contraceptive agents; YLP12 and testis specific antigen-1 (TSA-1). A dodecamer sequence designated YLP12 is a peptide sequence that have been identified to specifically localise on the acrosome and tail of spermatozoa [55]. It is known to recognise ZP3 component of human ZP proteins, to involve in sperm-ZP binding and the antibodies against synthetic 12-mer peptide based on YLP12 sequence was reported to specifically inhibit human sperm-ZP binding [56]. The antibody anti-YLP12, in other study, was reported to show a concentration-dependent inhibition of acrosome reaction but did not affect the sperm motility [57]. Immunisation of murine model with synthetic YLP12 produced antibodies affected fertility by reducing sperm capacitation, acrosome reaction and sperm-oocyte binding in an *in-vitro* assay but, immunised murine remained fertile and were capable of delivering the equal number of pups compared to control [55]. In contrast, other study reported that a sperm-specific YLP12 DNA vaccine injected intradermally in female mice caused anti fertility effects [53].

A study reported that TSA-1 is localised to the regions of acrosome, equatorial, mid-piece and tail of human sperm. An *in-vitro* test discovered that TSA-1 concentration-dependently inhibits human sperm acrosome reaction [58].

2.4 Various ASA that immobilise sperm

Sperm tail is widely known as an organelle of motility. Proteomic study showed that proteins extracted from tail fraction of sperm can be classified according to their functions into two main groups: proteins related to metabolism and energy production from endogenous sources, and those related to tail structure and motility [59]. These groups however, are at the end function together to support sperm motility.

*Ep*ididymal *p*rotease *in*hibitor (Eppin) is expressed in the testis and epididymis tissue and on the acrosome and tail of human sperm [60–62]. An in-vitro assay showed that the monkey anti-eppin antibodies decreased the progressive motility of human spermatozoa in terms of distance travelled and speed [62]. Other study suggested that blockade of Eppin epitope by anti-eppin antibody would halt the acrosome reaction through reduction of ionophore-induced calcium influx [60]. Further pre-clinical trial was performed *in-vivo* in non-human primates and showed that Eppin immunised *Macaca radiate* developed high titers to Eppin (78%) and all of these immune-converted monkeys were sterile [63].

Heparin-binding serpin, protein C inhibitor (PCI), is a nonspecific serpin that inactivates many plasmatic and extravascular serine proteases. Mutant male mice lacking PCI gene are infertile but apparently healthy. Histologic examination showed that Sertoli cells and their barrier were destroyed. The resulting sperm are malformed, lack of tail and deformed head and immobilised, similar to those seen in some cases of men infertility [64], thus the effect of PCI on testicle tissues is apparently cytotoxic. In *in-vivo* fertilisation experiments, only 0.5% (n = 416) eggs are fertilised by sperm of mutant male compared to the rate of 92% (n = 415) of eggs develop into blastocysts when intact mice is used [64].

The 80 kDa human sperm antigen (HAS) is known to present on the head of the human and rat spermatozoa, in the testes and epididymis but not in other somatic tissues. Active immunisation of male and female rats with 80 kDa HSA caused infertility in all the immunised animals [65]. Further, active immunisation of male rabbits, rat and marmosets with synthetic peptide-1 of HSA induced reversible infertility in 100, 100% and 6 of 7 of the respective animals [66]. It strongly indicates that antibodies anti-HSA have potential as immuno-contraceptive agents. Additionally, anti-HSA antibody induced *in-vitro* agglutination of human, rat and monkey sperm [67].

Two proteins, A-kinase anchoring protein 3 (AKAP 3) and especially AKAP 4, are proteins abundantly present in fibrous sheath of mid-piece tail of human and mice sperms [68, 69]. AKAP 3 is synthesised earlier during round spermatid formation and involves in the arrangement of the basic structure of the sperm tail, while AKAP 4 is expressed later during late phase of spermatid formation and plays role in the maturation of sperm tail structure [69]. A study showed that male mice lacking AKAP4 was not implicated in sperm numbers but, progressive motility of its sperm was failed and the male mice were infertile [70].

rSMP-B, following its discovery from mid-piece and tail of rabbit sperm [71], was identified to present on the same regions of human sperm [72]. Antibody-anti rSMP-B possessed immobilising activities against human and mouse spermatozoa, but no agglutinating activity, *in-vitro* [72].

Lactate dehydrogenase-C4 subunit (LDH-C4) was expressed specifically in the testis and most abundant in human sperm. Courtesy of Human Protein Atlas, www.proteinatlas.org [49]. Its high activity in the testis is associated with human sperm biogenesis and motility [73]. An *in-vitro* assessment of sperm from LDH-C4 immunised mature male baboon (*Papio sp.*) indicated that sperm binding capacity to Zona pellucida is reduced in seroconverted animal model [74].

Etomoxir is not an ASA. It is a mitochondrial carnitine palmitoyltransferase inhibitor which block serial reaction that transport fatty acid from cytosol into intermembrane space of mitochondria, thus halt the oxidation and energy production from the substrate [75, 76]. The incubation of sperm with etomoxir results in a decreased sperm motility in concentration-dependent manner but does not affect the sperm viability [59]. A systemic usage of Etomoxir for contraceptive is not applicable, as the substance is hepatotoxic [77]. However, more studies with Etomoxir could shed more light of contraceptive targeting sperm antigens responsible for energy production.

3. PCSK4 as a potential sperm antigen for ASA contraceptive developments

3.1 Biochemistry of PCSK4

One sperm antigen potential for development of contraceptive ASA is the proprotein convertase subtilisin/kexin type 4 (PCSK4) [78–81]. PCSK4 is an enzyme protein expressed in abundant on the outer surface of acrosomal plasma membrane of mammalian spermatozoa (**Figure 1**). It has a molecular weight of 45 kDa [79, 83, 84]. Biochemically it plays role in the proteolytic activation of precursor proteins in the cellular secretory pathway and physiologically it has a specific important role in mammalian reproductive process [79, 83–85]. PCSK4 gene is a 9 kilobase (kb) DNA, consists of 15 exon and 14 intron which in humans it is located in the chromosome 19 [78, 80, 85]. It is a protein associated with bacterial subtilisin and yeast kexin where its biosynthesis takes place in endoplasmic reticulum in the form of a multi-domain preprotein [78, 80]. PCSK4 is one among nine family members of calcium-dependent serin endoproteinase *Proprotein Convertase Subtilisin/Kexin* (PCSK) [79, 83–85]. These nine family members of PCSK are: PCSK1 and PCSK2 which are expressed in endocrine and neuroendocrine cells; PCSK3, PCSK5, PCSK6 and PCSK7 are widely expressed by different types of cells; PCSK4 is specifically presented by gonadal and placental cells and; PCSK8 and PCSK9 which play roles in the synthesis pathways of cholesterol and lipid acid [79, 80, 86–88]. PCSK 1 to 7 belong to sub-family of kexin while PCSK8 and PCSK9 belong to sub-family of pirolysin and proteinase-K, respectively [79, 80, 86]. PCSK 1 to 3 are also known

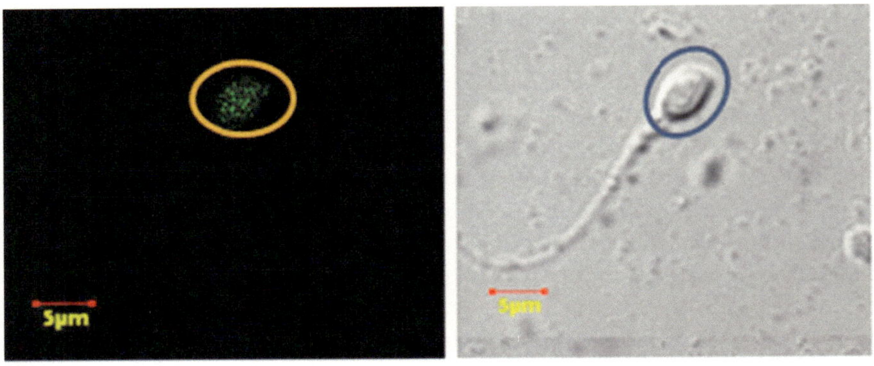

Figure 1.
Using monoclonal antibody anti-human PCSK4 and rodamin as staining, PCSK4 molecules are detected in abundant on the membrane surface of the head of human spermatozoa under Laser Scanning Microscope *(LSM) examination [82].*

as, consecutively, PC1/3, PC2 and furin, while PCSK 5 to 9 are also recognised as PC5/6, PACE4, PC7, SKI-1/SIP and NARC-1, respectively [89].

PCSK4 is synthesised as a zymogen, proPCSK4, in the endoplasmic reticulum [81]. Its maturation process remains unclear but suggested to be by an autocatalytic process that cleaves the molecule at two sites situated between prodomain and the catalytic domain [80]. PCSK4 proprotein contains five domains located consecutively, i.e. the signal peptide (SP) domain, prodomain, catalytic domain, a domain of 150 amino acids called P (Protease) domain or homo B domain and the C-terminal domain which carries transmembrane domain [80]. The SP domain of PCSK4 contains signal peptide which directs precursor proteins toward the secretory pathway. The Prodomain acts as an intra-molecule chaperone and regulator of the catalytic activity of the enzyme, removal of this domain is essential for the activity of the enzyme [90]. The primary and secondary cleavage sites of proPCSK4 are situated between prodomain and catalytic domain. Catalytic domain of PCSK4 is the active site of the enzyme and carries Asp-His-Ser catalytic triad characteristics of serin proteinase [80].

The P domain of PCSK4 plays an important role for proper folding, contains beta fold sandwich of galactose bond domain capable of mediating carbohydrates, phospholipids or membrane receptors. This P domain acts as a regulator site of ultimate enzyme activities under influences of optimum pH and calcium, but also in stabilising the structure of catalytic domain [80, 90]. It helps to balance asymmetric surface at the region of catalytic domain bond, owing to the specific characteristic of multi-basic residues of this enzyme (the consensus of substrate order is Arg-X-Lys-Arg-Arg, where X can be an amino acid; the site of peptide dihydrolysis) [80, 83, 91]. The C-terminal variable domain influences intracellular localisation, in-out recycle of proteins and protein–protein interactions. N-glycosylation sites are located at P domain and at C-terminal domain [80].

Expressions of PCSK4 are discovered in abundant in reproductive organs, especially in testis. In testis, they can be found in epididymic and germinal cells i.e. in acrosomal granules of round spermatids, in acrosomal ridges of elongated spermatids and on the acrosomal plasma membrane of spermatozoa [80, 81, 84, 92]. The PCSK4 or named as proprotein convertase PC4 in a study, is also expressed in the human placenta and macrophage-like cells in the ovary [87, 88].

3.2 Physiological roles of PCSK4

Intracellularly, PCSKs takes action in the limited endoproteolytic regulation mechanism of the secretory pathway. Limited endoproteolysis constitutes the post-translational modifications of proteins by which cells diversify and regulate gene products [78]. Endoproteolytic process occurs during modifications to activate many precursor proteins in biological cell functions including zymogen activations, formations of peptide hormones, complement activations, blood clotting and blood clot lysing, angiogenesis and tissue re-modelling. Secretory pathway processes of eukaryotic cells are mainly assisted by carboxyl residues of Lys or Arg (P1) in the order R/K – (X)n – X/K/R – R (where: X = amino acids other than Cys; n = 1, 3, or 5; K or R = the place of P2 amino acid) [78, 86, 91].

PCSK4 present in acrosome region of sperm thus, is hypothesised to play role in capacitation and acrosome reaction [80, 84]. SPCSK4-null sperm has normal appearance, normal motility competence and undergo normal capacitation process but, following capacitation they suffer reduced hyperactivated motility [93]. Post-capacitation hyperactivity is a qualitative characteristics of sperm which thought to be important to assist sperm penetrating zona pellucida of an egg. PCSK4-null sperms show a reduced fertilisation competence *in-vitro* and the embryo resulted from PCSK4-null sperm fails to develop further [93].

3.3 Substrates of PCSK4

Two molecules have been known as the natural substrates of PCSK4; pro-pituitary adenylate cyclase-activating protein (proPACAP) and Insulin-like growth factor II (IGF-II) [87, 94]. The proPACAP has two active isoforms; PACAP38 and PACAP27 residues. PACAPs are expressed in hypothalamus, in extra-hypothalamic regions of the brain, in the granulosa cells of the developing ovarian follicles of the rat and transiently in rat spermatid cap but, are absent at the other stages of spermatogenesis. They are also expressed in Sertoli cells and Leydig cells. Gonadal PCSK4 is the only enzyme that activates proPACAP both in the testis and the ovary of the mice [94]. A study reported that PACAP null female mice failed to implant its embryo to the uterus [95], suggesting proPACAP activation conducted by PCSK4 is pivotal in embryonic implantation. PCSK4 null male mice lack of PACAP activation and produce normal but incompetent sperm. It leads to the hypothesised that PACAP may not important in maturation process of the sperm but involves in the production of molecules required for the functional mature sperm [94].

Other substrate of PCSK4, IGF-II, is discovered in placenta and its inactivity has been shown to be involved in the pathophysiology of intrauterine growth restriction (IUGR) of human foetus; a major cause of perinatal death. In this pathway, Placental PCSK4 activates pro-IGF-II to form a half-matured IGF-II and successively mature IGF-II as a result of the cleavage of its terminal basic residues by carboxypeptidases [87]. Inhibition of Placental PCSK4 by a PCSK4-specific inhibitor blocks pro-IGF-II processing resulting a reduced trophoblast cell migration [87], likely due to reduced effectivity of trans-placental diffusional exchange leading to reduced nutritional supply [96]. The locality and functionality of the two substrates of PCSK4 indicate that PCSK4 are physiologically important during zona penetration and embryonic development.

3.4 Inhibitors of PCSK4

Studies in model animals showed that individuals with PCSK4 expression disorder have significantly lower fertilisation capability [79]. In our study, intact male *Rattus norvegicus* previously injected with antibody anti-PCSK4 was allowed to fertile female rats and it showed that the number of off-springs delivered by these female rats significantly declined in accordance with the increased doses of antibody anti-PCSK4 injected [82]. These indicate that inactivation of PCSK4 by injectable anti-PCSK4 could prevent conception.

The use of synthetic PCSK4 inhibitors could also serve as an option for contraception. A synthetic inhibitor of PCSK has been developed based on the knowledge, that prodomain removal is essential for activation of the enzyme. Binding of this domain to PCSK4 active enzyme could hypothetically inactivate the enzyme. A peptide, mimicking prodomain sequence near its primary activation site, was engineered and an *in-vitro* assay using a recombinant PCSK4 showed that PCSK4-mediated proteolysis was efficiently blocked by synthetic prodomain $rPC4_{101–116}$ peptide [90].

Other potent synthetic PCSK4-inhibitors: tetrapeptide chloromethyl ketone and the Dec-RVKR/K-cmk (Decanoyl-RVKR/K-chloromethyl ketone) were reported to inhibit PCSK4 more potently than synthetic prodomain $rPC4_{101–116}$ peptide [90]. Another substance, synthetic enediyne amino acid containing peptides, was developed and reported to inhibit PCSK4 activity *in-vitro* [97]. Further, dimeric form of CRES was reported to moderately block the PCSK4 activity to human proIGF-2 in human placental trophoblast cell line [98].

4. Future development of ASA contraceptives

Only a few of aforementioned ASA underwent animal models *in-vivo* study. Among are EQT, FA-1, YLP12, *Eppin*, PCI, HSA, AKAP 4 and PCSK4. None of these molecules however, shows full inhibition of fertilisation in animal models, whereas YLP12 contraceptive studies reported various results from partial to lack of inhibition of fertility to animal models [37, 53, 63–65, 82] [53, 55, 70]. Therefore, further efforts are needed to make ASA contraceptive become reality.

Future development of ASA contraceptives might include the studies of under-explored proteins such as those involve in the energy production in the mitochondria of sperm. Proteomic approach assistance, in this regard, have enabled the discovery of large number of novel proteins [59] and allows further investigations of single protein of interest.

On the other hand, as the usage of single molecule have been impractical, alternative of future ASA development might include the study of efficacy of multivalent vaccines, in order to boost the final effective contraception effect as well as reducing potential toxic effect of high dose administration of a single substance. Study of multivalent vaccine targeting proteins of acrosomal sperm has been actually initiated. In the study, immunised monkeys recognised the five antigens used: ESP, SLLP-1, SAMP 32, SP-10 and SAMP 14, with the highest IgG average absorbance values were to ESP, SAMP 32 and SP-10 but at IgG lower values for SLLP-1 and SAMP 14 [99]. Further, capacitated sperm treated with sera from immunised monkeys showed fusion inhibition but only in two of five individuals [99]. This was a sound study that used proteins which were pre-tested to not cross react to each other. But the study used molecules that never had undergone *in-vivo* study so individual effect of the vaccine component was unknown. In addition, a study of FA-1 and YLP12 mixed vaccine in mice further support the more potential of multivalent vaccine in inducing contraceptive effects compared to monovalent vaccine [54].

The *in-vivo* study of anti-PSCK4 administration demonstrated in our laboratory indicates that it is possible to efficaciously administer contraceptive agents in the form of antiserum rather than injecting them to an individual for a few times as immunisation [82]. In the future, this approach might be more practical if the molecule could reach therapeutic concentration in the seminal plasma once the semen ejaculated thus well mixed with sperm along their journey to egg, mimicking *in-vitro* incubation of sperm with its inhibitors prior to a fertilisation challenge with eggs.

Topical applications such as intravaginal administration might be strategy of choice in the antisperm contraceptive application especially for molecules which have been known to be toxic when administered systemically such as etomoxir. Topical intra-ampullar oviduct administration of antisperm agent in animal model has proven that topical ASA contraceptive application can be efficacious [37].

5. Conclusions

Existing contraceptive methods have been widely practiced by couples globally. However, some side effects limit the broader utilisation. Although ASA is a promising method of contraception it is not yet practical. More studies should be done in order to enable ASA to replace common contraceptive methods.

Acknowledgements

Authors would like to thank to Biochemistry Laboratory of University of Brawijaya for the provision of facilities that allows the writing of this manuscript.

Conflict of interest

We authors declare that there is no conflict of interest related to the preparation of this manuscript.

Author details

Dahril Dahril[1], Widi Nugroho[2] and Aulanni'am Aulanni'am[3]*

1 Sub Division of Urology, Faculty of Medicine, Zainoel Abidin Hospital, Syiah Kuala University, Banda Aceh, Indonesia

2 Laboratory of Veterinary Public Health, Faculty of Veterinary Medicine, University of Brawijaya, Malang, East Java, Indonesia

3 Laboratorium of Biochemistry, Faculty of Veterinary Medicine, University of Brawijaya, Malang, East Java, Indonesia

*Address all correspondence to: aulani@ub.ac.id

References

[1] Crosigani P. Hormonal contraseption: What is new? Human Reproduction Update. 2002;**8**(4):359-371

[2] Division UNP. World Population Prospects the 2010 Revision. United Nations Population Division: New York, United Nations; 2010

[3] Page ST, Amory JK, Bremner WJ. Advances in male contraception. Endocrine Reviews. 2008;**29**(4):465-493

[4] Division UNP. World Population Prospects the 2000 Revision. United Nations Population Division: New York, United Nations; 2000

[5] Suri A. Sperm-based contraceptive vaccines: Current status, merits and development. Expert Reviews in Molecular Medicine. 2005;**7**(18):1-16

[6] Boserup E. The Conditions of Agricultural Growth: The Economics of Agrarian Change under Population Pressure. New York: Routledge; 2017

[7] DeFries RS, Rudel T, Uriarte M, Hansen M. Deforestation driven by urban population growth and agricultural trade in the twenty-first century. Nature Geoscience. 2010;**3**(3):178

[8] Coccia M. General causes of terrorism: High population growth in problematic society. 2017. Available at SSRN: https://ssrn.com/abstract=2951293

[9] Naz RK. Antisperm immunity for contraception. Journal of Andrology. 2006;**27**(2):153-159

[10] Glasier A. Acceptability of contraception for men: A review. Contraception. 2010;**82**(5):453-456

[11] Meriggiola MC, Costantino A, Cerpolini S, Bremner WJ, Huebler D, Morselli-Labate AM, et al. Testosterone undecanoate maintains spermatogenic suppression induced by cyproterone acetate plus testosterone undecanoate in normal men. The Journal of Clinical Endocrinology and Metabolism. 2003;**88**(12):5818-5826

[12] Baird DT, Glasier AF. Science, medicine, and the future. Contraception. BMJ. 1999;**319**(7215):969-972

[13] Lara-Torre E, Spotswood L, Correia N, Weiss PM. Intrauterine contraception in adolescents and young women: A descriptive study of use, side effects, and compliance. Journal of Pediatric and Adolescent Gynecology. 2011;**24**(1):39-41

[14] Meriggiola M, Marcovina S, Paulsen C, Bremner W. Testosteron enanthate at the dose 200 mg/week decreases hdl-cholesterol levels in healthy men. International Journal of Andrology. 2006;**18**:237-242

[15] Namekawa T, Imamoto T, Kato M, Komiya A, Ichikawa T. Vasovasostomy and vasoepididymostomy: Review of the procedures, outcomes, and predictors of patency and pregnancy over the last decade. Reproductive Medicine and Biology. 2018;**17**(4):343-355

[16] Bhindi B, Wallis CJD, Nayan M, Farrell AM, Trost LW, Hamilton RJ, et al. The association between vasectomy and prostate Cancer: A systematic review and meta-analysisThe association between vasectomy and prostate Cancer the association between vasectomy and prostate Cancer. JAMA Internal Medicine. 2017;**177**(9):1273-1286

[17] Husby A, Wohlfahrt J, Melbye M. Vasectomy and Prostate Cancer Risk: A 38-Year Nationwide Cohort Study. Journal of the National Cancer Institute. 2020;**112**(1):djz099

[18] Nayan M, Hamilton RJ, Macdonald EM, Li Q, Mamdani MM, Earle CC, et al. Vasectomy and risk of prostate cancer: Population based matched cohort study. BMJ. 2016;**355**:i5546

[19] Yatim W. Reproduksi dan Embriologi. ke-3 ed. Bandung: Tarsito; 1994

[20] Moudgal N, Jeyakumar M, Krishnamurthy H, Sridhar S, Krihsnamurthy H, Martin F. Development of male contraceptive vaccine - a perspective. Human Reproduction Update. 1997;**3**(4):335-346

[21] Naz R. Immunization with sperm antigens to induce contraception. In: Krause WKH, Naz RK, editors. Immune Infertility. Berlin Heidelberg: Springer; 2009. pp. 197-207

[22] Talwar GP, Vyas HK, Purswani S, Gupta JC. Gonadotropin-releasing hormone/human chorionic gonadotropin β based recombinant antibodies and vaccines. Journal of Reproductive Immunology. 2009;**83**(1):158-163

[23] Kaur K, Prabha VJ. Immunocontraceptives: New approaches to fertility control. BioMed Research International. 2014;**2014**:868196

[24] Talwar GP, Nand KN, Gupta JC, Bandivdekar AH, Sharma RS, Lohiya NK. Current status of a unique vaccine preventing pregnancy. Frontiers in Bioscience. 2017;**9**:321-332

[25] Naz RK. Antisperm contraceptive vaccines: Where we are and where we are going? American Journal of Reproductive Immunology. 2011;**66**(1):5-12

[26] Gupta S, Bansal P. Vaccines for immunological control of fertility. Reproductive Medicine and Biology. 2010;**9**(2):61-71

[27] Naz RK. Contraceptive vaccines: Success, status, and future perspective. American Journal of Reproductive Immunology. 2011;**66**(1):2-4

[28] Chamley LW, Clarke GN. Antisperm antibodies and conception. Seminars in Immunopathology. 2007;**29**(2):169-184

[29] Naz RK. Human synthetic peptide vaccine for contraception targeting sperm. Archives of Andrology. 2004;**50**(2):113-119

[30] Frayne J, Hall L. The potential use of sperm antigens as targets for immunocontraception; past, present and future. Journal of Reproductive Immunology. 1999;**43**(1):1-33

[31] Naz RK. Antisperm contraceptive vaccine. In: Immune Infertility. Switzerland: Springer; 2017. pp. 249-261

[32] Primakoff P, Myles DG. Cell–cell membrane fusion during mammalian fertilization. FEBS Letters. 2007;**581**(11):2174-2180

[33] Ellerman DA, Brantúa VS, Martínez SP, Cohen DJ, Conesa D, Cuasnicú PS. Potential contraceptive use of epididymal proteins: Immunization of male rats with epididymal protein DE inhibits sperm fusion ability. Biology of Reproduction. 1998;**59**(5):1029-1036

[34] Hao Z, Wolkowicz MJ, Shetty J, Klotz K, Bolling L, Sen B, et al. SAMP32, a testis-specific, isoantigenic sperm acrosomal membrane-associated protein. Biology of Reproduction. 2002;**66**(3):735-744

[35] Shetty J, Wolkowicz MJ, Digilio LC, Klotz KL, Jayes FL, Diekman AB, et al. SAMP14, a novel, acrosomal membrane-associated, glycosylphosphatidylinositol-anchored member of the Ly-6/urokinase-type plasminogen activator receptor superfamily with a role in sperm-egg interaction. The

Journal of Biological Chemistry. 2003;**278**(33):30506-30515

[36] Anderson DJ, Abbott AF, Jack RM. The role of complement component C3b and its receptors in sperm-oocyte interaction. Proceedings of the National Academy of Sciences. 1993;**90**(21):10051-10055

[37] Yoshinaga K, Saxena D, Oh-Oka T, Tanii I, Toshimori K. Inhibition of mouse fertilization in vivo by intra-oviductal injection of an anti-equatorin monoclonal antibody. Reproduction. 2001;**122**(4):649-655

[38] Wolkowicz M, Digilio L, Klotz K, Shetty J, Flickinger C, Herr J. Equatorial segment protein (ESP) is a human alloantigen involved in sperm-egg binding and fusion. Journal of Andrology. 2008;**29**(3):272-282

[39] Inoue N, Ikawa M, Isotani A, Okabe M. The immunoglobulin superfamily protein Izumo is required for sperm to fuse with eggs. Nature. 2005;**434**(7030):234

[40] Inoue N, Ikawa M, Okabe M. The mechanism of sperm-egg interaction and the involvement of IZUMO1 in fusion. Asian Journal of Andrology. 2011;**13**(1):81-87

[41] Ito C, Yamatoya K, Yoshida K, Fujimura L, Hatano M, Miyado K, et al. Integration of the mouse sperm fertilization-related protein equatorin into the acrosome during spermatogenesis as revealed by super-resolution and immunoelectron microscopy. Cell and Tissue Research. 2013;**352**(3):739-750

[42] Cho C. Mammalian ADAMs with Testis-Specific or-Predominant Expression. In: N.M. Hooper, U. Lendeckel, editors. The ADAM Family of Proteases. US, Boston, MA: Springer; 2005. pp. 239-59

[43] Cho C, Bunch DOD, Faure J-E, Goulding EH, Eddy EM, Primakoff P, et al. Fertilization defects in sperm from mice lacking fertilin β. Science. 1998;**281**(5384):1857-1859

[44] Choi H, Jin S, Kwon JT, Kim J, Jeong J, Kim J, et al. Characterization of mammalian ADAM2 and its absence from human sperm. PLoS One. 2016;**11**(6):e0158321

[45] Kishida K, Harayama H, Kimura F, Murakami T. Individual differences in the distribution of sperm acrosome-associated 1 proteins among male patients of infertile couples; their possible impact on outcomes of conventional in vitro fertilization. Zygote. 2016;**24**(5):654-661

[46] Hasegawa A, Shigeta M, Shibahara H. Sperm immobilizing antibody and its target antigen. In: Immune Infertility. Switzerland: Springer; 2017. pp. 173-184

[47] Wolkowicz MJ, Shetty J, Westbrook A, Klotz K, Jayes F, Mandal A, et al. Equatorial segment protein defines a discrete Acrosomal subcompartment persisting throughout Acrosomal Biogenesis1. Biology of Reproduction. 2003;**69**(3):735-745

[48] Bianchi E, Doe B, Goulding D, Wright GJ. Juno is the egg Izumo receptor and is essential for mammalian fertilization. Nature. 2014;**508**(7497):483

[49] Uhlén M, Fagerberg L, Hallström BM, Lindskog C, Oksvold P, Mardinoglu A, et al. Tissue-based map of the human proteome. Science. 2015;**347**(6220):1260419

[50] Kadam AL, Fateh M, Naz RK. Fertilization antigen (FA-1) completely blocks human sperm binding to human zona pellucida: FA-1 antigen may be a sperm receptor for zona pellucida

in humans. Journal of Reproductive Immunology. 1995;**29**(1):19-30

[51] Naz R, Rosenblum B, Menge A. Characterization of a membrane antigen from rabbit testis and sperm isolated by using monoclonal antibodies and effect of its antiserum on fertility. Proceedings of the National Academy of Sciences. 1984;**81**(3):857-861

[52] Naz R, Ahmad K. Molecular identities of human sperm proteins that bind human zona pellucida: Nature of sperm-zona interaction, tyrosine kinase activity, and involvement of FA-1. Molecular Reproduction and Development. 1994;**39**(4):397

[53] Naz RK. Effect of fertilization antigen (FA-1) DNA vaccine on fertility of female mice. Molecular Reproduction and Development. 2006;**73**(11):1473-1479

[54] Williams J, Samuel A, Naz RK. Presence of Antisperm antibodies reactive with peptide epitopes of FA-1 and YLP12 in sera of Immunoinfertile women. American Journal of Reproductive Immunology. 2008;**59**(6):518-524

[55] Naz RK, Chauhan SC. Human sperm-specific peptide vaccine that causes long-term reversible Contraception1. Biology of Reproduction. 2002;**67**(2):674-680

[56] Zhu X, Naz RK, Kadam AL. Identification of human sperm peptide sequence involved in egg Bindingfor Immunocontraception1. Biology of Reproduction. 2000;**62**(2):318-324

[57] Naz RK, Chauhan S, Trivedi R.Monoclonal antibody against human sperm-specific YLP 12 peptide sequence involved in oocyte binding. Archives of Andrology. 2002;**48**(3):169-175

[58] Santhanam R, Naz RK. Novel human testis-specific cDNA: Molecular cloning, expression and immunobiological effects of the recombinant protein. Molecular Reproduction and Development. 2001;**60**(1):1-12

[59] Amaral A, Castillo J, Estanyol JM, Ballescà JL, Ramalho-Santos J, Oliva R. Human sperm tail proteome suggests new endogenous metabolic pathways. Molecular & Cellular Proteomics. 2013;**12**(2):330-342

[60] Zhang J, Ding X, Bian Z, Xia Y, Lu C, Wang S, et al. The effect of anti-eppin antibodies on ionophore A23187-induced calcium influx and acrosome reaction of human spermatozoa. Human Reproduction. 2009;**25**(1):29-36

[61] Richardson RT, Sivashanmugam P, Hall SH, Hamil KG, Moore PA, Ruben SM, et al. Cloning and sequencing of human Eppin: A novel family of protease inhibitors expressed in the epididymis and testis. Gene. 2001;**270**(1):93-102

[62] Widgren EE, Richardson RT, O'Rand MG, Beyler S. Inhibition of human sperm motility by contraceptive anti-Eppin antibodies from infertile male monkeys: Effect on cyclic adenosine Monophosphate1. Biology of Reproduction. 2009;**80**(2):279-285

[63] O'rand M, Widgren E, Sivashanmugam P, Richardson R, Hall S, French F, et al. Reversible immunocontraception in male monkeys immunized with eppin. Science. 2004;**306**(5699):1189-1190

[64] Uhrin P, Dewerchin M, Hilpert M, Chrenek P, Schöfer C, Zechmeister-Machhart M, et al. Disruption of the protein C inhibitor gene results in impaired spermatogenesis and male infertility. The Journal of Clinical Investigation. 2000;**106**(12):1531-1539

[65] Bandivdekar AH, Vernekar VJ, Moodbidri SB, Koide SS. Characterization of 80 kDa human sperm antigen responsible for Immunoinfertility. American Journal of Reproductive Immunology. 2001;**45**(1):28-34

[66] Khobarekar BG, Vernekar V, Raghavan V, Kamada M, Maegawa M, Bandivdekar AH. Evaluation of the potential of synthetic peptides of 80 kDa human sperm antigen (80 kDaHSA) for the development of contraceptive vaccine for male. Vaccine. 2008;**26**(29-30):3711-3718

[67] Vernekar VJ, Bandivdekar AH, Raghavan VP, Kamada M, Koide SS. Studies with synthetic peptides of 80 kDa human sperm antigen (80 kDa HSA). American Journal of Reproductive Immunology. 2004;**51**(2):106-111

[68] TURNER RM, MUSSE MP, Mandal A, Klotz K, JAYES FC, HERR JC, et al. Molecular genetic analysis of two human sperm fibrous sheath proteins, AKAP4 and AKAP3, in men with dysplasia of the fibrous sheath. Journal of Andrology. 2001;**22**(2):302-315

[69] Brown PR, Miki K, Harper DB, Eddy EM. A-kinase anchoring protein 4 binding proteins in the fibrous sheath of the sperm flagellum. Biology of Reproduction. 2003;**68**(6):2241-2248

[70] Miki K, Willis WD, Brown PR, Goulding EH, Fulcher KD, Eddy EM. Targeted disruption of the Akap4 gene causes defects in sperm flagellum and motility. Developmental Biology. 2002;**248**(2):331-342

[71] Wang L, Miao S, Cao S, Wu B, Koide S. Isolation and characterization of a rabbit sperm tail protein. Archives of Andrology. 1986;**16**(1):55-66

[72] Takikawa M, Kamada M, Maegawa M, Yamano S, Irahara M, Aono T, et al. Evaluation of two sperm antigens, rSMP-B and YWK-II, as targets for immunocontraception. Zygote. 2001;**9**(2):145-151

[73] Sawane MV, Kaore SB, Gaikwad RD, Patil PM, Patankar SS, Deshkar AM. Seminal LDH-C4 isoenzyme and sperm mitochondrial activity: A study in male partners of infertile couples. Indian Journal of Medical Sciences. 2002;**56**(11):560-566

[74] Goldberg E, VandeBerg JL, Mahony MC, Doncel GF. Immune response of male baboons to testis-specific LDH-C4☆☆this work was supported by contraceptive Research and Development (CONRAD) program CICCR Grant #640510 to Northwestern University and by NIH Grant P51RR13986 to the southwest regional primate research center. The views expressed by the authors do not necessarily reflect those of the CONRAD program. Contraception. 2001;**64**(2):93-98

[75] Schmidt-Schweda S, Holubarsch C. First clinical trial with etomoxir in patients with chronic congestive heart failure. Clinical Science. 2000;**99**(1):27-35

[76] Ferrick DA, Neilson A, Beeson C. Advances in measuring cellular bioenergetics using extracellular flux. Drug Discovery Today. 2008;**13**(5-6):268-274

[77] Holubarsch CJ, Rohrbach M, Karrasch M, Boehm E, Polonski L, Ponikowski P, et al. A double-blind randomized multicentre clinical trial to evaluate the efficacy and safety of two doses of etomoxir in comparison with placebo in patients with moderate congestive heart failure: The ERGO (etomoxir for the recovery of glucose oxidation) study. Clinical Science. 2007;**113**(4):205-212

[78] Gyamera-Acheampong C, Mbikay M. Proprotein convertase

subtilisin/kexin type 4 in mammalian fertility: A review. Human Reproduction Update. 2009;**15**(2):237-247

[79] Gyamera-Acheampong C, Tantibhedhyangkul J, Weerachatyanukul W, Tadros H, Xu H, van de Loo JW, et al. Sperm from mice genetically deficient for the PCSK4 proteinase exhibit accelerated capacitation, precocious acrosome reaction, reduced binding to egg zona pellucida, and impaired fertilizing ability. Biology of Reproduction. 2006;**74**(4):666-673

[80] Acheampong CG. The Physiology and Biochemistry of the Fertility Enzyme Proprotein Convertase Subtilisin/Kexin Type 4. Ottawa Canada: University of Ottawa; 2009

[81] Gyamera-Acheampong C, Sirois F, Denis NJ, Mishra P, Figeys D, Basak A, et al. The precursor to the germ cell-specific PCSK4 proteinase is inefficiently activated in transfected somatic cells: Evidence of interaction with the BiP chaperone. Molecular and Cellular Biochemistry. 2011;**348**(1-2):43-52

[82] Simanjuntak D. Pengaruh Antibodi Convertase Tipe 4 (PCSK4) Membran Plasma Akrosom Spermatozoa Manusia Terhadap Hambatan kemampuan Fertilisasi In Vitro dan In Vivo pada Tikus (*Rattus norvegicus*) [PhD]. Surabaya, Indonesia: Airlangga University; 2016

[83] Seidah NG. The proprotein convertases, 20 years later. Methods in Molecular Biology. 2011;**768**:23-57

[84] Dahril D, Aulanni'am A, Hilmanto D, Purwatiningsih W. The characterization of proprotein convertase subtilisin/kexin type4 (PCSK4) on human sperm membran for developping male immunocontraception candidates. International Journal of ChemTech Research. 2014;**5**:2229-2234

[85] Seidah N, Prat A. Precursor convertases in the secretory pathway, cytosol and extracellular milieu. Essays in Biochemistry. 2002;**38**:79-94

[86] Basak A, Touré BB, Lazure C, Mbikay M, Chrétien M, Seidah NG. Enzymic characterization in vitro of recombinant proprotein convertase PC4. The Biochemical Journal. 1999;**343**(Pt 1):29-37

[87] Qiu Q, Basak A, Mbikay M, Tsang BK, Gruslin A. Role of pro-IGF-II processing by proprotein convertase 4 in human placental development. Proceedings of the National Academy of Sciences. 2005;**102**(31):11047-11052

[88] Tadros H, Chrétien M, Mbikay M. The testicular germ-cell protease PC4 is also expressed in macrophage-like cells of the ovary. Journal of Reproductive Immunology. 2001;**49**(2):133-152

[89] Gyamera-Acheampong C, Vasilescu J, Figeys D, Mbikay M. PCSK4-null sperm display enhanced protein tyrosine phosphorylation and ADAM2 proteolytic processing during in vitro capacitation. Fertility and Sterility. 2010;**93**(4):1112-1123

[90] Basak A, Shervani NJ, Mbikay M, Kolajova M. Recombinant proprotein convertase 4 (PC4) from Leishmania tarentolae expression system: Purification, biochemical study and inhibitor design. Protein Expression and Purification. 2008;**60**(2):117-126

[91] Bergeron F, Leduc R, Day R. Subtilase-like pro-protein convertases: From molecular specificity to therapeutic applications. Journal of Molecular Endocrinology. 2000;**24**:1-22

[92] Mishra P. Study of Inhibitor Effect of Epididymal CRES on PC4/PCSK4 Activity [Science]. Ottawa, Ontario, Canada: University of Ottawa; 2011

[93] Mbikay M, Tadros H, Ishida N, Lerner C, Lamirande ED, Chen A, et al. Impaired fertility in mice deficient for the testicular germ-cell protease PC4. Proceedings of the National Academy of Sciences of the United States of America. 1997;**94**:6842-6846

[94] Li M, Mbikay M, Arimura A. Pituitary Adenylate Cyclase-activating polypeptide precursor is processed solely by Prohormone Convertase 4 in the gonads. Endocrinology. 2000;**141**:3723-3730

[95] Isaac ER, Sherwood NM. Pituitary adenylate cyclase-activating polypeptide (PACAP) is important for embryo implantation in mice. Molecular and Cellular Endocrinology. 2008;**280**(1):13-19

[96] Sibley C, Coan P, Ferguson-Smith A, Dean W, Hughes J, Smith P, et al. Placental-specific insulin-like growth factor 2 (Igf2) regulates the diffusional exchange characteristics of the mouse placenta. Proceedings of the National Academy of Sciences. 2004;**101**(21):8204-8208

[97] Basak A, Goswami M, Rajkumar A, Mitra T, Majumdar S, O'Reilly P, et al. Enediynyl peptides and iso-coumarinyl methyl sulfones as inhibitors of proprotein convertases PCSK8/SKI-1/S1P and PCSK4/PC4: Design, synthesis and biological evaluations. Bioorganic & Medicinal Chemistry Letters. 2015;**25**(10):2225-2237

[98] Mishra P, Qiu Q, Gruslin A, Hidaka Y, Mbikay M, Basak A. In vitro regulatory effect of epididymal serpin CRES on protease activity of proprotein convertase PC4/PCSK4. Current Molecular Medicine. 2012;**12**(8):1050-1067

[99] Kurth BE, Digilio L, Snow P, Bush LA, Wolkowicz M, Shetty J, et al. Immunogenicity of a multi-component recombinant human acrosomal protein vaccine in female Macaca fascicularis. Journal of Reproductive Immunology. 2008;**77**(2):126-141